AF780418

Drug Metabolism and Toxicological Mechanisms

Drug Metabolism and Toxicological Mechanisms

Guest Editors

Qi Wang
Youbo Zhang
An Zhu

MDPI

Basel • Beijing • Wuhan • Barcelona • Belgrade • Novi Sad • Cluj • Manchester

Guest Editors
Qi Wang
School of Public Health
Peking University
Beijing
China

Youbo Zhang
School of Pharmaceutical
Sciences
Peking University
Beijing
China

An Zhu
School of Basic Medical
Sciences
Fujian Medical University
Fuzhou
China

Editorial Office
MDPI AG
Grosspeteranlage 5
4052 Basel, Switzerland

This is a reprint of the Special Issue, published open access by the journal *Toxics* (ISSN 2305-6304), freely accessible at: https://www.mdpi.com/journal/toxics/special_issues/B13QU3I118.

For citation purposes, cite each article independently as indicated on the article page online and as indicated below:

Lastname, A.A.; Lastname, B.B. Article Title. *Journal Name* **Year**, *Volume Number*, Page Range.

ISBN 978-3-7258-5189-8 (Hbk)
ISBN 978-3-7258-5190-4 (PDF)
https://doi.org/10.3390/books978-3-7258-5190-4

© 2025 by the authors. Articles in this book are Open Access and distributed under the Creative Commons Attribution (CC BY) license. The book as a whole is distributed by MDPI under the terms and conditions of the Creative Commons Attribution-NonCommercial-NoDerivs (CC BY-NC-ND) license (https://creativecommons.org/licenses/by-nc-nd/4.0/).

Contents

About the Editors

Qi Wang

Qi Wang is a Professor of Toxicology at School of Public Health, Peking University. Qi Wang earned her PhD in Medicinal Chemistry from Peking University. Her research has been funded by the National Key Research and Development Program, the National Natural Science Foundation of China (NSFC), and the Ministry of Education of China. She has published over 100 papers in journals including *Phytomedicine* and *Science of the Total Environment*. Her research focuses on the mechanisms of drug metabolism and toxicity, computational toxicology, PBK modeling, and human health risk assessment.

Youbo Zhang

Youbo Zhang is an Associate Professor and Master's Supervisor at Peking University's School of Pharmaceutical Science. Youbo Zhang holds a Ph.D. from Peking University, and previously worked as a postdoctoral fellow at National Institutes of Health (NIH), USA. He is also a researcher at Henan Engineering Research Center for Technology of Medicinal and Edible Traditional Chinese Medicine, the High-Tech Leading Talent Xuzhou City, Jiangsu Province, and the director of Huanshenghui (Beijing) Biotechnology Research Institute. He is the member of Chinese Medicine Chemistry Committee, and Chinese Medicine Analysis Committee, China Association of Chinese Medicine. His research interests include the analysis of active constituents in traditional Chinese medicine and their metabolic mechanisms, and regulatory mechanisms of metabolic diseases based on nuclear receptors. He has led or participated in over 10 research projects, including those funded by the National Natural Science Foundation of China, the National Key R&D Program of China, and the Beijing Natural Science Foundation, with total funding exceeding RMB 5 million. He has published more than 70 SCI-indexed papers in renowned journals such as *Acta Pharmaceutica Sinica B (APSB)*, *Free Radical Biology and Medicine*, and *Drug Metabolism and Disposition (DMD)*.

An Zhu

An Zhu is an Associate Professor and Master's Supervisor at the School of Basic Medical Sciences, Fujian Medical University. He received his Bachelor's and Master's degrees in Medicine from Lanzhou University between 2009 and 2017, and earned his Ph.D. in Medicine from Peking University in 2020. His research focuses on pharmacology and toxicology. He teaches courses such as Medical Microbiology and Medical Molecular Biology. He has presided over several research projects, including the National Natural Science Foundation of China Youth Program, the Fujian Provincial Natural Science Foundation, the Fujian Science and Technology Innovation Joint Fund Project. He serves as a Guest Editor for *Toxics* and *Frontiers in Genetics*, a Youth Editorial Board member of *Epigenetics Insights*, and a reviewer for over 40 SCI journals, including *Phytomedicine*. He has published 54 papers, 32 of which as the first or corresponding author. He is a committee member of the Chinese Medicine Toxicology and Safety Research Branch of the China Association of Chinese Medicine, the Supervisor of the Fujian Association of Bioengineering, and High-Level Talent in Fujian Province.

toxics

MDPI

Editorial

Drug Metabolism and Toxicological Mechanisms

Qi Wang [1,*], Youbo Zhang [2,*] and An Zhu [3,*]

1 Department of Toxicology, School of Public Health, Peking University, Beijing 100191, China
2 State Key Laboratory of Natural and Biomimetic Drugs, School of Pharmaceutical Sciences, Peking University, Beijing 100191, China
3 Key Laboratory of Gastrointestinal Cancer (Fujian Medical University), Ministry of Education, Fuzhou 350108, China
* Correspondence: wangqi@bjmu.edu.cn (Q.W.); ybzhang@bjmu.edu.cn (Y.Z.); zhuan@fjmu.edu.cn (A.Z.)

The metabolism of drugs and xenobiotics is a cornerstone of pharmacology and toxicology, governing the efficacy, safety, and environmental impact of therapeutic agents [1]. Drug metabolism involves enzymatic transformations that convert lipophilic compounds into water-soluble metabolites for excretion, primarily mediated by cytochrome P450 (CYP) enzymes, UDP-glucuronosyltransferases (UGTs), and transporters [2]. These processes occur in two phases, functionalization (Phase I) and conjugation (Phase II), followed by excretion [3]. While metabolism is essential for detoxification, it can also generate reactive intermediates that contribute to organ damage, carcinogenesis, or immune-mediated toxicity [4]. Understanding these dual roles—detoxification versus toxification—is critical for drug development and personalized medicine.

Variability in drug metabolism, driven by genetic polymorphisms (e.g., CYP2D6 and CYP2C19), age, disease states, and environmental factors (e.g., diet and pollutants), complicates toxicity prediction. For instance, slow metabolizers of codeine due to CYP2D6 deficiencies risk opioid toxicity from unchecked conversion to morphine, while ultra-rapid metabolizers face overdose risks [5]. Similarly, drug–drug interactions (DDIs) involving enzyme induction or inhibition—such as grapefruit juice's inhibition of CYP3A4—can alter therapeutic outcomes [6,7]. These examples underscore the need for precision toxicology frameworks that account for individual and population-level variability.

Historically, toxicology relied on observational and empirical methods, but modern approaches integrate mechanistic insights from molecular biology, omics technologies (genomics, proteomics, and metabolomics), and computational models. Despite progress, challenges persist in predicting idiosyncratic reactions, rare adverse events, and long-term environmental impacts. Traditional animal models often fail to replicate human-specific metabolic pathways, spurring innovations like organ-on-a-chip systems, 3D organoids, and humanized mouse models [8]. Meanwhile, regulatory agencies increasingly demand mechanistic data to complement traditional safety assessments, reflecting a paradigm shift toward "adversity pathways" and quantitative risk modeling.

This Special Issue addresses these complexities by showcasing 12 peer-reviewed articles (11 original research papers and 1 review) that span molecular mechanisms, clinical toxicology, preclinical studies, and regulatory innovation. Contributions explore themes such as enzyme polymorphisms, environmental toxicants, and AI-driven toxicity prediction. Collectively, they highlight three transformative trends: (1) the integration of multi-omics to unravel metabolic networks, (2) the adoption of advanced in vitro and in silico models to reduce animal testing, and (3) the application of big data to bridge gaps between preclinical findings and clinical outcomes. In summary, this Special Issue reflects the dynamic evolution of drug metabolism research, emphasizing mechanistic clarity, technological innovation, and translational relevance.

 https://doi.org/10.3390/toxics13060464

1. An Overview of Published Articles

The study by Tian et al. (contribution 1) systematically elucidated the hepatotoxic mechanisms of mesaconitine (MA) through in vivo zebrafish models, revealing dose-dependent impairment of hepatic development characterized by reduced liver size, neutrophil infiltration, and ROS accumulation. Transcriptomic profiling and molecular validation demonstrated that MA exposure triggered endoplasmic reticulum stress through oxidative damage, activating the unfolded protein response (UPR) via upregulation of key chaperones. Prolonged UPR activation drives hepatocyte apoptosis through caspase-dependent pathways. These findings established a ROS-UPR–apoptosis axis as the molecular basis for MA-induced liver injury, bridging the gap between *Aconitum* alkaloid exposure and hepatic dysfunction. The use of transgenic zebrafish lines allowed real-time visualization of liver injury progression, neutrophil infiltration, and apoptosis dynamics, highlighting the unique advantages of zebrafish in mechanistic toxicology. This study not only advanced zebrafish-based toxicology assessment methodologies but also provided essential safety data for the clinical application of traditional medicines.

The study by Trakulsrichai et al. (contribution 2) systematically described the epidemiological features, clinical manifestations, therapeutic strategies, and prognostic factors of ethephon poisoning through a retrospective analysis of clinical data from 252 patients in the Ramathibodi Poison Center database. The study found that 21.4% of individuals exposed to ethephon exhibited no apparent symptoms, and gastrointestinal symptoms constituted the most frequently reported clinical manifestations at 55.6% in all cases. Furthermore, the mortality rate remained relatively low, representing 0.8% of the total ethephon-exposed population. However, advanced-age intentional ingestion and early neurological symptoms such as impaired consciousness were significantly associated with adverse outcomes. As a study with a large reported sample size, this research comprehensively elucidated the clinical characteristics of ethephon poisoning, addressing a critical lack of human data for this field. Furthermore, by integrating epidemiological and toxicological perspectives, the study validated the World Health Organization classification of ethephon as slightly hazardous, supporting its safety assessment. Future investigations can explore the metabolic mechanisms of ethephon and its association with atypical cholinergic manifestations. The authors not only systematically delineated the clinical profile of ethephon poisoning but also advanced precision medicine through prognostic analysis. This work established a benchmark for pesticide toxicity management and toxicological research, serving as a valuable reference for both clinical practice and public health initiatives.

The study by Lin et al. (contribution 3) investigated the mechanisms underlying the effects of the environmental endocrine disruptor bisphenol S (BPS) on hepatic lipid metabolism, revealing the biological processes through which BPS promotes lipid accumulation via oxidative stress-mediated molecular pathways. The research team utilized two hepatocellular cell models, HepG2 and SK-Hep-1, combined with cell viability assays, oxidative stress indicator analyses, and measurement of lipid metabolism-related gene and protein expression to systematically characterize the metabolic disturbances in hepatocytes exposed to BPS. The results demonstrated that BPS significantly suppressed the expression of PPARα and CPT1B, key regulators of fatty acid oxidation, while upregulating the expression of SREBP1C and FASN, genes associated with lipid synthesis. Oxidative stress further exacerbated lipid droplet deposition, ultimately leading to hepatic lipid metabolism imbalance. By systematically dissecting the molecular mechanisms through which BPS disrupts lipid synthesis and degradation pathways via oxidative stress in hepatic cell models, this study identified the critical regulatory role of the PPARα/SREBP1C-FASN axis. Additionally, the identified targets, such as PPARα and SREBP1C, provide new directions for developing interventions targeting lipid metabolism disorders. Through multi-timepoint and multi-concentration gradient exposure experiments, the authors dynamically elucidated the dose–response relationship and time-dependent toxicity of BPS, significantly enhancing the credibility of the conclusions.

The study by Gonçalves et al. (contribution 4) systematically investigated the regulatory effects of ethanol intake on paracetamol, also named acetaminophen (APAP)-induced hepatotoxicity, using a C57BL/6 mouse model. The findings revealed that acute ethanol (AE) exacerbated APAP-induced liver injury by elevating CYP2E1 activity, TBARS, and GSSG, manifested as expanded necrotic areas, increased ALT/AST levels, and upregulated inflammatory cytokines. In contrast, chronic ethanol (CE) significantly mitigated liver damage by enhancing UGT1A1 gene expression, restoring glutathione homeostasis, and reducing carbonylated protein levels, with hepatic pathological features resembling those of the control group. Proteomic profiling further demonstrated that the CE group clustered with the control group in protein expression patterns, whereas the AE group aligned with the APAP group, suggesting that chronic ethanol consumption may confer protective effects through metabolic adaptation mechanisms. By integrating histopathological, oxidative stress, gene expression, and proteomic analyses, the study elucidated the critical regulatory role of the UGT1A1/CYP2E1 axis, providing molecular mechanistic evidence for understanding ethanol–drug metabolic interactions. Additionally, the identified UGT1A1 upregulation mechanism highlighted novel therapeutic targets for hepatoprotective strategies. The authors dynamically dissected molecular networks underlying liver injury through proteomics, enhancing the credibility of conclusions. This work established a paradigm for research on drug–alcohol interactions, offering significant guidance for rational medication practices and toxicological risk assessment.

The study by Yin et al. (contribution 5) systematically investigated the acute toxicity and cardiotoxicity of the natural phenolic acid compound protocatechuic aldehyde (PCA) in juvenile zebrafish. Through exposure experiments with different concentration gradients (50–80 μg/mL) of PCA, the study found that high concentrations (70 and 80 μg/mL) of PCA caused severe malformations in zebrafish larvae, including spinal curvature, pericardial edema, significant reduction in locomotor activity, and cardiac structural abnormalities and functional dysfunction through phenotypic observation, behavioral analysis, cardiac function assessment, and histopathological evaluation. Further analysis using network pharmacology predictions and RT-PCR validation revealed that the inhibition of genes such as *PIK3CA*, *PARP1*, and *GSK3β* mediated cardiotoxicity through regulation of the PI3K/AKT/GSK3β signaling pathway. This study provides a comprehensive evaluation of PCA's toxic effects in a zebrafish model, offering important theoretical insights for safety assessments of PCA-containing drugs and the development of low-toxicity pharmaceuticals.

The study by Yang et al. (contribution 6) investigated the nephrotoxicity and mechanisms of *Cassiae semen* aqueous extracts (CSAEs) through a 28-day repeated-dose experiment in rats. The study revealed that CSAEs induced dose-dependent increases in serum creatinine and blood urea nitrogen levels, accompanied by morphological alterations in rat kidneys. Using molecular docking and experimental validation, the authors identified that key CSAE components, namely, obtusifolin, aurantio-obtusin, and obtusin, exhibited strong binding affinity to F-actin, ROCK1, and Rac1, with the RhoA-ROCK pathway identified as the regulatory mechanism mediating CSAE nephrotoxicity. Immunofluorescence staining confirmed disrupted renal cell membranes and brush borders, establishing F-actin as a primary toxicity target. Further experiments demonstrated that CSAEs dose-dependently suppressed mRNA expression of RhoA-ROCK pathway genes such as *ROCK1* and *cofilin* and reduced GTP-RhoA protein and phosphorylated ROCK/cofilin levels, leading to actin depolymerization, cytoskeletal destabilization, and subsequent nephrotoxicity. This study linked *Cassiae semen* toxicity to aberrant actin cytoskeleton remodeling, offering novel insights into the mechanisms of natural product-induced nephrotoxicity.

The study by Kim et al. (contribution 7) evaluated the risk of optic neuropathy (ON) and visual impairment induced by ethambutol in tuberculosis treatment in a retrospective cohort analysis of 204,598 ethambutol users in the Korean NHIS database from 2015 to 2021, tracked to 2022. The findings revealed that 2.6% of ethambutol-treated patients developed ON, with risk factors including female sex, older age, higher cumulative ethambutol doses, longer treatment duration, and systemic comorbidities such as diabetes, hypertension, hyperlipidemia, kidney and liver diseases, and malnutrition. Notably, concomitant isoniazid use demonstrated a protective effect with an OR value of 0.78, mediated by shortened ethambutol exposure, while deficiencies in vitamins B1, B6, and B12 exacerbated ethambutol-induced neurotoxicity. Despite limitations inherent to its retrospective design, the study provides critical guidance for monitoring and preventive strategies in ethambutol-treated patients, emphasizing the importance of personalized risk assessment and interventions. Overall, this research advances the understanding of ethambutol-associated ON and its interactions with isoniazid, systemic comorbidities, and nutritional status, and underscores the necessity of mitigating ON risks to optimize tuberculosis treatment protocols.

The study by Wan et al. (contribution 8) investigated how rutaecarpine affected APAP-induced liver toxicity. Mouse and liver cell models demonstrated that rutaecarpine aggravates liver injury, as evidenced by significantly elevated serum ALT and AST levels, extensive hepatic necrosis with substantial parenchymal damage on histopathological examination, and notable upregulation of inflammatory cytokines, including IL-6 and IL-1β. Mechanistic studies revealed that rutaecarpine induced CYP1A2 expression at both mRNA and protein levels, accelerating APAP metabolism to its toxic metabolite NAPQI. These effects were reversed by α-Naphthoflavone, a CYP1A2 inhibitor, confirming the enzyme's critical role in accelerating APAP metabolism. The study reveals the risks of combining rutaecarpine with APAP, providing critical insights for clinical drug safety and the rational use of traditional Chinese medicine (TCM) with synthetic drugs.

The study by Gao et al. (contribution 9) conducted a proteomic analysis on 20 laryngeal squamous cell carcinoma patient samples, uncovering the significant role of ribosome biogenesis pathways in tumor metastasis. Their study demonstrated a clear relationship between lymph node metastasis and the overexpression of ribosomal proteins (RPS10 and RPL24), heightened activity in protein synthesis pathways, and disrupted cell adhesion mechanisms, creating a network that promotes metastatic spread. In vitro experiments further revealed that the RNA polymerase I inhibitor CX-5461 exhibited anti-metastatic properties at non-cytotoxic concentrations by reversing epithelial–mesenchymal transition and reducing the levels of ribosomal proteins, thereby suppressing tumor cell invasion and migration. Despite the known DNA-damaging effects of CX-5461 posing challenges to its clinical use, both the authors and reviewers acknowledge the potential of developing therapeutic strategies with inhibitory activity against ribosome biogenesis pathways based on optimizing drug design and comprehensive safety evaluations. This study not only deepens our understanding of ribosomal dysregulation in LSCC metastasis but also emphasizes the significance of the pathology-based grouping approach in proteomic analysis in identifying potential cancer targets and providing personalized treatment recommendations.

The study by Wu et al. (contribution 10) conducted epigenetic, proteomic, and metabolomic analyses on the human trophoblast cell line HTR-8/SVneo, revealing the reproductive toxicity effects induced by oridonin. The study found that the Wnt/β-catenin signaling pathway, tight junction, thiamine metabolism, and amino acid degradation pathways were all involved in the toxic effects of oridonin on HTR-8/SVneo cells. Further in vitro experiments demonstrated that the toxic effects involved elevated intracellular Ca^{2+} levels, oxidative stress, the occurrence of mitochondrial dysfunction, DNA damage, and abnormal expression of molecules related to the Wnt/β-catenin signaling pathway and tight junction. These findings confirmed that the inhibition of the Wnt/β-catenin signaling pathway and disruption of the tight junction were key mechanisms underlying oridonin-induced cytotoxicity. Despite oridonin's significant pharmacological potential in anti-inflammatory, anti-tumor, and antibacterial applications, its reproductive toxicity poses a critical limitation to its clinical use. By deeply elucidating the toxic mechanisms of oridonin, it is possible to provide a theoretical basis for optimizing its clinical application strategies, thereby maximizing its therapeutic potential while ensuring safety. This study not only provides a deeper understanding of oridonin's reproductive toxicity mechanisms through a multi-omics approach but also underscores the value of integrated multi-omics analysis in identifying toxicity targets. It establishes a novel research framework for evaluating the safety of active compounds in TCM.

The study by Bian et al. (contribution 11) investigated the biochemical and toxicological changes following insulin overdose using a rat model, aiming to identify specific molecular markers for forensic diagnosis. Here, 20 IU/kg insulin aspart induced severe hypoglycemia, convulsions, and metabolic disturbances, including reduced glucose and glycogen levels, along with elevated lactate. Key findings revealed potassium redistribution due to activated Na^{+}-K^{+}-ATPase and stimulation of the PI3K-AKT pathway in skeletal muscle, promoting GLUT4 translocation, suggesting that detecting GLUT4 and Na^{+}-K^{+}-ATPase proteins on the skeletal muscle cell membrane can provide valuable auxiliary diagnostic information for forensic identification of insulin overdose. The study proposes the ratio of insulin to C-peptide as a forensic marker for identifying exogenous insulin overdose, addressing the challenges in postmortem insulin detection. This work bridges clinical insights with forensic applications, offering valuable tools for postmortem diagnosis, particularly useful when physical evidence of injection is absent.

The study by Mohammed et al. (contribution 12) conducted a comprehensive review focusing on the toxicity mechanisms, clinical presentations, and diagnostic and treatment approaches for methanol poisoning, emphasizing the importance of preventive measures. Methanol is metabolized into formaldehyde and formic acid, leading to severe metabolic acidosis and multiorgan damage, particularly affecting the central nervous system and vision. The article highlighted that clinical manifestations vary by age and exposure type. Diagnosis relies on clinical evaluation, laboratory tests, and advanced techniques like gas chromatography. Methanol poisoning results in severe metabolic acidosis and multiorgan damage due to the accumulation of formic acid, leading to significant morbidity and mortality. Effective clinical management includes timely administration of antidotes like fomepizole or ethanol and hemodialysis for severe cases. This article provides a comprehensive perspective on understanding methanol poisoning, from its pathogenesis to clinical management, offering valuable guidance for healthcare providers.

2. Conclusions

The articles in this Special Issue collectively advance our understanding of drug metabolism and toxicity, offering novel insights and tools to address longstanding challenges. A study investigated CYP450 isoforms to reveal disparities in drug response and toxicity risks. Several papers dissect mechanisms of organ-specific toxicity, such as hepatotoxicity from acetaminophen and nephrotoxicity from *Cassiae* semen aqueous extracts. Environmental toxicology is also well represented, with studies on the impacts of pollutants on metabolic pathways. Emerging technologies are another highlight. Mechanistic toxicology has seen significant progress. Papers elucidating mitochondrial dysfunction, oxidative stress, and immune-mediated injury provide frameworks for predicting organ-specific toxicity. Such mechanisms offer biomarkers for early toxicity detection and targets for protective interventions.

The rise of alternatives to animal experimentation marks a paradigm shift in toxicology. Zebrafish (*Danio rerio*) and *Caenorhabditis elegans* (*C. elegans*) have become invaluable models for high-throughput drug toxicity screening and mechanistic studies [9]. These tools not only enhance predictive accuracy but also align with global efforts to promote the 3Rs (Replacement, Reduction, and Refinement) in toxicology. Their unique biological features, combined with advanced genetic and molecular techniques, enable rapid hypothesis testing while reducing reliance on mammalian systems. Zebrafish have gained prominence due to their genetic tractability, optical transparency during early development, and high genetic similarity to humans (87%). These attributes facilitate real-time observation of organogenesis and physiological responses to toxicants. For instance, zebrafish mutants like space cadet—which exhibit aberrant escape responses due to disrupted Mauthner cell connectivity—provide insights into neurotoxicant effects on behavior [10]. Meanwhile, *C. elegans* offers a tractable system to study metabolic perturbations, as seen in research linking mitochondrial dysfunction to drug-induced oxidative stress [11]. Its short lifecycle of 3 days, fully mapped genome, and conserved metabolic pathways make it ideal for high-throughput screens. These models not only reduce reliance on mammals but also enable rapid hypothesis testing in drug metabolism and toxicology [12].

TCMs present unique challenges due to their complex compositions and potential for herb–drug interactions. Metabolomics has emerged as a powerful tool to unravel TCM toxicity, as demonstrated in studies. Similarly, UPLC-Q-TOF/MS-based analyses of toxicity identified detoxification mechanisms, highlighting the synergy between modern technology and traditional knowledge [13]. Such research aligns with global efforts to standardize TCM safety assessments while preserving their therapeutic potential.

Some research methods are not covered in this Special Issue, and these techniques are also worthy of application in drug toxicology and metabolism studies. The integration of advanced technologies is a milestone. Organ-on-a-chip platforms replicate human tissue interactions, enabling real-time monitoring of metabolite kinetics and toxicity [14]. In parallel, AI models trained on multi-omics datasets demonstrate remarkable accuracy in predicting idiosyncratic reactions, bridging gaps between in vitro assays and clinical outcomes [15]. These tools are poised to revolutionize preclinical testing, reducing reliance on animal models and accelerating drug discovery. Additionally, the rise of biologics and gene therapies demands new metabolic paradigms, as traditional small-molecule pathways may not apply. Regulatory science must also evolve. While mechanistic data are increasingly valued, standardization of novel methodologies such as organoids and AI models is needed for regulatory acceptance. Global collaboration, as seen in the FDA Emerging Technology Program, can harmonize guidelines and foster innovation [16].

Looking ahead, the field must embrace interdisciplinary collaboration. Integrating pharmacogenomics, environmental science, and computational toxicology will yield holistic models of metabolic networks. Public health initiatives, such as biobanking and global toxicity databases, can enhance predictive power and equity in drug safety. In closing, this Special Issue not only catalogs current achievements but also charts a course for future inquiry. By prioritizing mechanistic depth, technological innovation, and translational impact, the toxicology community can mitigate adverse drug reactions, safeguard environmental health, and usher in an era of precision medicine.

Data Availability Statement: Data sharing is not applicable (only appropriate if no new data is generated or the article describes entirely theoretical research).

Conflicts of Interest: The authors declare no conflicts of interest.

List of Contributions:

1. Tian, J.; Zhuang, Y.; Liu, Y.; Zheng, Y.; Liu, X.; Lin, S.; Zheng, C.; Wu, Z. ROS-Mediated Unfolded Protein Response Activation Drives Hepatocyte Apoptosis in Mesaconitine-Induced Liver Injury. *Toxics* **2025**, *13*, 155. https://doi.org/10.3390/toxics13030155.
2. Trakulsrichai, S.; Chuayaupakarn, K.; Tansuwannarat, P.; Rittilert, P.; Tongpoo, A.; Sriapha, C.; Wananukul, W. Ethephon Poisoning: Clinical Characteristics and Outcomes. *Toxics* **2025**, *13*, 115. https://doi.org/10.3390/toxics13020115.
3. Lin, K.-X.; Wu, Z.-Y.; Qin, M.-L.; Zeng, H.-C. Bisphenol S Induces Lipid Metabolism Disorders in HepG2 and SK-Hep-1 Cells via Oxidative Stress. *Toxics* **2025**, *13*, 44. https://doi.org/10.3390/toxics13010044.
4. Gonçalves, A.C.; Coelho, A.M.; da Cruz Castro, M.L.; Pereira, R.R.; da Silva Araújo, N.P.; Ferreira, F.M.; Machado Júnior, P.A.; Pio, S.; Vital, C.E.; Bezerra, F.S.; et al. Modulation of Paracetamol-Induced Hepatotoxicity by Acute and Chronic Ethanol Consumption in Mice: A Study Pilot. *Toxics* **2024**, *12*, 857. https://doi.org/10.3390/toxics12120857.
5. Yin, J.; Wang, H.; Zhao, F.; Liang, D.; Yang, W.; Zhang, D. The Acute Toxicity and Cardiotoxic Effects of Protocatechuic Aldehyde on Juvenile Zebrafish. *Toxics* **2024**, *12*, 799. https://doi.org/10.3390/toxics12110799.
6. Yang, J.; Xiao, S.; Li, L.; Zhu, A.; Xiao, W.; Wang, Q. Actin Dysregulation Mediates Nephrotoxicity of Cassiae Semen Aqueous Extracts. *Toxics* **2024**, *12*, 556. https://doi.org/10.3390/toxics12080556.
7. Kim, J.; Ahn, S.J. Risk Factors of Optic Neuropathy in Ethambutol Users: Interaction with Isoniazid and Other Associated Conditions of Toxic Optic Neuropathy. *Toxics* **2024**, *12*, 549. https://doi.org/10.3390/toxics12080549.
8. Wan, M.; Gao, H.; Liu, X.; Zhang, Y. Rutaecarpine Aggravates Acetaminophen-Induced Acute Liver Injury by Inducing CYP1A2. *Toxics* **2024**, *12*, 515. https://doi.org/10.3390/toxics12070515.
9. Gao, M.; Liu, T.; Hu, K.; Chen, S.; Wang, S.; Gan, D.; Li, Z.; Lin, X. Ribosomal Dysregulation in Metastatic Laryngeal Squamous Cell Carcinoma: Proteomic Insights and CX-5461's Therapeutic Promise. *Toxics* **2024**, *12*, 363. https://doi.org/10.3390/toxics12050363.
10. Wu, Q.; Gao, X.; Lin, Y.; Wu, C.; Zhang, J.; Chen, M.; Wen, J.; Wu, Y.; Tian, K.; Bao, W.; et al. Integrating Epigenetics, Proteomics, and Metabolomics to Reveal the Involvement of Wnt/β-Catenin Signaling Pathway in Oridonin-Induced Reproductive Toxicity. *Toxics* **2024**, *12*, 339. https://doi.org/10.3390/toxics12050339.
11. Bian, C.; He, X.; Wang, Q.; Zheng, Z.; Zhang, Y.; Xiong, H.; Li, Y.; Zhao, M.; Li, J. Biochemical Toxicological Study of Insulin Overdose in Rats: A Forensic Perspective. *Toxics* **2024**, *12*, 17. https://doi.org/10.3390/toxics12010017.
12. Alrashed, M.; Aldeghaither, N.S. Almutairi, S.Y.; Almutairi, M.; Alghamdi, A.; Alqahtani, T.; Almojathel, G.H.; Alnassar, N.A. Alghadeer, S.M.; Alshehri, A.; et al. The Perils of Methanol Exposure: Insights into Toxicity and Clinical Management. *Toxics* **2024**, *12*, 924. https://doi.org/10.3390/toxics12120924.

References

1. Solanki, M. Cytochrome P450 2J2: Potential Role in Drug Metabolism and Cardiotoxicity. *Drug Metab. Dispos.* **2018**, *46*, 1053–1065. [CrossRef] [PubMed]
2. Zhang, M. The Potential Impact of CYP and UGT Drugmetabolizing Enzymes on Brain Target Site Drug Exposure. *Drug Metab. Rev.* **2024**, *56*, 1–30. [CrossRef] [PubMed]
3. Doan, T.N.K. Differential Effects of 1α,25-Dihydroxyvitamin D3 on the Expressions and Functions of Hepatic CYP and UGT Enzymes and Its Pharmacokinetic Consequences In Vivo. *Pharmaceutics* **2020**, *12*, 1129. [CrossRef] [PubMed]
4. Ahmed Laskar, A.; Younus, H. Aldehyde Toxicity and Metabolism: The Role of Aldehyde Dehydrogenases in Detoxification, Drug Resistance and Carcinogenesis. *Drug Metab. Rev.* **2019**, *51*, 42–64. [CrossRef] [PubMed]

5. Kinnunen, M. Updated Clinical Pharmacokinetics and Pharmacodynamics of Oxycodone. *Clin. Pharmacokinet.* **2019**, *58*, 705–725. [CrossRef] [PubMed]
6. Fuhr, L.M. Physiologically Based Pharmacokinetic Modeling of Bergamottin and 6,7-Dihydroxybergamottin to Describe CYP3A4 Mediated Grapefruit-Drug Interactions. *Clin. Pharmacol. Ther.* **2023**, *114*, 470–482. [CrossRef] [PubMed]
7. Sobczak, Ł.; Goryński, K. Pharmacological Aspects of Over-the-Counter Opioid Drugs Misuse. *Molecules* **2020**, *25*, 3905. [CrossRef] [PubMed]
8. Esposito, A. Three-Dimensional In Vitro Cell Cultures as a Feasible and Promising Alternative to Two-Dimensional and Animal Models in Cancer Research. *Int. J. BIiol Sci.* **2024**, *20*, 5293–5311. [CrossRef] [PubMed]
9. Lin, Y. Toosendanin-Induced Liver Damage through Irreparable DNA Damage and Autophagy Flow Blockade. *Phytomedicine* **2025**, *140*, 156586. [CrossRef] [PubMed]
10. Ferdous, J. Retinoic Acid Prevents Synaptic Deficiencies Induced by Alcohol Exposure during Gastrulation in Zebrafish Embryos. *NeuroToxicology* **2017**, *62*, 100–110. [CrossRef] [PubMed]
11. Liu, J.-L.; Hekimi, S. The Impact of Mitochondrial Oxidative Stress on Bile Acid-Like Molecules in *C. elegans* Provides a New Perspective on Human Metabolic Diseases. *Worm* **2014**, *2*, e21457. [CrossRef] [PubMed]
12. Zhu, A. Oxidation and Antioxidation of Natural Products in the Model Organism *Caenorhabditis elegans*. *Antioxidants* **2022**, *11*, 705. [CrossRef] [PubMed]
13. Dong, H. UPLC-Q-TOF/MS-Based Metabolomic Studies on the Toxicity Mechanisms of Traditional Chinese Medicine Chuanwu and the Detoxification Mechanisms of Gancao, Baishao, and Ganjiang. *Chin. J. Nat. Med.* **2015**, *13*, 687–698. [CrossRef] [PubMed]
14. Mina, S.G. Assessment of Drug-Induced Toxicity Biomarkers in the Brain Microphysiological System (MPS) Using Targeted and Untargeted Molecular Profiling. *Front Big Data* **2019**, *2*, 23. [CrossRef] [PubMed]
15. Cui, H. scGPT: Toward Building a Foundation Model for Single-Cell Multi-Omics Using Generative AI. *Nat. Methods* **2024**, *21*, 1470–1480. [CrossRef] [PubMed]
16. Zane, D. Development and Regulatory Challenges for Peptide Therapeutics. *Int. J. Toxicol.* **2020**, *40*, 108–124. [CrossRef] [PubMed]

Disclaimer/Publisher's Note: The statements, opinions and data contained in all publications are solely those of the individual author(s) and contributor(s) and not of MDPI and/or the editor(s). MDPI and/or the editor(s) disclaim responsibility for any injury to people or property resulting from any ideas, methods, instructions or products referred to in the content.

toxics

MDPI

Article

ROS-Mediated Unfolded Protein Response Activation Drives Hepatocyte Apoptosis in Mesaconitine-Induced Liver Injury

Jin Tian [1,†], Yubin Zhuang [2,†], Yinuo Liu [1], Yihong Zheng [1], Xuyang Liu [1], Shiyu Lin [1], Chenhua Zheng [3,*] and Zekai Wu [1,*]

1 Key Laboratory of Gastrointestinal Cancer, Ministry of Education, School of Basic Medical Sciences, Fujian Medical University, Fuzhou 350122, China; tianjin1128@fjmu.edu.cn (J.T.); liuyinuo@stu.fjmu.edu.cn (Y.L.); zhengyihong@stu.fjmu.edu.cn (Y.Z.); lxydsgyx@163.com (X.L.); linshiyudmvyx@163.com (S.L.)
2 Laboratory Animal Center, Fujian Medical University, Fuzhou 350122, China; zyb880@fjmu.edu.cn
3 Experiment Teaching Center of Basic Medical Sciences, School of Basic Medical Sciences, Fujian Medical University, Fuzhou 350122, China
* Correspondence: zhengchenhua@fjmu.edu.cn (C.Z.); zekaiwu@fjmu.edu.cn (Z.W.)
† These authors contributed equally to this work.

Abstract: Mesaconitine (MA), a predominant diterpenoid alkaloid isolated from Aconitum species, exhibits notable pharmacological properties but is simultaneously associated with significant toxicological concerns, with its hepatotoxic mechanisms remaining largely unelucidated. In this study, zebrafish embryos were systematically exposed to MA to investigate its effects on hepatic development and function. Comprehensive analyses of liver morphology, inflammatory response, oxidative stress, and apoptotic pathways were conducted. MA induced dose-dependent hepatotoxicity, manifesting in a significant reduction in liver size and a marked downregulation of liver-specific genes, including *tfa*, *cp*, *hhex*, and *fabp10a*. The presence of oxidative stress was substantiated by elevated reactive oxygen species (ROS) levels, while hepatic inflammation was characterized by enhanced neutrophil infiltration and the upregulation of proinflammatory mediators, particularly *il1b* and *tnfa*. A global transcriptome analysis revealed the substantial upregulation of unfolded protein response (UPR)-associated genes, notably *hsp90b1*, *hspa5*, and *hspb9*, indicating that MA-induced oxidative stress triggered endoplasmic reticulum (ER) stress and subsequent UPR activation. Prolonged ER stress ultimately resulted in hepatocyte apoptosis, as demonstrated by the increased expression of the pro-apoptotic genes *casp3a*, *casp3b*, and *baxa*. These findings elucidate the molecular mechanisms underlying MA-induced hepatotoxicity and identify potential therapeutic targets for preventing and treating liver injury associated with Aconitum alkaloid exposure.

Keywords: mesaconitine (MA); hepatotoxicity; inflammation; oxidative stress; apoptosis; unfolded protein response (UPR)

1. Introduction

Traditional Chinese medicines derived from Aconitum species, such as *Aconitum carmichaelii Debx.* (Fuzi), exhibit analgesic, anti-inflammatory, antidepressant, and vasodilatory properties [1–3]. However, natural products extracted from Aconitum plants, particularly Aconitum alkaloids, possess potent toxic effects. Current research on the toxicity of Aconitum alkaloids primarily focuses on their impact on the cardiovascular and central nervous systems, with limited studies addressing hepatotoxicity mechanisms. Preclinical studies have demonstrated clear dose-dependent hepatotoxicity associated with Aconitum alkaloids [4]. Moreover, several investigations into the toxicity resulting from a single or prolonged oral administration of Aconitum extract in rodents have reported instances of liver injury [5,6]. Consequently, it is imperative to conduct a systematic study of the hepatotoxicity mechanisms of Aconitum alkaloids to enable their safe clinical application.

MA is one of the principal diterpenoid alkaloids found in Aconitum species, exhibiting significant pharmacological effects while also being highly toxic. MA can penetrate the blood–brain barrier through proton-coupled organic cation antiporter mechanisms, leading to neurotoxicity [7]. Studies have demonstrated that MA induces neurotoxicity in zebrafish and HT22 cells, resulting in oxidative stress and mitochondrial dysfunction [8]. Additionally, MA significantly reduces the survival rate of H9C2 rat cardiomyocytes by inducing calcium influx, which subsequently decreases the mitochondrial membrane potential and causes nuclear damage [9]. Following MA exposure, cardiomyocytes from SD rats exhibit marked coagulative necrosis, with abnormal levels of polyunsaturated fatty acids (PUFAs) and altered expression of peroxisome proliferator-activated receptor α (PPARα) pathway-related proteins [10]. MA can induce cardiotoxicity and apoptosis, affecting cardiovascular-related genes such as *tbx5*, *gata4*, and *nkx2.5* in embryonic zebrafish [11]. Furthermore, a post-mortem analysis of patients who succumbed to Aconitine alkaloid poisoning revealed higher concentrations of MA in the liver and kidneys, reaching 960.9 ng/g and 776.9 ng/g, respectively [12]. In rats, MA has been shown to cause hepatocyte necrosis and inflammatory cell infiltration [13]. A network toxicological analysis indicated that MA affects pathways such as HIF-1, MAPK, PI3K-Akt, and FoxO signaling by modulating targets including ALB, AKT1, CASP3, and IL2. These findings provide partial insight into MA's hepatoxicity; however, the exact mechanisms of this, particularly in vivo, remain to be elucidated.

In this study, using zebrafish as a model organism, we uncovered MA's hepatotoxic effects. Our findings demonstrated that exposure to varying concentrations of MA significantly impaired liver development in zebrafish embryos, as evidenced by reduced liver size, the increased infiltration of neutrophils into the liver, elevated levels of ROS, and enhanced hepatocyte apoptosis. To elucidate the underlying mechanisms of MA-induced hepatotoxicity, we performed transcriptome sequencing on control and MA-treated zebrafish embryos. By constructing a comprehensive molecular profile, we discovered a significant upregulation of genes associated with UPR, including *hsp90b1*, *hspa5*, and *hspb9*, in response to MA treatment. These findings suggested that MA induced oxidative stress and hepatocyte apoptosis through the activation of ER stress and the UPR signaling pathway. Collectively, this study not only revealed novel molecular mechanisms underlying MA-induced hepatotoxicity but also provided valuable insights into potential diagnostic and therapeutic strategies for liver dysfunction associated with MA exposure.

2. Materials and Methods

2.1. Zebrafish Husbandry

Wild-type zebrafish (AB strain); transgenic lines *Tg(mpx:EGFP)* which specifically label neutrophils; and *Tg(fabp10a:dsred)* which specifically label hepatocytes were obtained from the China Zebrafish Resource Center (CZRC) in Wuhan, China. The zebrafish were maintained at a temperature of 28 ± 0.5 °C under a light/dark cycle of 14 h of light and 10 h of dark. Water changes were performed twice daily to ensure optimal water quality, and the fish were fed freshly hatched brine shrimp twice per day. All procedures adhered to the guidelines established by the Animal Care and Use Committee of Fujian Medical University.

2.2. Chemical Exposure

To assess MA's toxicity, healthy embryos at 3 dpf were transferred into six-well plates, with a density of 40 embryos per well, and subsequently treated with MA (Must Bio-Technology, Chengdu, China). The exposure concentrations of MA utilized in this study were 0 μM, 2.5 μM, 5 μM, and 7.5 μM.

2.3. Toxicity Analysis of MA

The number of dead and deformed zebrafish embryos was recorded at 24 h post treatment (24 hpt) and 48 hpt, from which the survival rate and malformation rate were calculated. Heart rate was measured at 48 hpt. Using a microscope for observation, we manually counted the number of heartbeats over a 1 min period. Images were captured using a fluorescence stereomicroscope (Nikon, Shinagawa-ku, Japan), following anesthesia with a 0.02% tricaine solution. Liver size was assessed using *Tg(fabp10a:dsred)* transgenic zebrafish larvae at 48 hpt. Additionally, *Tg(mpx:EGFP)* transgenic zebrafish larvae at 48 hpt were selected for neutrophil counting within the liver region. The pericardial area and liver size were analyzed utilizing the ImageJ software (version number: 1.53t).

2.4. Oxidative Stress Detection

Zebrafish larvae at 48 hpt underwent treatment with the DCFH-DA fluorescent probe (Beyotime, Shanghai, China) and were incubated in the dark at 28.5 °C for 30 min before thorough washing with PBS. After standardizing exposure values across samples, fluorescence images were captured using a fluorescence stereomicroscope. The fluorescence intensity of the liver region for each group was quantified using the ImageJ software.

2.5. Quantitative Real-Time PCR (qRT-PCR)

Total RNA was extracted from zebrafish larvae employing TRIzol reagent (Invitrogen, CA, USA, Xiamen, China), following a previously reported protocol [14]. RNA was reverse-transcribed into cDNA utilizing a reverse transcription kit (Accurate Biology, Changsha, China). qRT-PCR analysis was conducted using SYBR Green Pro Taq HS Premix (Accurate Biology, Changsha, China), with cDNA serving as the template. The reactions were conducted on an Agilent AriaMX Real-Time PCR System (Agilent Santa Clara, CA, USA). The sequences of PCR primers are detailed in Table 1. The relative quantification analysis of target gene expression levels employed the $2^{-\Delta\Delta Ct}$ method [15].

Table 1. Primer sequences of qRT-PCR in zebrafish.

Designed qRT-PCR Primer Sequences (5′ to 3′)			
	Gene	**Forward**	**Reverse**
Reference gene	*actb2*	CCCAAACCCAAGTTCAGCCA	ACCCACGATGGATGGGAAGA
Apoptosis-related genes	*baxa*	TGGCAAGTTCAACTGGG-GAA	ATAACTGCGGATTCCGTCCC
	casp3a	CCCAGTGGAGGCAGATTTCC	AGCATTGAGAC-GATGCAGGG
	casp3b	ACAACACCAGAAGCAGGACTT	TTTGCATCGCTTTGTCTGGC
Liver Development-related genes	*cp*	CGCTTCTGGAACCGTCAGTC	CTCGTTGCCTGGGCTTTCTT
	fabp10a	CCACCATGGACGGCAAGAAG	GACTGTCAGCGTCTCCACCA
	hhex	AATCCTCCGTCCACCGGTAA	GGGTGAACTGATGCTCGTCC
	tfa	GACTGCAGCTGCTCACACAA	TCTGCCTCTCACTCTCTGGG
Unfolded protein response-related genes	*hspa5*	CAGATCTGGCCAAAATGCGG	ATGACGGAGTGATGCGGTTT
	hspb9	TCCTCAACCTTCTCCAGGCT	CCTGGGACTCAGCAGATGAC
	hsp90b1	TCTGTGCACTTTTGGCGTTC	TCGATTCACTTCTGCCTGGA
Inflammation-related genes	*il1b*	TCTGCTCAGCCTGTGTGTTT	GAGACCCGCTGATCTCCTTG
	il6	ACTCAGAGACGAGCAGTTTGA	GCGGTCTGAAGGTTTGAGGA
	tnfa	TCACGCTCCATAAGACCCAG	AAATGGATGGCAGCCTTGGA

2.6. Transcriptome Sequencing

Total RNA was extracted from zebrafish larvae in both the control group and 5 μM MA-treated group, followed by sequencing performed by Seqhealth Technology Co., Ltd. (Wuhan, China). Sequencing was conducted using the Novaseq6000 platform (Illumina, San Diego, CA, USA) with a read length of 150 base pairs. The DESeq2 software (version number: 1.28.1) package was employed to analyze differentially expressed genes (DEGs). Gene Ontology (GO) and Kyoto Encyclopedia of Genes and Genomes (KEGG) analyses were performed using the DAVID database. A heatmap was generated on https://www.bioinformatics.com.cn (last accessed on 10 December 2024).

2.7. Cell Apoptosis Detection

Acridine orange (AO) staining was utilized to identify apoptotic cells in zebrafish larvae. An AO dye solution at a concentration of 5 μg/mL was administered to each group and incubated at 28.5 °C for 20 min. Subsequently, the larvae were washed twice with PBS for three minutes each time. Zebrafish larvae were then photographed under a fluorescence stereomicroscope, and the fluorescence intensity within the liver region of each group was quantified using the ImageJ software.

2.8. Statistical Analysis

Statistical analyses were performed using GraphPad Prism 9.0. Group differences were assessed through one-way ANOVA for multiple group comparisons. Data are expressed as means ± standard deviation (SD). Statistical significance relative to the control group is denoted as $p < 0.05$ (*), $p < 0.01$ (**) or $p < 0.001$ (***).

3. Results

3.1. Effects of MA on Zebrafish Embryos Development

To investigate the effects of MA on zebrafish embryo survival and development, embryos at 3 dpf were exposed to MA at concentrations of 0 μM, 2.5 μM, 5 μM, and 7.5 μM for a duration of 48 h. The survival rates and morphological abnormalities were observed and recorded at 24 hpt and 48 hpt. Additionally, the heart rate and pericardial cavity area were measured at 48 hpt to assess developmental impacts. The results showed that with the increase in treatment time and MA concentration, the embryos' survival rate decreased, and their malformation rate significantly increased (Figure 1A,B). MA concentrations of less than 2.5 μM did not cause the zebrafish larvae to die. The survival rates at MA concentrations of 5 μM and 7.5 μM were 89.74% and 55.26%, respectively. Moreover, increasing the MA concentration resulted in pericardial edema and elevated heart rates, highlighting its cardiotoxic effects, which align with previous studies' findings (Figure 1C–E).

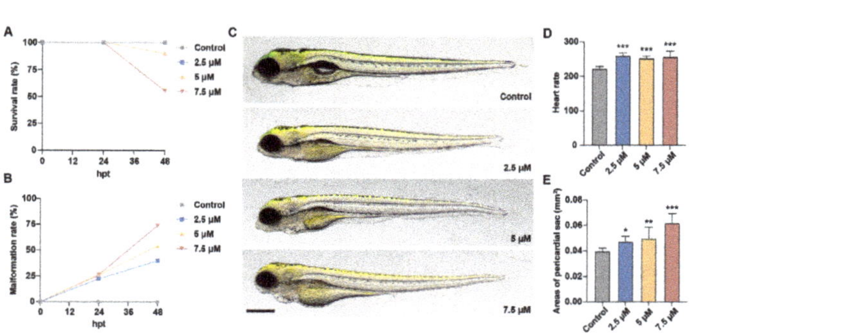

Figure 1. Effects of MA on zebrafish embryo survival and development. (**A**,**B**) Survival rate (**A**) and malformation rate (**B**) of zebrafish larvae exposed to 0 μM, 2.5 μM, 5 μM, and 7.5 μM of MA at 24 hpt

and 48 hpt. (**C**) Representative images of control and MA-treated zebrafish larvae. Scale bar: 400 μm. (**D**,**E**) Statistical analysis of heart rate (**D**) and pericardial cavity area (**E**) of control and MA-treated zebrafish larvae at 48 hpt. One-way ANOVA–Dunnett test; * $p < 0.05$, ** $p < 0.01$, *** $p < 0.001$. Error bars represent standard deviation.

3.2. MA Impaired Liver Development in Zebrafish Embryos

To investigate MA's effects on liver development, we utilized the Tg(fabp10:DsRed) transgenic zebrafish line to observe the liver morphology. Compared with the control group, the fluorescent area of the liver region in the MA-treated groups was significantly reduced (Figure 2A,B). We further analyzed liver development gene expression using qRT-PCR and found that genes related to liver development, such as tfa, cp, hhex, and fabp10a, were significantly downregulated (Figure 2C–F). These findings indicate that MA exerts toxic effects on liver development in a dose-dependent manner.

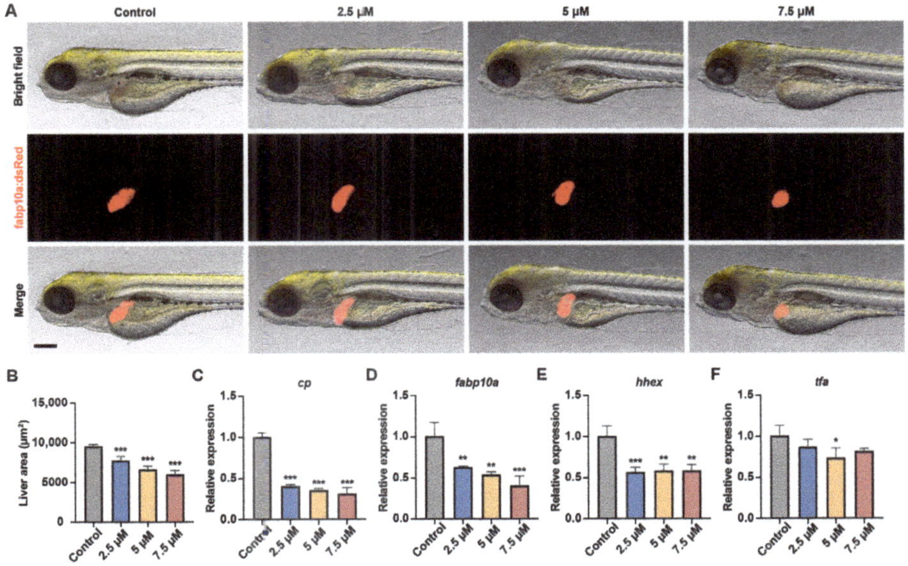

Figure 2. MA impaired liver development in zebrafish embryos. (**A**) Representative images of the Tg(*fabp10a:DsRed*) transgenic zebrafish larvae in the control and MA-treated groups at 48 hpt. Scale bar: 200 μm. (**B**) Statistical analysis of the liver area of zebrafish larvae. (**C**–**F**) qRT-PCR showing the effects of MA treatment on the expression of *cp* (**C**), *fabp10a* (**D**), *hhex* (**E**), and *tfa* (**F**) in zebrafish larvae. One-way ANOVA–Dunnett test; * $p < 0.05$, ** $p < 0.01$, *** $p < 0.001$. Error bars represent standard deviation.

3.3. MA Induced Liver Inflammation in Zebrafish Embryos

Neutrophils play a crucial role in maintaining immune system function and responding to infections. After tissue damage, neutrophils rapidly migrate to the damaged area, releasing cytokines and ROS to trigger inflammatory responses [16]. To investigate whether MA induced inflammation in the liver region, we used the *Tg*(*mpx:EGFP*) transgenic zebrafish line to observe changes in the number of neutrophils in the liver area. As shown in Figure 3A,B, the neutrophil number significantly increased in the MA-treated groups compared to that in the control group, displaying a clear dose-dependent relationship. In addition, we further analyzed the expression of inflammatory mediators such as *il6*, *il1b*, and *tnfa* in the zebrafish embryos The results revealed a significant upregulation of *il1b* and *tnfa* (Figure 3C–E). These findings indicate that MA treatment induces inflammation in the liver region of zebrafish larvae.

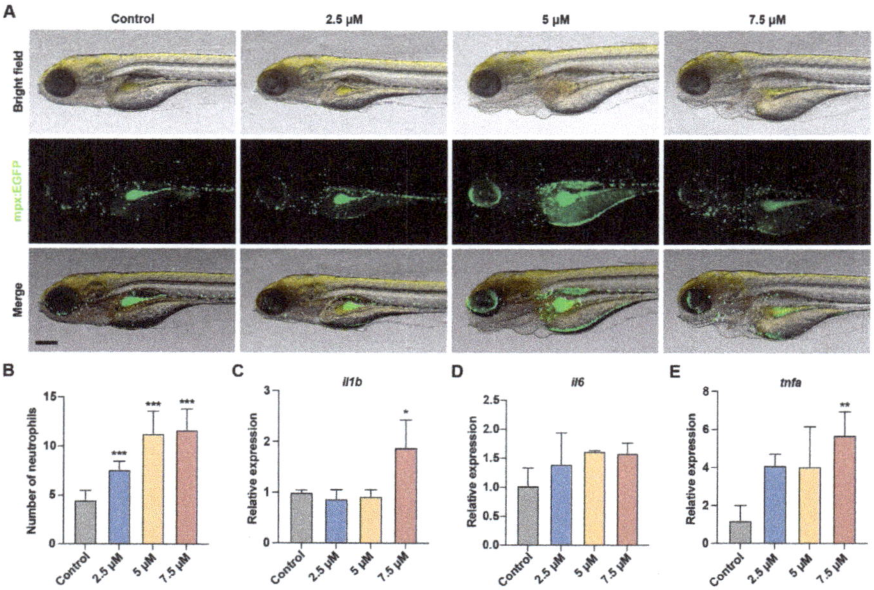

Figure 3. MA Induces liver inflammation in zebrafish embryos. (**A**) Representative images of the *Tg(mpx:EGFP)* transgenic zebrafish larvae in the control and MA-treated groups at 48 hpt. Scale bar: 200 μm. (**B**) Statistical analysis of the number of neutrophils in the liver area of zebrafish larvae. (**C–E**) qRT-PCR showing the effects of MA treatment on the expression of *il1b* (**C**), *il6* (**D**), and *tnfa* (**E**) in zebrafish larvae. One-way ANOVA–Dunnett test, * $p < 0.05$, ** $p < 0.01$, *** $p < 0.001$. Error bars represent standard deviation. The white dashed line indicates the liver region.

3.4. *MA Induced Oxidative Stress Response in Zebrafish Embryos*

Cells naturally produce ROS as byproducts of normal metabolism. However, when cells are exposed to internal or external stress, ROS production increases, disrupting the balance between oxidative and antioxidant systems and ultimately leading to oxidative stress [17]. To verify whether MA induces oxidative stress in hepatocytes, we used DCFH-DA probes to measure the ROS levels in the liver region. The results showed a significant increase in fluorescence intensity in the liver area of zebrafish embryos treated with MA (Figure 4A,B). This indicates that ROS levels were markedly elevated in the treatment groups, confirming that MA induces oxidative stress in hepatocytes.

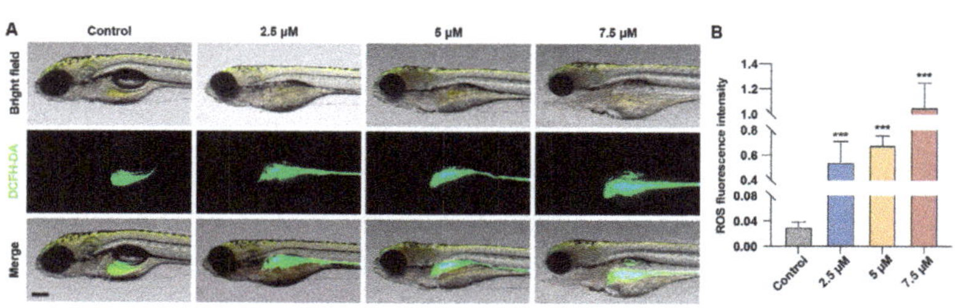

Figure 4. MA induces oxidative stress response. (**A**) Representative images of ROS staining results of control and MA-treated zebrafish larvae at 48 hpt using DCFH-DA probes. Scale bar: 200 μm. (**B**) Statistical analysis of fluorescence intensity in the liver area. One-way ANOVA–Dunnett test; *** $p < 0.001$. Error bars represent standard deviation. The white dashed line indicates the liver region.

3.5. MA Induced UPR in Zebrafish Embryos

To investigate the mechanisms underlying MA-induced liver toxicity, we conducted transcriptome sequencing on zebrafish embryos at 5 dpf to analyze the DEGs between the control and MA-treated groups. A principal component analysis (PCA) of the sequencing data revealed a clear separation between the gene expression profiles of the control and MA-treated embryos (Figure 5A). We utilized 17,549 genes with non-zero variance as input variables for the PCA. Principal Component 1 (PC1) accounted for 44. 07% of the total variance, while PC2 explained 15. 54%. A total of 345 DEGs were identified in the MA-treated group, including 184 upregulated and 161 downregulated genes (Figure 5B), indicating significant alterations in liver gene expression following MA exposure. To further explore the functions of these DEGs, a GO analysis was performed, identifying associated biological processes (BPs), cellular components (CCs), and molecular functions (MFs). The results revealed that the upregulated genes were primarily associated with BPs such as protein refolding, heat response, muscle contraction, bacterial response, and chaperone cofactor-dependent protein refolding (Figure 5C). The CC terms were enriched in the endoplasmic reticulum lumen, extracellular vesicles, chylomicrons, low-density lipoprotein (LDL) particles, and endoplasmic reticulum chaperone complexes. The MF terms included ATP-dependent protein folding, unfolded protein binding, heat shock protein binding, protein folding chaperones, and hormone receptor binding. The downregulated genes were mainly involved in BPs such as the mitotic cell cycle, microtubule depolymerization, neuron projection development, neurofilament bundle assembly, and signal transduction regulation. The CCs were primarily located in the intermediate filaments, microtubules, cytoskeleton, axons, and synapses. The MFs mainly included structural components of the cytoskeleton, tubulin binding, extracellular matrix structural constituent, chromatin binding, and GTP binding (Figure 5D). To identify the metabolic pathways in which these DEGs play critical roles, we performed a KEGG pathway enrichment analysis to further elucidate their biological functions. Following MA treatment, the protein processing pathway in the endoplasmic reticulum was significantly upregulated, consistent with the results of our GO enrichment analysis (Figure 5E). Genes associated with phototransduction, gap junctions, and motor proteins were downregulated (Figure 5F). Collectively, these findings suggested that MA activated UPR in the zebrafish embryos.

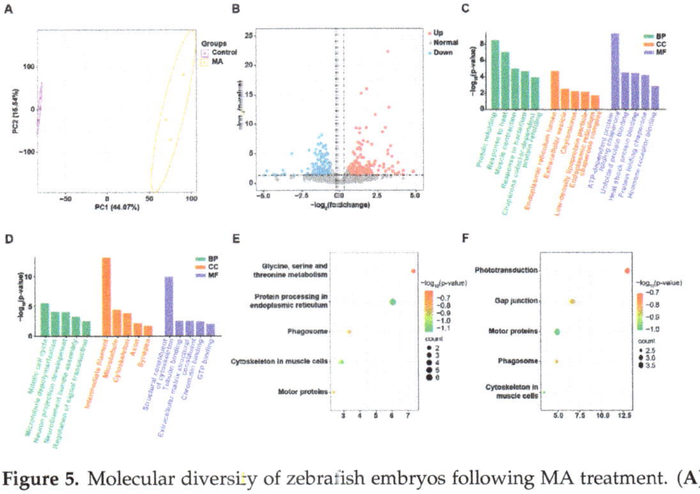

Figure 5. Molecular diversity of zebrafish embryos following MA treatment. (**A**) PCA analysis of RNA sequencing results showing differences in gene expression between control and MA-treated zebrafish

embryos. (**B**) Volcano plot showing differentially expressed genes between control and MA-treated embryos. Significance was defined as a fold change greater than 1.5 or less than 0.67, with a *p*-value less than 0.05. (**C**,**D**) Representative GO terms of upregulated (**C**) and downregulated (**D**) genes after MA treatment. (**E**,**F**) Representative KEGG entries for upregulated (**E**) and downregulated (**F**) genes after MA treatment.

To investigate the mechanism by which oxidative stress induces UPR, we analyzed the changes in HSP expression between the control and MA-treated groups. The heatmap showed that HSP gene expression was upregulated in the MA-treated group (Figure 6A). We further validated these findings using qRT-PCR, which confirmed the significant increase in *hsp90b1*, *hspa5*, and *hspb9* expression levels (Figure 6B–D).

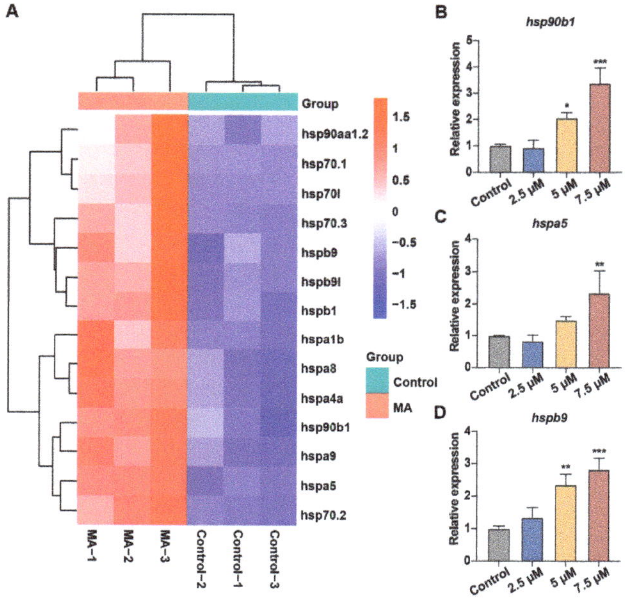

Figure 6. MA induced UPR in zebrafish embryos. (**A**) Heatmap showing scaled expression levels of hsp family genes in the control and MA-treated groups. (**B**–**D**) qRT-PCR analysis showing increased expression levels of *hsp90b1* (**B**), *hspa5* (**C**), and *hspb9* (**D**) in zebrafish larvae treated with MA compared to the control group. One-way ANOVA–Dunnett test; * $p < 0.05$, ** $p < 0.01$, *** $p < 0.001$. Error bars represent standard deviation.

3.6. MA Induces Hepatocytes Apoptosis in Zebrafish Embryos

Persistent ER stress, which fails to restore ER homeostasis, activates pro-apoptotic pathways and ultimately leads to apoptosis [18]. To evaluate hepatocyte apoptosis, we employed acridine orange, a cell-permeable nucleic acid-binding fluorochrome that exhibits green fluorescence upon binding to DNA in apoptotic cells when visualized under fluorescence microscopy. A quantitative analysis revealed that MA exposure induced a significant dose-dependent increase in the fluorescence intensity within the hepatic region compared to the control group, indicating substantial hepatocyte apoptosis (Figure 7A,B). Furthermore, the molecular analysis demonstrated the significant upregulation of key pro-apoptotic genes, including *casp3a*, *casp3b*, and *baxa* (Figure 7C–E). These findings collectively demonstrate that MA exposure induces dose-dependent hepatotoxicity characterized by enhanced hepatocyte apoptosis.

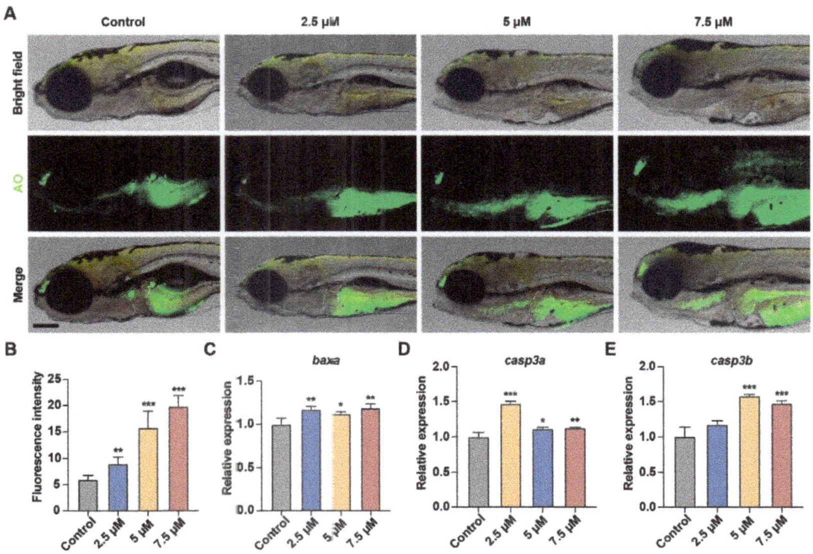

Figure 7. MA induces hepatocyte apoptosis in zebrafish embryos. (**A**) Representative images of AO staining results in control and MA-treated zebrafish larvae at 48 hpt. Scale bar: 200 μm. (**B**) Statistical analysis of fluorescence intensity in the liver area. (**C–E**) qRT-PCR showing the effects of MA treatment on the expression of *baxa* (**C**), *casp3a* (**D**), and *casp3b* (**E**) in zebrafish larvae. One-way ANOVA–Dunnett test; * $p < 0.05$, ** $p < 0.01$, *** $p < 0.001$. Error bars represent standard deviation. The white dashed line indicates the liver region.

4. Discussion

In this study, we used zebrafish as a model organism to explore MA's toxic effects on the liver. Our findings demonstrated that exposure to varying MA concentrations significantly impaired liver development in zebrafish embryos, as evidenced by the reduced liver size, increased infiltration of neutrophils into the liver, elevated ROS levels, and enhanced hepatocyte apoptosis. Moreover, we observed a significant upregulation of UPR-associated genes, including *hsp90b1*, *hspa5*, and *hspb9*, in response to MA treatment. These findings suggest that MA induced oxidative stress and hepatocyte apoptosis through the activation of endoplasmic reticulum stress and the UPR signaling pathway.

We initially investigated the developmental toxicity of MA exposure in zebrafish embryos. Both the mortality and malformation rates showed a positive correlation with the MA concentration. The pericardial area expansion correlated with increasing MA concentrations. While the heart rate showed a slight elevation, the changes were not markedly concentration-dependent. The increased heart rate may reflect enhanced energy metabolic demands, suggesting that MA accelerates zebrafish metabolism. These findings indicate that MA induces organ toxicity in zebrafish through both cardiotoxic and metabolic pathways, which aligns with previously reported observations of MA-induced cardiotoxicity.

To visually assess the MA-induced hepatotoxicity in vivo, we examined the liver size changes in *Tg(fabp10a:dsRed)* transgenic zebrafish, which specifically labels hepatocytes. At 5 dpf, we observed that the liver fluorescence area decreased with an increase in the MA concentration. Previous studies have shown that *tfa* is involved in tissue factor synthesis in the liver [19]; *cp* encodes ceruloplasmin, a glycoprotein primarily synthesized in the liver that transports copper ions and iron oxides, participates in iron metabolism and oxidative stress regulation, and maintains hepatocyte survival and function through oxidative stress repair [20]. *hhex* is crucial for liver specification, liver bud growth, and cell differentiation [21], while *fabp10a* encodes a fatty acid-binding protein (FABP) family member essential for hepatic fatty acid metabolism [22]. To further confirm that MA hindered liver development and metabolism, resulting in liver toxicity, we selected four genes, *tfa, cp, hhex,* and *fabp10a,* for qPCR detection. The results revealed the downregulation of all four genes, indicating suppressed liver development and metabolism. These findings suggest that one of MA's hepatotoxic mechanisms involves the inhibition of genes essential for liver development and metabolism, resulting in reduced liver growth and impaired hepatic metabolic function.

In this study, we quantified the neutrophil numbers in the hepatic region to test whether MA induces hepatocellular damage and triggers an inflammatory response [23]. The statistical data showed that neutrophils significantly accumulated in the zebrafish liver area, with their numbers increasing in a concentration-dependent manner with MA treatment, supporting our previous findings regarding MA-induced hepatic injury. To further investigate the mechanism of the MA-induced inflammatory response at the transcriptional level, we examined the expression of inflammatory genes *il1b, tnfa,* and *il6* using qRT-PCR. The results revealed the significant upregulation of both *il1b* and *tnfa,* while *il6* showed an increasing trend without reaching statistical significance. Previous studies have established that *il1b* encodes the proinflammatory cytokine IL-1β, which regulates immune and inflammatory responses [24]. *tnfa* encodes TNF-α, a proinflammatory cytokine involved in immune regulation, inflammatory response, apoptosis, and anti-tumor processes [25]. Similarly, *il6* encodes IL-6, which enhances neutrophil function and immune cell activity while promoting and regulating the secretion of cytokines, adhesion molecules, and inflammatory mediators such as nitric oxide [26]. These findings indicate that MA induces inflammatory gene expression, promotes neutrophil recruitment to injury sites, and thereby activates the inflammatory response.

ROS are highly reactive oxygen-containing molecules that play crucial roles in cell signaling and physiological processes. Certain toxins can trigger excessive ROS generation, leading to oxidative stress, cellular damage, and cytotoxicity [27]. To investigate the MA-induced hepatotoxicity, we measured the ROS levels in zebrafish exposed to various MA concentrations using the DCFH-DA fluorescent probe. The results demonstrated a significant positive correlation between the fluorescence intensity in the liver region and the MA concentration, indicating that MA stimulates ROS production and disrupts the oxidation–antioxidation balance. This oxidative stress leads to hepatocellular damage and dysfunction, which may contribute to the observed reduction in the zebrafish liver size.

To further investigate MA's hepatotoxicity, we performed transcriptome sequencing of the control and MA-treated zebrafish and identified the increased expression of several HSP family genes, including *hsp90b1, hspa5,* and *hspb9.* The HSP gene family encodes heat shock proteins that protect cells from stress-induced damage and function as molecular chaperones in protein folding, assembly, transport, and degradation. These proteins prevent protein misfolding and aggregation [28], playing crucial roles in the UPR [29]. The UPR is a cellular stress response mechanism activated by the accumulation of unfolded or misfolded proteins in the endoplasmic reticulum. The upregulation of HSP genes and subsequent increase in heat shock protein levels indicate that zebrafish activate anti-damage and UPR mechanisms to counter MA-induced cellular damage and protein synthesis disruption. To validate these findings, we performed a qRT-PCR analysis of the aforementioned genes. The results confirmed the upregulation of multiple HSP family genes following the MA treatment, suggesting that MA exposure causes protein and cellular damage while triggering the UPR. These findings indicate that MA interferes with normal protein folding in the hepatocyte endoplasmic reticulum, leading to misfolded protein accumulation and subsequent hepatotoxicity.

The ROS-triggered UPR can induce apoptosis [29,30], potentially contributing to zebrafish liver shrinkage. Using AO staining to detect cell apoptosis, we observed that the fluorescence intensity increased in a concentration-dependent manner with MA treatment, indicating MA-induced hepatocyte apoptosis. We focused on *casp3a*, *casp3b*, and *baxa*, which are apoptotic genes with broad regulatory roles in programmed cell death, hypothesizing their involvement in MA-mediated hepatocyte apoptosis [31–33]. To validate this hypothesis, we performed a qRT-PCR analysis of these genes. The results demonstrated the upregulation of all three apoptotic genes, providing strong experimental support for our hypothesis. These findings indicate that MA promotes hepatocyte apoptosis through the upregulation of key apoptotic genes including *casp3a*, *casp3b*, and *baxa*, further demonstrating its hepatotoxic effects.

5. Conclusions

Our findings demonstrate that MA induces hepatotoxicity in zebrafish, as evidenced by a reduced liver size, increased neutrophil infiltration, elevated ROS level, upregulation of UPR, and enhanced hepatocyte apoptosis. This study expands our understanding of MA's toxic profile and elucidates the underlying mechanisms of its hepatotoxicity. Given MA's use as a pharmaceutical component, these findings highlight the importance of careful dosage control to minimize potential adverse effects and underscore the need for appropriate risk management strategies in its clinical application.

Author Contributions: Conceptualization, Z.W., J.T. and Y.Z. (Yubin Zhuang); methodology, C.Z., Y.Z. (Yihong Zheng) and Y.L.; software, J.T.; validation, X.L. and S.L.; formal analysis, J.T.; investigation, J.T., Y.Z. (Yihong Zheng) and C.Z.; resources, C.Z.; data curation, Y.Z. (Yubin Zhuang); writing—original draft preparation, J.T., Y.Z. (Yubin Zhuang), C.Z., Y.Z. (Yihong Zheng) and Y.L.; writing—review and editing, Z.W. and Y.L.; visualization, Y.Z. (Yubin Zhuang); supervision, Z.W.; project administration, Z.W.; funding acquisition, Z.W. and Y.Z. (Yubin Zhuang). All authors have read and agreed to the published version of the manuscript.

Funding: This work was supported by Natural Science Foundation of Fujian Province (2024J01490), Fujian Provincial Education Research Projects for Young and Middle-aged Teachers (JAT210123), Startup Fund for scientific research, Fujian Medical University (2023QH1019), and Fujian Medical University High-level Talent Research Startup Funding Project (XRCZX2023003).

Institutional Review Board Statement: For animal research, all procedures adhered to the guidelines established by the Animal Care and Use Committee of Fujian Medical University (IACUC FJMU 2023-Y-0824).

Informed Consent Statement: Not applicable.

Data Availability Statement: The RNA-seq data are available on the NCBI Sequence Read Archive (SRA) database: PRJNA1202211. Other materials used in this study are available from the corresponding authors on reasonable request.

Conflicts of Interest: The authors declare no conflicts of interest.

Abbreviations

The following abbreviations are used in this manuscript:

MA	Mesaconitine
PUFAs	Polyunsaturated fatty acids
PPARα	Peroxisome proliferator-activated receptor α
ROS	Reactive oxygen species
UPR	Unfolded protein response

CZRC	China Zebrafish Resource Center
DEGs	Differentially expressed genes
GO	Gene Ontology
KEGG	Kyoto Encyclopedia of Genes and Genomes
AO	Acridine orange
SD	Standard deviation
PCA	Principal component analysis
BP	Biological processes
CC	Cellular components
MF	Molecular functions
LDL	Low-density lipoprotein
ER	Endoplasmic reticulum
HSP	Heat shock protein
FABP	Fatty acid binding protein

References

1. Sun, Z.; Yang, L.; Zhao, L.; Cui, R.; Yang, W. Neuropharmacological Effects of Mesaconitine: Evidence from Molecular and Cellular Basis of Neural Circuit. *Neural Plast.* **2020**, *2020*, 8814531. [CrossRef]
2. Mitamura, M.; Horie, S.; Sakaguchi, M.; Someya, A.; Tsuchiya, S.; Van de Voorde, J.; Murayama, T.; Watanabe, K. Mesaconitine-induced relaxation in rat aorta: Involvement of Ca^{2+} influx and nitric-oxide synthase in the endothelium. *Eur. J. Pharmacol.* **2002**, *436*, 217–225. [CrossRef]
3. Nesterova, Y.V.; Povetieva, T.N.; Suslov, N.I.; Semenov, A.A.; Pushkarskiy, S.V. Antidepressant activity of diterpene alkaloids of Aconitum baicalense Turcz. *Bull. Exp. Biol. Med.* **2011**, *151*, 425–428. [CrossRef] [PubMed]
4. Yang, M.; Ji, X.; Zuo, Z. Relationships between the Toxicities of Radix Aconiti Lateralis Preparata (Fuzi) and the Toxicokinetics of Its Main Diester-Diterpenoid Alkaloids. *Toxins* **2018**, *10*, 391. [CrossRef] [PubMed]
5. Zhou, H.; Zhang, P.; Hou, Z.; Xie, J.; Wang, Y.; Yang, B.; Xu, Y.; Li, Y. Research on the Relationships between Endogenous Biomarkers and Exogenous Toxic Substances of Acute Toxicity in Radix Aconiti. *Molecules* **2016**, *21*, 1623. [CrossRef]
6. Tan, Y.; Ko, J.; Liu, X.; Lu, C.; Li, J.; Xiao, C.; Li, L.; Niu, X.; Jiang, M.; He, X.; et al. Serum metabolomics reveals betaine and phosphatidylcholine as potential biomarkers for the toxic responses of processed Aconitum carmichaelii Debx. *Mol. Biosyst.* **2014**, *10*, 2305–2316. [CrossRef]
7. Li, T.F.; Gong, N.; Wang, Y.X. Ester Hydrolysis Differentially Reduces Aconitine-Induced Anti-hypersensitivity and Acute Neurotoxicity: Involvement of Spinal Microglial Dynorphin Expression and Implications for Aconitum Processing. *Front. Pharmacol.* **2016**, *7*, 367. [CrossRef] [PubMed]
8. Lin, X.; Zhang, J.; Wu, Z.; Shi, Y.; Chen, M.; Li, M.; Hu, H.; Tian, K.; Lv, X.; Li, C.; et al. Involvement of autophagy in mesaconitine-induced neurotoxicity in HT22 cells revealed through integrated transcriptomic, proteomic, and m6A epitranscriptomic profiling. *Front. Pharmacol.* **2024**, *15*, 1393717. [CrossRef]
9. Song, L.; Mi, S.; Zhao, Y.; Liu, Z.; Wang, J.; Wang, H.; Li, W.; Wang, J.; Zu, W.; Du, H. Integrated virtual screening and in vitro studies for exploring the mechanism of triterpenoids in Chebulae Fructus alleviating mesaconitine-induced cardiotoxicity via TRPV1 channel. *Front. Pharmacol.* **2024**, *15*, 1367682. [CrossRef]
10. Chen, Q.; Deng, X.; Zhang, K.; Kang, Y.; Jiao, M.; Zhang, J.; Wang, C.; Li, F. Changes to PUFA-PPAR pathway during mesaconitine induced myocardial coagulative necrosis. *Food Chem. Toxicol.* **2023**, *177*, 113831. [CrossRef] [PubMed]
11. Liu, F.; Han, X.; Li, N.; Liu, K.; Kang, W. Aconitum alkaloids induce cardiotoxicity and apoptosis in embryonic zebrafish by influencing the expression of cardiovascular relative genes. *Toxicol. Lett.* **2019**, *305*, 10–18. [CrossRef] [PubMed]
12. Niitsu, H.; Fujita, Y.; Fujita, S.; Kumagai, R.; Takamiya, M.; Aoki, Y.; Dewa, K. Distribution of Aconitum alkaloids in autopsy cases of aconite poisoning. *Forensic Sci. Int.* **2013**, *227*, 111–117. [CrossRef] [PubMed]
13. Chen, Q.; Zhang, K.; Jiao, M.; Jiao, J.; Chen, D.; Yin, Y.; Zhang, J.; Li, F. Study on the Mechanism of Mesaconitine-Induced Hepatotoxicity in Rats Based on Metabonomics and Toxicology Network. *Toxins* **2022**, *14*, 486. [CrossRef] [PubMed]
14. Wu, Z.; Shi, Y.; Cui, Y.; Xing, X.; Zhang, L.; Liu, D.; Zhang, Y.; Dong, J.; Jin, L.; Pang, M.; et al. Single-cell analysis reveals an Angpt4-initiated EPDC-EC-CM cellular coordination cascade during heart regeneration. *Protein Cell* **2023**, *14*, 350–368. [CrossRef]
15. Livak, K.J.; Schmittgen, T.D. Schmittgen, Analysis of Relative Gene Expression Data Using Real-Time Quantitative PCR and the $2^{-\Delta\Delta CT}$ Method. *Methods* **2001**, *25*, 402–408. [CrossRef]
16. Rosales, C. Neutrophils at the crossroads of innate and adaptive immunity. *J. Leukoc. Biol.* **2020**, *108*, 377–396. [CrossRef] [PubMed]
17. Sies, H. Oxidative stress: A concept in redox biology and medicine. *Redox Biol.* **2015**, *4*, 180–183. [CrossRef] [PubMed]

18. Tagawa, Y.; Hiramatsu, N.; Kasai, A.; Hayakawa, K.; Okamura, M.; Yao, J.; Kitamura, M. Induction of apoptosis by cigarette smoke via ROS-dependent endoplasmic reticulum stress and CCAAT/enhancer-binding protein-homologous protein (CHOP). *Free Radic. Biol. Med.* **2008**, *45*, 50–59. [CrossRef]
19. Kopec, A.K.; Luyendyk, J.P. Coagulation in liver toxicity and disease: Role of hepatocyte tissue factor. *Thromb. Res.* **2014**, *133* (Suppl. S1), S57–S59. [CrossRef] [PubMed]
20. Johannesson, T.; Kristinsson, J.; Torsdottir, G.; Snaedal, J. Ceruloplasmin (Cp) and iron in connection with Parkinson's disease (PD) and Alzheimer's disease (AD). *Laeknabladid* **2012**, *98*, 531–537.
21. Jin, Q.; Hu, Y.; Gao, Y.; Zheng, J.; Chen, J.; Gao, C.; Peng, J. Hhex and Prox1a synergistically dictate the hepatoblast to hepatocyte differentiation in zebrafish. *Biochem. Biophys. Res. Commun.* **2023**, *686*, 149182. [CrossRef] [PubMed]
22. Wang, Y.; Peng, H.; Yu, H. Bixafen causes hepatotoxicity and pancreas toxicity in zebrafish (*Danio rerio*). *Ecotoxicology* **2023**, *32*, 837–844. [CrossRef] [PubMed]
23. Liew, P.X.; Kubes, P. The Neutrophil's Role During Health and Disease. *Physiol. Rev.* **2019**, *99*, 1223–1248. [CrossRef]
24. Raziyeva, K.; Kim, Y.; Zharkinbekov, Z.; Kassymbek, K.; Jimi, S.; Saparov, A. Immunology of Acute and Chronic Wound Healing. *Biomolecules* **2021**, *11*, 700. [CrossRef] [PubMed]
25. Idriss, H.T.; Naismith, J.H. TNF alpha and the TNF receptor superfamily: Structure-function relationship(s). *Microsc. Res. Tech.* **2000**, *50*, 184–195. [CrossRef] [PubMed]
26. Tanaka, T.; Narazaki, M.; Kishimoto, T. IL-6 in inflammation, immunity, and disease. *Cold Spring Harb. Perspect. Biol.* **2014**, *6*, a016295. [CrossRef]
27. Filomeni, G.; De Zio, D.; Cecconi, F. Oxidative stress and autophagy: The clash between damage and metabolic needs. *Cell Death Differ.* **2015**, *22*, 377–388. [CrossRef] [PubMed]
28. Zininga, T.; Ramatsui, L.; Shonhai, A. Heat Shock Proteins as Immunomodulants. *Molecules* **2018**, *23*, 2846. [CrossRef] [PubMed]
29. Brenner, C.; Galluzzi, L.; Kepp, O.; Kroemer, G. Decoding cell death signals in liver inflammation. *J. Hepatol.* **2013**, *59*, 583–594. [CrossRef] [PubMed]
30. Hetz, C.; Zhang, K.; Kaufman, R.J. Mechanisms, regulation and functions of the unfolded protein response. *Nat. Rev. Mol. Cell Biol.* **2020**, *21*, 421–438. [CrossRef] [PubMed]
31. Tucker, M.B.; MacKenzie, S.H.; Maciag, J.J.; Ackerman, H.D.; Swartz, P.; Yoder, J.A.; Hamilton, P.T.; Clark, A.C. Phage display and structural studies reveal plasticity in substrate specificity of caspase-3a from zebrafish. *Protein Sci.* **2016**, *25*, 2076–2088. [CrossRef] [PubMed]
32. Li, D.D.; Ling, S.C.; Wu, K.; Luo, Z. Identification of Five Key Genes Involved in Intrinsic Apoptotic Pathway From Yellow Catfish Pelteobagrus fulvidraco and Their Transcriptional Responses to High Fat Diet (HFD). *Front. Physiol.* **2019**, *10*, 921. [CrossRef] [PubMed]
33. Tsujimoto, Y. Role of Bcl-2 family proteins in apoptosis: Apoptosomes or mitochondria? *Genes Cells* **1998**, *3*, 697–707. [CrossRef]

Disclaimer/Publisher's Note: The statements, opinions and data contained in all publications are solely those of the individual author(s) and contributor(s) and not of MDPI and/or the editor(s). MDPI and/or the editor(s) disclaim responsibility for any injury to people or property resulting from any ideas, methods, instructions or products referred to in the content.

toxics

MDPI

Article

Ethephon Poisoning: Clinical Characteristics and Outcomes

Satariya Trakulsrichai [1,2,*], Kanokrat Chuayaupakarn [1,3], Phantakan Tansuwannarat [2,4], Panee Rittilert [2], Achara Tongpoo [2], Charuwan Sriapha [2] and Winai Wananukul [2,5]

1 Department of Emergency Medicine, Faculty of Medicine Ramathibodi Hospital, Mahidol University, Bangkok 10400, Thailand; kanokrat.mc3@gmail.com
2 Ramathibodi Poison Center, Faculty of Medicine Ramathibodi Hospital, Mahidol University, Bangkok 10400, Thailand; phantakan.tans@gmail.com (P.T.); rittilert@gmail.com (P.R.); achara.ton@mahidol.ac.th (A.T.); charuwan.sri@mahidol.edu (C.S.); winai.wan@mahidol.edu (W.W.)
3 Emergency Department, Maharaj Nakhon Si Thammarat Hospital, Nakhon Si Thammarat 80000, Thailand
4 Chakri Naruebodindra Medical Institute, Faculty of Medicine Ramathibodi Hospital, Mahidol University, Samut Prakan 10540, Thailand
5 Department of Medicine, Faculty of Medicine Ramathibodi Hospital, Mahidol University, Bangkok 10400, Thailand
* Correspondence: satariya.tra@mahidol.ac.th

Abstract: Ethephon (2-chloroethylphosphonic acid) is a generally used plant growth regulator, but the data on its toxic effects, especially in humans, are very limited. This study was conducted to describe the clinical characteristics, management, and outcomes of patients exposed to products containing ethephon. We performed an 8-year retrospective study using data from the Ramathibodi Poison Center database (2013–2020), which included 252 patients. Most patients were male, with a median age of 32 years. Almost all patients were exposed through ingestion, mainly in unintentional circumstances. The clinical presentations included local effects, gastrointestinal (GI), neurological, and respiratory symptoms. Some patients required hospital admission; specifically, seven patients received inotropic drugs, and six were intubated with ventilator support. Most patients had either no or only minor clinical effects. However, six patients experienced moderate/severe effects, and two patients died. Age, intentional exposure, and the presence of initial neurological symptoms could prognosticate moderate to fatal outcomes. In conclusion, exposure to ethephon predominantly resulted in no or minor effects, and GI symptoms were the most common clinical manifestation. The cholinergic toxic syndrome was not frequently observed. The mortality rate was very low. Patients presenting with factors associated with worse outcomes should be monitored closely for clinical deterioration and appropriately managed.

Keywords: 2-chloroethylphosphonic acid; plant growth regulator; plant hormone; mortality rate

1. Introduction

Ethephon (2-chloroethylphosphonic acid) is a commonly used plant growth regulator to promote fruit ripening, abscission, flower induction, and other responses [1,2]. After being metabolized by the plant, it is converted into ethylene, a potent regulator of plant growth and maturity. It is frequently used in agriculture for plenty of crops, including wheat, coffee, rice, and cotton [1].

Ethephon is a cholinesterase or acetylcholinesterase (AChE) inhibitor. Previous animal and human studies demonstrate that the plasma and erythrocyte cholinesterase were inhibited at all doses [2–5].

Symptoms indicating inhibition of cholinesterase activity were described in animals and human volunteers [5,6]. The reported toxic effects also include corrosive effects following acute oral, inhalation, and dermal exposure [2,3]. Based on studies conducted on animals [7–11], repeated exposure to this substance has been found to cause hepatotoxicity and nephrotoxicity, as well as potentially harmful effects on reproduction and fetal development. Ethephon is widely used in many countries [12]. It is marketed and available in Thailand as well, especially as a soluble concentrate (SL) formulation. The clinical data and studies regarding ethephon poisoning in humans are currently very limited.

Numerous patients exposed to ethephon-containing products in Thailand have been referred to the Ramathibodi Poison Center (RPC) for consultations. Therefore, this study was carried out to describe the clinical characteristics, treatment, and outcomes of patients with a history of acute exposure to ethephon-containing products by analyzing data from the RPC database.

2. Materials and Methods

2.1. Study Design

We performed an 8-year retrospective cross-sectional study by using data from the RPC database (RPC Toxic Exposure Surveillance System) from January 2013 to December 2020. The primary objective of this study was to outline the clinical characteristics and outcomes of patients exposed to products containing ethephon. The secondary objective was to indicate the prognostic factors contributing to moderate to fatal outcomes.

2.2. Study Setting and Population

RPC is a tertiary teaching hospital poison center that provides consultations via telephone for healthcare providers and the public 24 h a day with approximately 15,000–29,000 calls/year during the study period. Follow-up calls are arranged to evaluate the patient's clinical progress and outcomes and provide further treatment recommendations if the patient's condition changes. All data were recorded in the RPC database, and the team of senior information scientists and clinical toxicologists finally reviewed and validated the data.

We included the patients who were exposed to products containing ethephon through every route and were referred to the RPC for consultations in our study. The poisoning from ethephon-containing products was diagnosed based on a history of exposure to the products. The exposure was indicated by identifying the ingredients listed on the bottles if the container was brought to the hospital or by obtaining the brand name and detailed list of ingredients from the patients. The patients who co-ingested herbs, illicit drugs, pesticides, or other chemicals were excluded. We also excluded patients who overdosed on pharmaceutical drugs.

We collected patients' data, including demographic data, medical history, clinical information, laboratory results, treatments, clinical course during hospitalization, and clinical outcomes.

2.3. Definitions

The estimated amount of ingestion is as follows: a teaspoon of the product equals 5 milliliters (mL), a mouthful is 25 mL (in adults), and a cup/glass is 250 mL [13,14].

This study defines hypotension and fever/high temperature as a systolic blood pressure < 90 mmHg and body temperature > 37.7 °C [15,16]. Abnormal heart rates, defined as bradycardia and tachycardia, occur when heart rates are below 60 and above 100 beats per minute, respectively [17]. The normal vital signs for pediatric patients were determined based on the normal range for their age [18].

Acute kidney injury was noted following the Kidney Disease: Improving Global Outcomes (KDIGO) Clinical Practice Guideline for Acute Kidney Injury [19]. Patients without preexisting conditions were presumed to have normal kidney function prior to exposure. Hypernatremia was defined as a serum sodium level > 145 mEq/L, while hyponatremia was defined as a serum sodium level < 135 mEq/L [20]. The definitions for hyperkalemia and hypokalemia were serum potassium levels > 5.0 mEq/L and <3.5 mEq/L, respectively [20]. Metabolic acidosis was defined as arterial pH < 7.40 and serum bicarbonate < 24 mEq/L [21], or as documented in a patient's records. A high anion gap is defined as being >12 mEq/L [21]. The Glasgow Coma Scale (GCS) is scored between 3 and 15 [22]. The definitions and terms for grading the severity and effects of acute poisoning that are used in the RPC database were derived from the Poisoning Severity Score [23,24].

2.4. Statistical Analysis

The study data were collected and statistically analyzed using Microsoft Office 2019 (version 17, Redmond, WA, USA) and STATA software (StataCorp, College Station, TX, USA), respectively. Continuous data are reported as the mean and standard deviation when they are normally distributed; otherwise, the median with minimum and maximum range is presented. For categorical data, the frequency and percentage were reported. For normally distributed continuous data, a Student's *t*-test was used for comparisons between groups, while a Mann–Whitney U test was employed for non-normally distributed data. Categorical data were analyzed to identify differences between groups using either a chi-square test or Fisher's exact test. Logistic regression was used for univariate analysis, and the forward selection method was used for multivariate analysis. A *p*-value of less than 0.05 was considered statistically significant.

3. Results

There were a total of 258 consultations regarding exposure to ethephon-containing products. After the exclusion of patients with co-ingestion of other substances, 252 patients were included in our study. Table 1 presents the clinical characteristics of all the patients. A total of 166 patients (65.9%) were male; the median age was 32 years (range, 0.9–86). Patients were from every region in Thailand, with the most commonly reported cases arising from the eastern region (36.1%). Almost all patients were exposed through ingestion (98.8%), while three were exposed through inhalation. No patients were exposed via dermal contact. Accidental exposure accounted for 83.3% (n = 210), while intentional exposure or suicidal attempts were delineated in 16.7% (n = 42). The median duration from exposure to hospital visits was 60 min. The median amount ingested was 25 mL.

The clinical effects at presentation are summarized in Table 2. The clinical presentations mostly were gastrointestinal (GI) symptoms (55.6%). A total of 54 patients (21.4%) had no obvious symptoms. At presentation, 35 patients (13.9%) had tachycardia, 8 patients (3.2%) had bradycardia, and 2 patients (0.8%) had a high temperature. One patient (0.4%) had hypotension. Five patients (2%) had a Glasgow Coma Scale (GCS) score of less than 15 (range 3–14).

The results of the initial laboratory tests for electrolyte levels and kidney function are presented in Table 3. Most patients had normal results of initial laboratory tests. Two patients had hypernatremia (serum sodium of 148 and 149 mEq/L), and one patient had hyponatremia (serum sodium of 124 mEq/L). A total of 16 patients experienced hypokalemia (with a serum potassium range of 2.7–3.4 mEq/L), and 2 patients had hyperkalemia (serum potassium of 5.3 and 6.1 mEq/L). A high anion gap metabolic acidosis was reported in two patients with anion gaps of 25 and 33 mEq/L.

Table 1. Clinical characteristics of all patients.

Clinical Characteristics (Number of Patients with Data Available)	*n* (%)
Sex	
Male	166 (65.9)
Female	86 (34.1)
Age (years), median (min–max)	32 (0.9–86)
Region	
Central *	31 (12.3)
North	8 (3.2)
North-East	44 (17.5)
East	91 (36.1)
West	19 (7.5)
South	59 (23.4)
Duration from exposure to hospital visits (minutes), median (min-max) (248 patients)	60 (5–8640)
Amount of ingestion (milliliters), median (min-max) (219 patients)	25 (0.2–500)

* Including Bangkok.

Table 2. Clinical presentations of all patients.

Clinical Presentations *	*n* (%)
No apparent symptoms	54 (21.4)
Local symptoms	
-Oral mucosa irritation	89 (35.3)
-Dermal or ocular irritation	2 (0.8)
Gastrointestinal (GI) symptoms **	140 (55.6)
Neurologic symptoms ***	23 (9.1)
Respiratory symptoms ****	4 (1.6)

* Some patients presented with > 1 symptom. ** Nausea/vomiting (110 patients), abdominal pain (61 patients), hypersalivation (13 patients), diarrhea (9 patients), GI bleeding (5 patients), and constipation (2 patients). *** Dizziness (10 patients), drowsiness (7 patients), and headache (2 patients). **** Dyspnea (4 patients) and chest discomfort (1 patient).

Table 3. Results of initial laboratory tests for electrolyte levels and kidney function of all patients.

Laboratory Results (Number of Patients with Data Available)	Value
Serum sodium (mEq/L), mean ± SD (50 patients)	139.1 ± 3.8
Serum potassium (mEq/L), mean ± SD (56 patients)	3.8 ± 0.6
Serum chloride (mEq/L), mean ± SD (50 patients)	104.7 ± 4.3
Serum bicarbonate (mEq/L), mean ± SD (50 patients)	22.1 ± 5.0
Serum blood urea nitrogen (mg/dL), mean ± SD (39 patients)	11.7 ± 3.5
Serum creatinine (mg/dL), mean ± SD (39 patients)	0.9 ± 0.3

A total of 244 patients (96.8%) had no or minor effects. Some 108 patients (42.9%) were admitted to hospitals, with a median length of hospital stay of 2 days, ranging from 1 to 14 days. The lengths of hospital stay of 17 admitted patients were not documented in our database for the reason that they recovered from poisoning and then were not followed up by the RPC until their discharge. Two patients developed AKI during hospitalization. Supportive care was the main treatment for almost all of patients, and they were finally discharged.

Eight patients (3.2%) had moderate, severe and fatal outcomes (Table 4). Seven of the patients were male, and six of them intentionally ingested ethephon. The maximum amount of ingestion was 300 mL (Patient 7). Six patients were admitted to the intensive care unit. Six patients underwent an endotracheal intubation with mechanical ventilator support. Seven patients received inotropes. The most common complication during hospitalization was pneumonia, noted in four patients. Two patients died, resulting in a mortality rate of 0.8%.

The dead patients are summarized as follows (Table 4).

The first dead case (Patient 1, Table 4) was a 40-year-old male with multiple underlying diseases, including alcohol dependence. He intentionally ingested a product containing ethephon in an unknown amount. At the scene, he had hypersalivation, nausea, and vomiting. One hour after exposure, he arrived at the emergency department with altered consciousness, a low GCS score (E2V2M5), and sinus bradycardia. The initial venous blood gas (VBG) showed acute respiratory acidosis. Approximately 1 h later, his electrocardiogram demonstrated pulseless electrical activity. Subsequently, cardiopulmonary resuscitation (CPR), intravenous (IV) adrenaline, and endotracheal intubation were performed. Hypersecretion was observed, and IV atropine was administered to treat this condition. Four hours later, he regained consciousness and received IV thiamine, dextrose, and norepinephrine. One day after admission, he developed pneumonia and upper GI bleeding. On the second day of hospitalization, he experienced hypotension and eventually died.

The second dead case (Patient 2, Table 4) was an 80-year-old male with a history of hypertension and coronary artery disease. He accidentally ingested 25 mL of ethephon. Thirty minutes after ingestion, he had no apparent symptoms. Hypokalemia (serum potassium of 2.66 mEq/L) was initially observed. He was treated with an IV antiemetic drug and IV fluids with a potassium chloride supplement. He developed tachypnea, fever (body temperature 38.5 °C), and crepitation of both lungs. He was then intubated with ventilator support. He experienced diarrhea several times (>20 times), sinus tachycardia (heart rate 166 bpm), depressed consciousness (GCS score: E4VTM5), and oliguria. His treatment included comprehensive supportive care and consulting a gastroenterologist for severe diarrhea evaluation. On the sixth day of admission, his chest X-ray showed right lung infiltration, and VBG showed respiratory and metabolic acidosis. He was diagnosed with severe pneumonia with septic shock. IV meropenem and norepinephrine were administered. After 10 days of admission, he died from complications.

We compared the clinical manifestations between patients with no/minor and moderate/severe/fatal outcomes to analyze the factors associated with moderate, severe, and fatal outcomes/severities. The amount of ingestion, intentional exposure, neurological symptoms, and GCS score at presentation <15 showed statistically significant differences (Table 5).

Table 6 presents the univariate and multivariate analysis of factors associated with moderate, severe, and fatal outcomes/severities. In the multivariate analysis, age, intentional exposure, and the presence of neurological symptoms at presentation were associated with worse outcomes.

Table 4. Clinical characteristics and laboratory findings of patients with moderate, severe, and fatal outcomes.

Clinical Characteristics	Patient 1	Patient 2	Patient 3	Patient 4	Patient 5	Patient 6	Patient 7	Patient 8
Patient characteristics								
Sex/Age (years)	Male/40	Male/80	Male/55	Male/52	Male/26	Male/40	Male/41	Female/28
Underlying diseases	AD, HIV infection, MDD	HT, CAD	AD	No	No	AD	No	No
Duration after exposure to hospital visits (minutes)	60	30	30	60	60	60	60	120
Circumstances	Intentional	Accidental	Intentional	Intentional	Intentional	Accidental	Intentional	Intentional
Amount of ingestion (mL)	N/A	25	N/A	25	N/A	25	300	75
Clinical manifestations at presentation								
Local effects (yes/no) Oral mucosa irritation Salivation	 No Yes	 Yes No	 No No	 Yes No	 No Yes	 No No	 No Yes	 No Yes
GI symptoms (yes/no)	Yes	Yes	Yes	No	No	Yes	No	Yes
Neurologic symptoms (yes/no)	Yes	No	No	No	Yes (seizure)	Yes (tremor)	Yes	Yes
Respiratory symptoms (yes/no)	Yes	No	Yes	No	No	No	No	Yes
Systemic effects at presentation								
Vital signs: BT (°C), HR (/minute), RR (/minute), BP (mmHg)	 N/A 60 18 112/53	 N/A N/A N/A N/A	 N/A 70 N/A 70/30	 36.7 98 20 160/96	 36.6 78 18 160/90	 37.2 98 20 138/82	 37.5 108 20 137/87	 N/A 40 N/A N/A
GCS	9	15	15	15	7	15	12	6
Metabolic acidosis (yes/no) Anion gap (mEq/L)	Yes 33	No 5	Yes 25	No 4	No 10	Yes 22	No 9	N/A N/A
Acute kidney injury (yes/no) Serum BUN, Creatinine (mg/dL)	No 8, 1.1	Yes N/A	No N/A	No 13, 0.87	No 10, 0.8	Yes 7, 1.8	No N/A, 0.89	No N/A

Table 4. *Cont.*

Clinical Characteristics	Patient 1	Patient 2	Patient 3	Patient 4	Patient 5	Patient 6	Patient 7	Patient 8
Treatment (yes/no)								
Oxygen therapy	Yes	Yes	Yes	Yes	No	Yes	Yes	Yes
Endotracheal intubation	Yes	Yes	Yes	Yes	No	Yes	No	Yes
Administration of inotropes	Yes	Yes	Yes	No	Yes	Yes	Yes	Yes
Hospital clinical course								
Complication during hospitalization (yes/no)								
Pneumonia	Yes	Yes	No	No	No	Yes	No	Yes
Acute kidney injury	Yes	Yes	Yes	No	No	Yes	No	Yes
Hospital stays (days)	2	10	N/A	N/A	2	N/A	6	14
Outcomes	Death	Death	Severe	Moderate	Moderate	Severe	Moderate	Moderate

Abbreviations: AD, Alcohol dependence; MDD, major depressive disorder; HIV, human immunodeficiency virus; HT, hypertension; CAD, coronary artery disease; N/A, not applicable; mL, milliliters; BUN, blood urea nitrogen.

Table 5. Comparison of clinical manifestations between patients who had no/minor and moderate to fatal outcomes.

Clinical Manifestations (Number of Patients with Data Available)	No/Minor Outcomes (n = 244)	Moderate/Severe/Fatal Outcomes (n = 8)	p-Value
Sex: number of male: female (252 patients)	159:85	7:1	0.271
Age (years), median (min–max) (252 patients)	31 (0.92–86)	40.5 (26–80)	0.387
Amount of ingestion (milliliters), median (min–max) (n = 219)	25 (0–500)	50 (25–300)	0.035
Number of unintentional: intentional exposure (252 patients)	208:36	2:6	<0.001
Time to hospital (minutes)	60 (5–8640)	60 (30–60)	1.000
Clinical presentations			
Gastrointestinal symptoms	134 (54.9)	6 (75.0)	0.306
Neurologic symptoms	18 (7.4)	5 (62.5)	<0.010
Respiratory symptoms	3 (1.2)	1 (12.5)	0.122
Glasgow coma scale score < 15	3 (1.2)	2 (25.0)	0.008

Table 6. Univariate and multivariate analyses of factors associated with moderate, severe, and fatal outcomes.

Factors	Univariate Analysis			Multivariate Analysis		
	Odds Ratio (OR)	95%CI	p-Value	Odds Ratio (OR)	95%CI	p-Value
Sex	3.742	0.453–30.921	0.221	-	-	-
Age (years)	1.032	0.997–1.068	0.076	1.107	1.024–1.197	0.011
Amount of ingestion (milliliters)	1.006	0.999–1.012	0.093	-	-	-
Number of unintentional: intentional exposures	17.333	3.366–89.262	0.001	45.557	3.650–568.591	0.003
Time to hospital	0.995	0.983–1.007	0.392	-	-	-
Clinical presentations						
Gastrointestinal symptoms	2.463	0.487–12.445	0.276	-	-	-
Neurologic symptoms	20.926	4.624–94.697	<0.001	57.377	5.724–575.120	0.001
Respiratory symptoms	11.476	1.057–124.580	0.045	-	-	-
Glasgow coma scale score < 15	26.778	3.757–190.871	0.001	-	-	-

4. Discussion

In this study, we examined patients who had been exposed to ethephon to analyze their clinical characteristics and outcomes. According to the limited data on ethephon poisoning in humans within the literature in English, this study, which described 252 patients, is one of the largest conducted regarding ethephon poisoning. The findings of the study provide significant data that expand the existing knowledge on this poisoning. The importance of this study on the toxicity of ethephon is emphasized. The majority of the patients were exposed orally, mostly through accidental circumstances. Our findings suggest that the containers of these products might be easily accessible or that ethephon may be stored in other food containers, increasing the risk of accidental ingestion. In addition, unclear or absent labeling on the product bottles may have contributed to unawareness about their contents. This finding suggested that implementing safety measures, such as clear product labeling or appropriate containers, could be a strategy to prevent this poisoning.

Most patients presented with no apparent symptoms or mild clinical effects, with normal vital signs at presentation. The median lethal dose (LD50) of ethephon is >4000 mg/kg. The WHO recommended classification of pesticides by hazard categorizes ethephon as classification III (Slightly hazardous) [25]. Therefore, our findings supported this classification.

Local irritation was also observed in our patients, consistent with the findings of the previous study [2,3]. GI symptoms were the most common clinical finding in our study. Neurological symptoms, especially depressed consciousness, were occasionally reported. Although ethephon is an AChE inhibitor, prominent symptoms of cholinergic toxic syndrome were not commonly reported in our patients. Hypersecretion and diarrhea were observed in some patients. However, plasma and erythrocyte cholinesterase levels were not evaluated in these patients. Previous findings in animal studies involving repeated exposure revealed liver toxicity [7,8]. The patients in our study did not exhibit hepatotoxicity. Therefore, in acute poisoning, liver toxicity is not a clinical feature. The cornerstone of management was supportive care.

Six patients with worse outcomes (moderate to fatal final severities) were exposed through intentional ingestion. Intentional circumstances may lead to greater exposure than unintentional ones and contribute to significant clinical effects. In our study, two patients died. Although the mortality rate was very low, patients experiencing this poisoning could still be at risk of death. One patient died rapidly after intentional exposure, developing consciousness depression and complications. The other one accidentally ingested and died from complications of pneumonia 10 days later.

According to the multivariate analyses, we found that age, intentional exposure, and having neurological symptoms at presentation were prognostic factors associated with moderate, severe, or fatal outcomes. Therefore, elderly patients with intentional exposure or having neurological symptoms should be closely and carefully observed, monitored, and well managed. Adequate supportive care and appropriate management of laboratory abnormalities or complications during admission are essential for all patients.

The current study has several limitations, as follows. The data may not reflect the true incidences of poisoning and mortality in Thailand, as reporting exposure to ethephon-containing products to the RPC is not mandatory. The retrospective study design may have led to incomplete or unclear data. The medical histories were collected from patients or their relatives, who reported to the medical staff. These histories may not have been clearly or entirely documented. The diagnosis was primarily based on the patient's exposure history, without specific laboratory confirmation of ethephon exposure.

5. Conclusions

Ethephon poisoning commonly results in no effects or only mild symptoms. GI symptoms were the predominant clinical manifestations. It is important to note that cholinergic toxic syndrome is not a typical clinical feature associated with this type of poisoning. The mortality rate was very low. Supportive care may be considered as the main treatment. Age, intentional exposure, and neurological symptoms at presentation were prognostic factors for worse outcomes. Consequently, patients with these factors should be closely observed and monitored for clinical deterioration.

Author Contributions: Conceptualization, S.T. and K.C.; methodology, S.T. and K.C.; software, S.T., A.T. and C.S.; validation, S.T., K.C., P.T., P.R. and C.S.; formal analysis, S.T., K.C. and A.T.; investigation, S.T. and K.C.; resources, S.T. and W.W.; data curation, S.T. and K.C.; writing—original draft preparation, S.T. and K.C.; writing—review and editing, S.T.; visualization, S.T., P.T. and A.T.; supervision, S.T.; project administration, S.T. All authors have read and agreed to the published version of the manuscript.

Funding: This research received no external funding.

Institutional Review Board Statement: The study was conducted following the Declaration of Helsinki, and approved by the Institutional Ethics Committee of Ramathibodi Hospital Faculty of Medicine, Mahidol University (approval number COA. MURA2021/303).

Informed Consent Statement: Patient consent was not required according to the study's retrospective design and the anonymous reporting of confidential data obtained from the poison center database.

Data Availability Statement: The data in this article were presented at the North American Congress of Clinical Toxicology (NACCT) 2023, Montreal, Quebec, Canada, 29 September–1 October 2024, as a poster presentation with interim findings. The data are inaccessible to the public due to patient privacy concerns, but they can be obtained from the corresponding author upon reasonable request.

Acknowledgments: The authors thank Sasiporn Sitthisorn and Chanatpon Aonnuam, Department of Clinical Epidemiology and Biostatistics, Faculty of Medicine, Ramathibodi Hospital, Mahidol University, for their assistance in conducting the statistical analyses. We utilized a commercial AI program to assist in editing English and contributed to this text by responding to the AI prompts: Improve it.

Conflicts of Interest: The authors declare no conflicts of interest.

References

1. Ethephon. Available online: https://pubchem.ncbi.nlm.nih.gov/compound/Ethephon (accessed on 13 October 2024).
2. Ethephon. Available online: https://www3.epa.gov/pesticides/chem_search/reg_actions/reregistration/fs_PC-099801_1-Apr-95.pdf (accessed on 13 October 2024).
3. EFSA (European Food Safety Authority); Alvarez, F.; Arena, M.; Auteri, D.; Binaglia, M.; Castoldi, A.F.; Chiusolo, A.; Colagiorgi, A.; Colas, M.; Crivellente, F.; et al. Conclusion on peer review of the pesticide risk assessment of the active substance ethephon. *EFSA J.* **2023**, *21*, e07742. [CrossRef] [PubMed]
4. El-Okazy, A.M. The Effects of Combination of Gibberellic Acid—3 (GA3) and Ethephon (2-Chloroethyl Phosphonic Acid) (Plant Growth Regulators) on Some Physiological Parameters in Mice. *J. Egypt. Public Health Assoc.* **2008**, *83*, 67–86. [PubMed]
5. Pesticide Residues in Food—2002, Report of the Joint Meeting of the FAO Panel of Experts on Pesticide Residues in Food and the Environment, Rome, Italy; 16–25 September 2002. Available online: https://www.fao.org/fileadmin/templates/agphome/documents/Pests_Pesticides/JMPR/Reports_1991-2006/Report_2002.pdf (accessed on 29 October 2024).
6. Cetinkaya, M.A.; Baydan, E. Investigation of in vitro effects of ethephon and chlorpyrifos, either alone or in combination, on rat intestinal muscle contraction. *Interdiscip. Toxicol.* **2010**, *3*, 35–39. [CrossRef] [PubMed]
7. Bhadoria, P.; Nagar, M.; Bahrioke, V.; Bhadoria, A.S. Effect of ethephon on the liver in albino rats: A histomorphometric study. *Biomed J.* **2015**, *38*, 421–427. [CrossRef] [PubMed]
8. Bhadoria, P.; Nagar, M.; Bharihoke, V.; Bhadoria, A.S. Ethephon, an organophosphorous, a Fruit and Vegetable Ripener: Has potential hepatotoxic effects? *J. Fam. Med. Prim. Care* **2018**, *7*, 179–183. [CrossRef] [PubMed]
9. Mokhtari, T.; Hussein Osman, H.E.; El-Meghawry El-Kenawy, A.; Dashti, N. Ameliorative effect of virgin olive oil against nephrotoxicity following sub-chronic administration of ethephon in male rats. *J. Tradit. Complement. Med.* **2019**, *10*, 487–495. [CrossRef] [PubMed]
10. El Raouf, A.; Girgis, S. Mutagenic, teratogenic and biochemical effects of ethephon on pregnant mice and their fetuses. *Glob Vet.* **2011**, *6*, 251–257.
11. Huang, H.; Zhao, X.; Shi, X.; Tan, Q.; Zhang, R.; Yue, M.; Ma, R.; Chen, Q.; Zhao, S.; Yang, L. Effects of ethephon on serum levels of sex hormone, apoptosis, and cell cycle of ovaries in mice. *Endokrynol. Pol.* **2022**, *73*, 346–352. [CrossRef] [PubMed]
12. Ethephon. Available online: https://www.fao.org/fileadmin/templates/agphome/documents/Pests_Pesticides/JMPR/Evaluation94/ethephon.pdf (accessed on 13 October 2024).
13. Sriapha, C.; Trakulsrichai, S.; Tongpoo, A.; Pradoo, A.; Rittilert, P.; Wananukul, W. Acute Imidacloprid Poisoning in Thailand. *Ther. Clin. Risk Manag.* **2020**, *16*, 1081–1088. [CrossRef] [PubMed]
14. Trakulsrichai, S.; Sittiyuno, P.; Tansuwannarat, P.; Tongpoo, A. Emamectin Poisoning in Thailand: Clinical Characteristics and Outcomes. *Toxics* **2024**, *12*, 668. [CrossRef] [PubMed]
15. Nicks, B.A.; Gaillard, J.P. Approach to Nontraumatic Shock. In *Tintinalli's Emergency Medicine: A Comprehensive Study Guide*, 9th ed.; Tintinalli, J.E., Ma, O., Yealy, D.M., Eds.; McGraw-Hill Education: New York, NY, USA, 2020; pp. 57–63.

16. Ogoina, D. Fever, fever patterns and diseases called 'fever'—A review. *J. Infect. Public Health* **2011**, *4*, 108–124. [CrossRef] [PubMed]
17. Michaud, G.F.; Stevenson, W.G. Physiologic and Nonphysiologic Sinus Tachycardia. In *Harrison's Principles of Internal Medicine*, 20th ed.; Jameson, J., Fauci, A.S., Kasper, D.L., Eds.; McGraw-Hill Education: New York, NY, USA, 2018; pp. 4316–4318.
18. Nelson, L.S.; Howland, M.A.; Lewin, N.A.; Goldfrank, L.R.; Hoffman, R.S. Initial Evaluation of the Patient: Vital Signs and Toxic Syndromes. In *Goldfrank's Toxicologic Emergencies*, 11th ed.; Nelson, L.S., Howland, M.A., Lewin, N.A., Smith, S.W., Goldfrank, L.R., Hoffman, R.S., Eds.; McGraw-Hill Education: New York, NY, USA, 2019; pp. 33–41.
19. Kidney Disease: Improving Global Outcomes (KDIGO) Acute Kidney Injury Work Group. KDIGO Clinical Practice Guideline for Acute Kidney Injury. *Kidney Int. Suppl.* **2012**, *2*, 1–138.
20. Mount, D.B. Fluid and Electrolyte Disturbances. In *Harrison's Principles of Internal Medicine*, 20th ed.; Jameson, J., Fauci, A.S., Kasper, D.L., Eds.; McGraw-Hill Education: New York, NY, USA, 2018; pp. 789–817.
21. Charney, A.N.; Hoffman, R.S. Fluid, electrolyte, and Acid-Base Principles. In *Goldfrank's Toxicologic Emergencies*, 11th ed.; Nelson, L.S., Howland, M.A., Lewin, N.A., Eds.; McGraw Hill Education: New York, NY, USA, 2019; pp. 189–202.
22. Matis, G.; Birbilis, T. The Glasgow Coma Scale--a brief review. Past, present, future. *Acta Neurol. Belg.* **2008**, *108*, 75–89. [PubMed]
23. Persson, H.; Sjöberg, G.; Haines, J.; Pronczuk de Garbino, J. Poisoning Severity Score: Grading of acute poisoning. *J. Toxicol. Clin. Toxicol.* **1998**, *36*, 205–213. [CrossRef] [PubMed]
24. POISONING SEVERITY SCORE (PSS) IPCS/EAPCCT. Available online: https://cdn.who.int/media/docs/default-source/chemical-safety/intox/pss95699a36-61ab-4be6-848f-c1d894d21fbd.pdf?sfvrsn=5750967e_10 (accessed on 29 October 2024).
25. World Health Organization. *WHO Recommended Classification of Pesticides by Hazard and Guidelines to Classification*, 2019th ed.; World Health Organization: Geneva, Switzerland, 2020.

Disclaimer/Publisher's Note: The statements, opinions and data contained in all publications are solely those of the individual author(s) and contributor(s) and not of MDPI and/or the editor(s). MDPI and/or the editor(s) disclaim responsibility for any injury to people or property resulting from any ideas, methods, instructions or products referred to in the content.

toxics

MDPI

Article

Bisphenol S Induces Lipid Metabolism Disorders in HepG2 and SK-Hep-1 Cells via Oxidative Stress

Kai-Xing Lin [1,2], Zi-Yao Wu [1], Mei-Lin Qin [1] and Huai-Cai Zeng [1,2,*]

[1] Guangxi Key Laboratory of Environmental Exposomics and Entire Lifecycle Health, School of Public Health, Guilin Medical University, Guilin 541199, China; linkaixing922@163.com (K.-X.L.); ziyaowu@163.com (Z.-Y.W.); qmeilin2022@163.com (M.-L.Q.)

[2] Guangxi Health Commission Key Laboratory of Entire Lifecycle Health and Care, School of Public Health, Guilin Medical University, Guilin 541199, China

* Correspondence: zenghuaicai@glmc.edu.cn

Abstract: Bisphenol S (BPS) is a typical endocrine disruptor associated with obesity. To observe BPS effects on lipid metabolism in HepG2 and SK-Hep-1 human HCC cells, a CCK-8 assay was used to assess cell proliferation in response to BPS, and the optimal concentration of BPS was selected. Biochemical indices such as triglyceride (TG) and total cholesterol (T-CHO), and oxidative stress indices such as malondialdehyde (MDA) and catalase (CAT) were measured. ROS and MDA levels were significantly increased after BPS treatment for 24 h and 48 h ($p < 0.05$), indicating an oxidative stress response. Alanine aminotransferase (ALT), T-CHO, and low-density lipoprotein cholesterol (LDL-C) levels also increased significantly after 24 or 48 h BPS treatments ($p < 0.05$). RT-PCR and Western blot analyses detected mRNA or protein expression levels of peroxisome proliferator-activated receptor α (PPARα) and sterol regulatory element-binding protein 1c (SREBP1C). The results indicated that BPS could inhibit the mRNA expression of PPARα and carnitine palmitoyl transferase 1B (CPT1B), reduce lipid metabolism, promote mRNA or protein expression of SREBP1C and fatty acid synthase (FASN), and increase lipid synthesis. Increased lipid droplets were observed using morphological Oil Red O staining. Our study demonstrates that BPS may cause lipid accumulation by increasing oxidative stress and perturbing cellular lipid metabolism.

Keywords: oxidative stress; lipid metabolism; bisphenol S; metabolic disorders

1. Introduction

Bisphenol S (BPS) serves as a substitute for BPA and is incorporated in a variety of industrial and consumer products [1]. It exerts endocrine-disrupting effects and can seriously affect the endocrine system in various ways [2], leading to lipid metabolism disorders and serious damage to the human body [3]. The median value of BPS glucosinolates detected in the urine of the general population was 0.38 ng/mL [4], and the median urinary BPS concentration in the occupational population of cashiers exposed to thermal paper was 2.53 μg/L [5], much higher than that of the general population. During the seawater monitoring in the Pearl River Estuary in China, BPS was observed at a detection rate of 100%, and this was similar to that of BPA and BPF [6]. However, during the detection of biodegradation of bisphenol compounds in seawater, BPS exhibited higher stability and more difficult biodegradation than BPA and BPF [7]. Due to increasing levels of BPS exposure in the environment, its safety has attracted increasing attention.

 https://doi.org/10.3390/toxics13010044

Obesity has become increasingly prevalent. BPS is a typical endocrine disruptor closely linked to the occurrence of obesity [8]. Studies have demonstrated that BPS promotes weight gain in adults [9], and it is significantly associated with obesity [10]. Meng et al. [11,12] reported that BPS exposure may disrupt lipid and glucose metabolism in perinatal male and female mice, enhancing fatty acid and triglyceride (TG) production and elevating obesity risk. Another study indicated that BPS caused hepatic steatosis and lipid accumulation in mice as well as oxidative stress [13]. Serum BPS levels in humans are connected to oxidative stress and endocrine disorders [14]. Prior research has indicated that BPS increases reactive oxygen species levels in adipocyte progenitors and promotes fat synthesis [15]. Chen et al. [16] observed that improving oxidative stress can alleviate type 2 diabetes combined with non-alcoholic fatty liver disease.

In regulating the mechanism of liver lipid metabolism disorders, the PPAR signaling pathway plays an important role. For example, peroxisome proliferator-activated receptor α (PPARα) is a key regulator of liver beta-oxidation, which is involved in the main process of fatty acid metabolism in the liver, and it regulates downstream target genes, such as carnitine palmitoyl transferase 1 (CPT1) [17], to control mitochondrial fatty acid beta-oxidation. Overexpression of the novel biomarker for non-alcoholic fatty liver, MIR20B, significantly reduces the oxidation of free fatty acids by targeting PPARα, resulting in a significant upregulation of TG and cholesterol content in HepG2 cells treated with oleic acid [18]. Qiu et al. [19] demonstrated that BPS exposure induces chronic inflammatory stress in the liver. When carp livers were exposed to 100 mg/L of both BPS and BPA, the oxidative stress levels induced by BPS were significantly higher compared to those induced by BPA. This also illustrates that BPS is not necessarily a safe alternative to BPA and that its potential harm to organisms or the environment should be further studied. Current evidence suggests that BPS may affect the gene expression of liver lipid synthesis, transport, and metabolism through oxidative stress, leading to lipid accumulation and alleviating oxidative stress in HepG2 cells by affecting the sterol regulatory element-binding protein 1c (SREBP1C)/FASN pathway through PPARα [20]. Therefore, this study mainly examined proteins or genes related to liver lipid synthesis and metabolism, such as SREBP1C, fatty acid synthase (FASN), PPARα, carnitine palmitoyl transferase 1B(CPT1B), etc.

The impact of BPS on lipid metabolism in HepG2 and SK-Hep-1 cells remains unclear. Current research indicates that BPS causes oxidative stress, which alters the expression of genes in the liver linked to lipid production, transport, and metabolism and results in lipid accumulation. In vitro studies on human red blood cells revealed no discernible alteration in the levels of catalase (CAT) after treatment with 100 μg/mL BPS for 24 h [21]. Considering that different individuals exhibit different sensitivities to chemicals and that the HepG2 cell line's metabolome is unstable, a major transition may occur over time [22]. To this end, this study utilized the HepG2 and SK-Hep-1 human hepatocellular carcinoma cells to assess the responses to BPS treatment for 24 h and 48 h, respectively. A BPS concentration of 250 μmol/L was selected according to the results of CCK-8 experiments. Based on the detection of malondialdehyde (MDA), TG, total cholesterol (T-CHO), and other indicators, the staining results of Oil Red O assays, and reactive oxygen species assessments, the aim is to examine how lipid metabolism is affected by varying BPS treatment durations in the experimental cell lines, thus providing a reference for the study of the mechanisms of preventing environmental pollutants from causing obesity by inducing lipid accumulation.

2. Experimental Method

2.1. Cell Culture and Exposure

For cell culture, human hepatocellular carcinoma cells (HepG2 and SK-Hep-1) were rapidly thawed and inoculated into culture dishes containing 7 mL of complete medium and were incubated at 37 °C under 5% CO_2. Cell exposure refers to the transfer of two separate dishes of 80% grown cells to 10 mL centrifuge tubes, the addition of 6 mL of complete medium, the inoculation of cells into 6-well plates with a 0.5 mL density of cell volume per well, and the replacement of the complete medium with new complete medium when growth reaches 50%. After 24 h of BPS exposure, each well was filled with 3 mL of complete medium, and after 48 h of BPS exposure, each well was filled with 4 mL of complete medium. According to whether the cells were exposed to BPS or not, the two types of cells were divided into control and BPS-stained groups, respectively. An amount of 3 or 4 μL of DMSO was incorporated into the control group, and 3 or 4 μL of the 250 mmol/L BPS (Sigma, Shanghai, China) master batch was added to the BPS group, which ensured that the BPS was exposed at a final concentration of 250 μmol/L for 24 or 48 h. The final BPS concentration for cell exposure was 250 μmol/L.

2.2. CCK-8 Method Cell Viability Assays

HepG2 and SK-Hep-1 cells under optimal growth conditions were prepared into single cell suspensions, and 10 μL was extracted for cell counting to adjust the number of cells. After 24 or 48 h BPS exposure HepG2 cells were inoculated at a density of 3000 or 2000 cells per well, and SK-Hep-1 cells were inoculated at a density of 4000 or 3000 cells per well. After 50% of the cells adhered to the wall, the BPS stock solution was diluted into 0, 50, 150, 200, 250, 300, and 350 μmol/L solutions with complete medium and then added to each well at a total volume of 100 μL. The treated cells were cultured in a CO_2 incubator (Thermo Fisher Scientific, Waltham, MA, USA) for 24 or 48 h, and the 96-well plates were then removed to discard the original medium. Each well was then filled with complete medium with 10 μL of CCK-8 solution at a 10:1 ratio. Following a one-hour incubation period at 37 °C, absorbance values in each well were measured at 450 nm.

2.3. ROS Reactive Oxygen Detection

After cell treatments, the DCFH-DA probe was diluted to 10 μmol/L with preheated serum-free medium according to the instructions of the reactive oxygen species detection kit (Beijing Solarbio Science & Technology Co., Ltd., Beijing, China, CA1410). The original medium was removed, and the cells underwent two gentle PBS washes, were injected with DCFH-DA probe dilution solution in the dark and were incubated for 20 min at 37 °C in a cell incubator. Serum-free cell culture media was then used to wash the cells three times. After removing residual DCFH-DA, the cells were observed and captured on camera using an inverted microscope.

2.4. Oil Red O Staining

After the cells were exposed to BPS and cultured, they were washed twice with PBS buffer, fixed by adding Oil Red O (Beijing Solepol Science and Technology Co., Ltd., Beijing, China, G1262) fixative for 20 min, and the fixative was discarded and washed twice with distilled water. The process of Oil Red O staining was carried out sequentially according to the following steps: 60% isopropanol wash for 20 s, Oil Red O dip staining for 10 min, 60% isopropanol wash for 20 s, distilled water wash 3 times, hematoxylin staining for 1 min, distilled water wash 3 times, and dip staining with Oil Red O buffer for 1 min. Finally, after discarding the Oil Red O buffer, distilled water was added to cover the cells, and the lipid droplet production of the cells in each group was observed under an inverted microscope.

2.5. Measurement of Biochemical Indicators and Oxidative Stress Indicators

Because HepG2 cells and SK-Hep-1 cells are different in the 6-well plate, different levels of lysate are required. After cell exposure culture, 400 μL of cell lysate was added to a 6-well plate containing HepG2 cells, and 300 μL of cell lysate was added to a 6-well plate containing SK-Hep-1 cells for protein extraction. Intracellular TG (A110-1-1), T-CHO (A111-1-1), low-density lipoprotein cholesterol (LDL-C, A113-1-1), alanine aminotransferase (ALT, C009-2-1), malondialdehyde (MDA, BC0025), catalase (CAT, C009-1-1), and T-CHO (A111-1-1) were measured according to the kit's instructions. Following the detection of the indicators, a full wavelength scanning multifunction microplate reader (Thermo Scientific Varioskan LUX, Waltham, MA, USA) was used to quantify each kit. Every kit was acquired from the Nanjing Institute of Bioengineering, China.

2.6. Real-Time Quantitative PCR (qPCR) Analysis

TRIzol reagent (Ambion, Austin, TX, USA) was used to extract total RNA and determine its concentration, and reverse transcription was used to synthesize cDNA using a reverse transcription kit (Monad, Wuhan, China). The mRNA expression levels of PPARα, CD36, SREBP1C, and FASN were detected using a QuantStudio 6 Flex according to the instructions for the reagent. The primer sequences are presented in Table 1.

Table 1. Real-time quantitative PCR primer sequences.

Gene	Primer	Sequences (5′ → 3′)
FASN	Forward	CGGAGTCGCTTGAGTATA
	Reverse	CACAGGGACCGAGTAATG
PPARα	Forward	CAAGTGCCTGTCTGTCGG
	Reverse	CAGGTAGGCTTCGTGGAT
CD36	Forward	ATTCTCATGCCAGTCGGA
	Reverse	TTTGCTGCTGTTCTTTGC
SREBP1C	Forward	ACAGTGACTTCCCTGGCCTAT
	Reverse	GCATGGACGGGTACATCTTCAA
CPT1B	Forward	AGACTGTGCGTTCCTGTA
	Reverse	TTGGAGACGATGTAAAG
GAPDH	Forward	CAGGAGGCATTGCTGATGAT
	Reverse	GAAGGCTGGGGCTCATTT

2.7. Western Blotting

After extracting the cell protein, the BCA kit (Beyotime, Shanghai, China) was used to determine the cell protein content and adjust samples to the same concentration, and the protein sampling buffer was added and then heated at 100 °C for 5 min to prepare the protein samples. A total of 10 μL of the protein samples was aspirated and added to the concentrated gel wells, and after electrophoresis at 80 V to move the proteins to the separation gel, the voltage was increased to 120 V for 1 h. After transferring the protein to polyvinylidene fluoride, it was shaken at room temperature for 1 h, followed by the addition of a rapid containment solution, thus allowing the protein primary antibodies of sterol regulatory element binding protein (SREBP1C, 1:2500, Proteintech Group, Inc., Wuhan, China), fatty acid synthetase (FASN, 1:1000, servicebio, Wuhan, China), and GAPDH (1:2000, servicebio, Wuhan, China) to be incubated at 4 °C overnight. The following day, goat anti-rabbit or goat anti-mouse secondary antibodies were added to the solution, incubated for 1 h at room temperature and finally developed using a gel-imager.

2.8. Statistical Analysis

IBM SPSS Statistics 21 software and ImageJ were used for statistical analysis. Images were drawn using PRISM 8.0 and Adobe Illustrator CS6. The data are expressed as mean ± standard error ($\overline{x} \pm s$), and the test level was set as $\alpha = 0.05$.

3. Results

3.1. Selection of the Best BPS Concentration

Cell viability was measured by CCK-8 assay after 24 h and 48 h BPS treatment. With an increase in the exposure concentration, the survival rate of HepG2 and SK-Hep-1 cells diminished in a dose-dependent fashion (Figure 1A,B). At 250 μmol/L, the cell viability of HepG2 and SK-Hep-1 was between 70% and 80%. To simultaneously study the effect of BPS on HepG2 cells and SK-Hep-1 cells and to ensure that BPS exerts an effect on cells without excessive damage, we selected the 250 μmol/L BPS concentration for subsequent experiments.

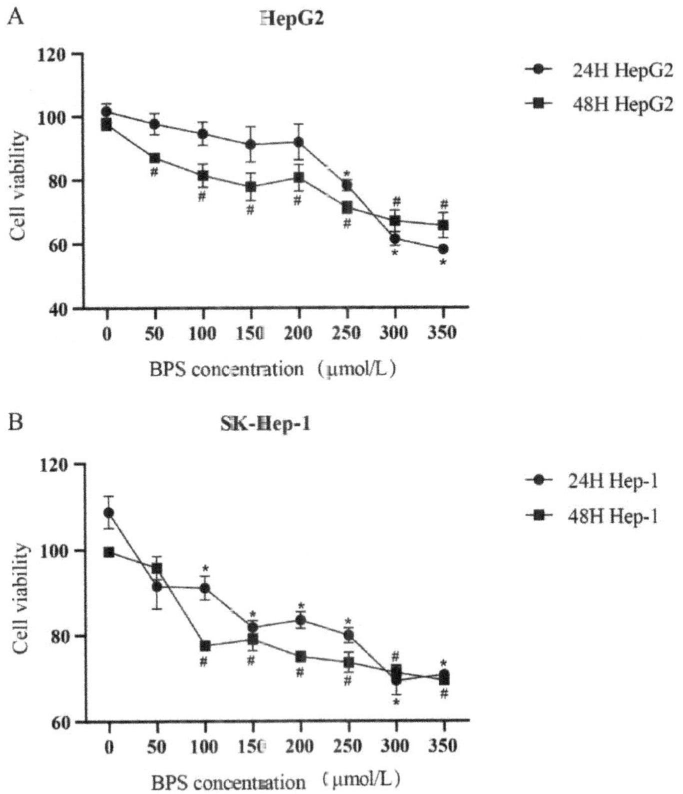

Figure 1. Effect of different concentrations of BPS on the viability of HepG2 and SK-Hep-1 cells. Note: (**A**,**B**) presents the alterations in cell viability following treatment with varying concentrations of BPS. "*" represent cell viability following a 24 h exposure to BPS relative to the 0 μmol/L group, $p < 0.05$. "#" represents cell viability following a 48 h exposure to BPS relative to the 0 μmol/L group, $p < 0.05$. n = 3, the same below.

3.2. Effect of BPS on ROS Levels in HepG2 Cells and SK-Hep-1 Cells

After BPS treatment for 24 h, the BPS-treated HepG2 and SK-Hep-1 cells produced an obvious oxidative stress response, and the intensity of oxidative stress within the SK-Hep-1 cells was more obvious (Figure 2A,B). After 48 h of BPS treatment, oxidative stress in both cell types was markedly elevated compared to the control group. Notably, the degree of oxidative stress in HepG2 cells treated with BPS was stronger than that in the BPS group treated with BPS for 24 h. Therefore, an increase in BPS exposure time would increase the degree of oxidative stress in HepG2 cells.

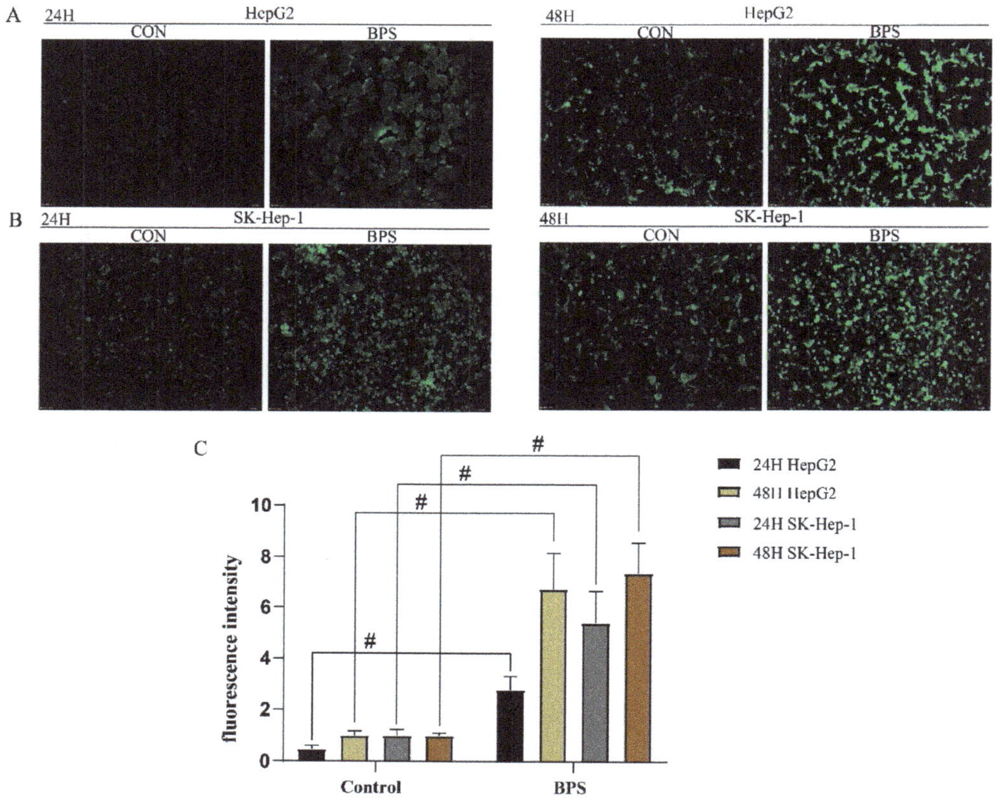

Figure 2. Effect of BPS treatment on ROS levels in HepG2 and SK-Hep-1 cells. Note: (**A**,**B**) shows the results of reactive oxygen species detection in HepG2 and SK-Hep-1 cells exposed to BPS for 24 h or 48 h conditions with a microscopic scale of 100 μm. (**C**) indicates reactive oxygen species fluorescence intensity quantification, and "#" represents the oxidative stress of cells after exposure compared to that of the control group, $p < 0.05$. n = 3.

3.3. BPS Induced Lipid Droplet Deposition in HepG2 and SK-Hep-1 Cells

The effects of BPS on the intracellular lipid content in HepG2 and SK-Hep-1 cells were observed under a microscope. Both HepG2 and SK-Hep-1 cells produced red lipid droplets after 24 h and 48 h of exposure (Figures 3 and 4A–H), and the production of lipid droplets in SK-Hep-1 cells exposed to BPS for 48 h was noticeably greater than that in the BPS group treated for 24 h.

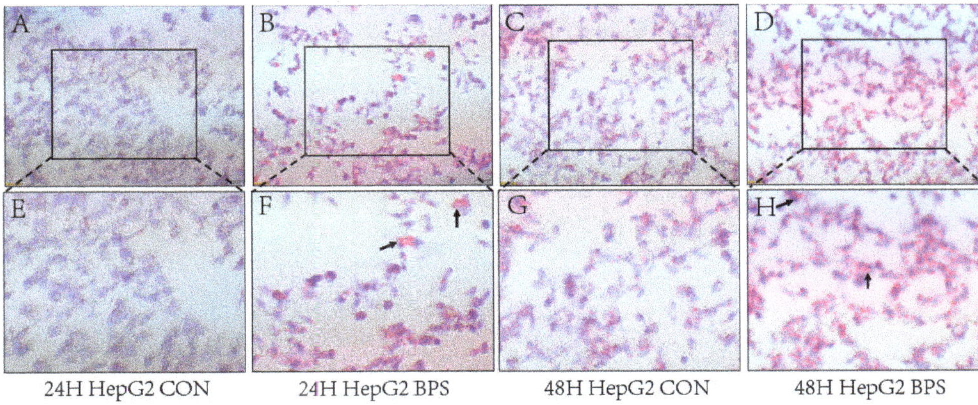

Figure 3. BPS-induced lipid droplet deposition in HepG2 cells. Note: (**A–D**) shows Oil Red O staining in HepG2 cells following BPS exposure for 24 h or 48 h with a microscopic scale of 50 μm. (**E–H**) presents the proportionally enlarged "□" window in (**A–D**), while "↑" in (**F**,**H**) refers to red fat droplets.

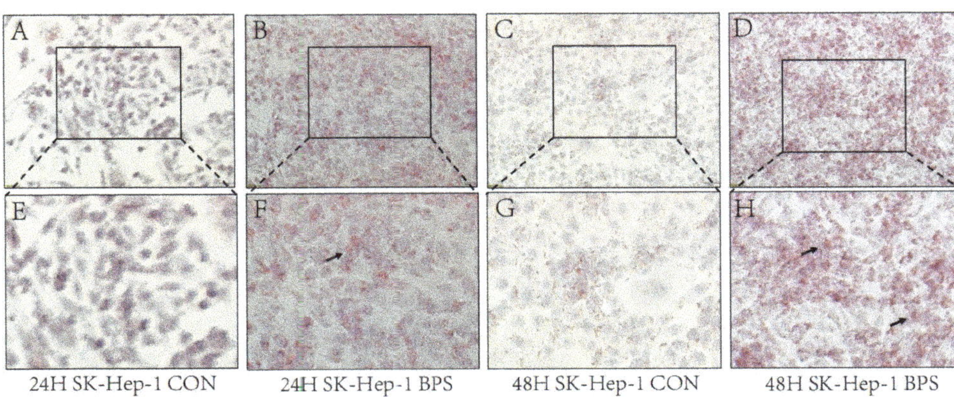

Figure 4. BPS-induced lipid droplet deposition in SK-Hep-1 cells. Note: (**A–D**) presents Oil Red O staining of SK-Hep-1 cells after exposure to BPS for 24 h or 48 h with a microscopic scale of 50 μm. (**E–H**) presents the proportionally enlarged "□" window in (**A–D**), while "↑" in (**F**,**H**) refers to the red fat droplets.

3.4. Effect of BPS on MDA and CAT Levels in HepG2 and SK-Hep-1 Cells

In contrast to the control group, a marked rise in MDA content was observed in both cells following 24 h and 48 h exposure ($p < 0.05$) (Figure 5A). The CAT content in SK-Hep-1 cells decreased after BPS treatment for 24 h; however, there was no statistically significant difference. After BPS treatment for 48 h, the CAT content significantly dropped ($p < 0.05$). The CAT content in HepG2 cells decreased after BPS treatment for 24 h, which was not statistically significant. But the CAT content increased significantly in HepG2 cells after BPS exposure for 48 h ($p < 0.05$) (Figure 5B).

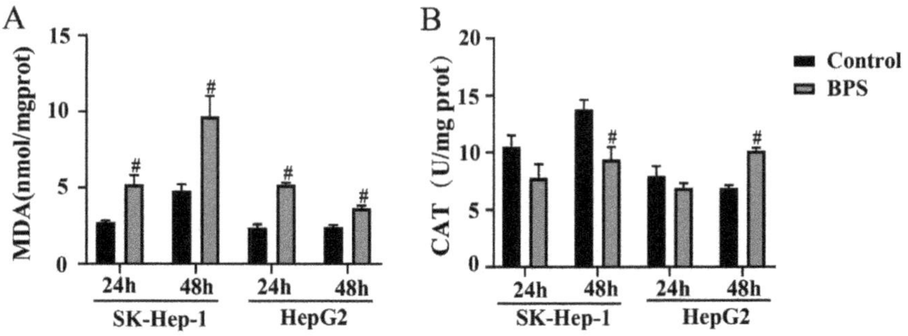

Figure 5. Effect of BPS on oxidative stress levels in HepG2 cells and SK-Hep-1 cells. Note: (**A**) shows the MDA levels within SK-Hep-1 and HepG2 cells following BPS treatments for 24 h and 48 h. (**B**) shows the CAT levels within SK-Hep-1 and HepG2 cells following BPS treatments for 24 h and 48 h; "#" represents BPS compared to the control group, $p < 0.05$. n = 3.

3.5. Effects of BPS on HepG2 and SK-Hep-1 Cell Damage and Metabolic-Related Indicators

After 24 h and 48 h of exposure, HepG2 cells' levels of TG and T-CHO were noticeably greater than those in the control group (Figure 6A,B). However, after 24 h of exposure, the SK-Hep-1 cells exhibited significantly reduced TG and T-CHO levels compared to the control group ($p < 0.05$), and after 48 h of exposure, T-CHO levels were markedly higher compared to the control group ($p < 0.05$). At 24 h following exposure, no significant difference in ALT levels was observed between both cell types relative to the control group; however, at 48 h following exposure, the ALT levels were markedly elevated compared to the control group (Figure 6C). When exposed for 24 h, the LDL-C level in both cell lines was markedly greater than that in the control group, and after 48 h, the LDL-C level in SK-Hep-1 cells was lower than that in the control group. After 48 h of BPS exposure, there was no discernible variation between the control group and HepG2 cells (Figure 6D).

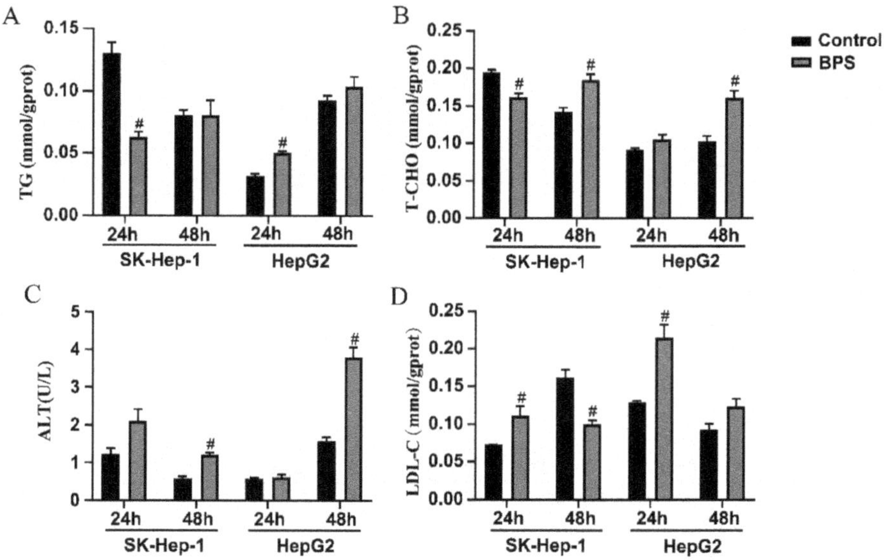

Figure 6. Effects of BPS on HepG2 and SK-Hep-1 cell damage and metabolic-related indicators. Note: (**A–D**) presents the results of TG, T-CHO, ALT, and LDL-C analyses after BPS exposure in SK-Hep-1 and HepG2 cells for 24 h and 48 h, respectively. "#" represents BPS compared to the control group, $p < 0.05$. n = 3.

3.6. Effects of BPS on PPARα, CPT1B, CD36, SREBP1C, and FASN mRNA Levels in HepG2 and SK-Hep-1 Cells

Following 24 h of BPS exposure, in contrast to the control, the mRNA expression levels of PPARα and CPT1B in HepG2 cells were significantly downregulated ($p < 0.05$), while the mRNA expression levels of SREBP1C and FASN were significantly upregulated ($p < 0.05$) (Figure 7A). SK-Hep-1 cells exhibited a marked decrease in the mRNA expression of PPARα, SREBP1C, and FASN, and there was a significant upregulation of CD36 mRNA expression ($p < 0.05$) (Figure 7C). After 48 h of BPS exposure, CPT1B mRNA expression in HepG2 cells was markedly reduced ($p < 0.05$) (Figure 7B), while the mRNA expressions of CD36 were significantly upregulated ($p < 0.05$) (Figure 7B). The mRNA levels of other genes did not change markedly. The mRNA expressions of PPARα and CPT1B in SK-Hep-1 cells were markedly downregulated, while the mRNA expressions of SREBP1C and FASN were significantly upregulated ($p < 0.05$) (Figure 7D).

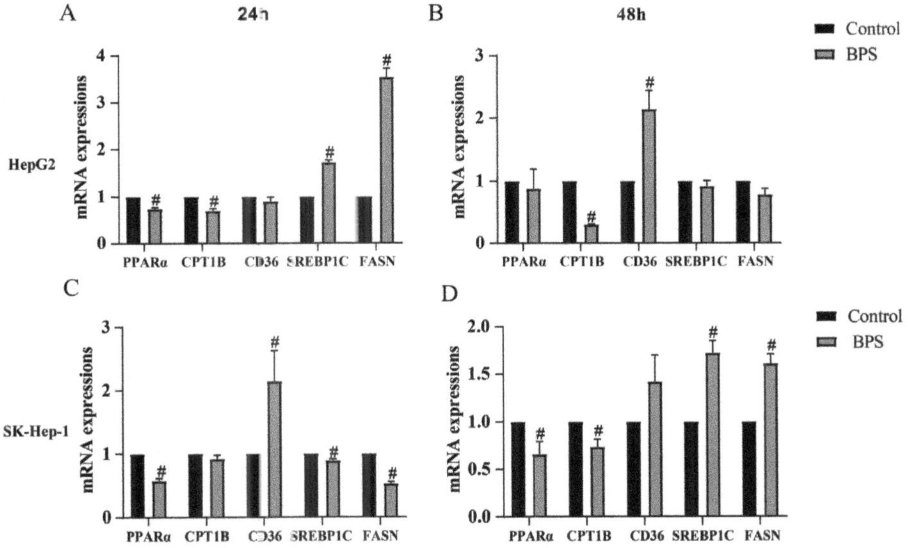

Figure 7. Effect of BPS on the expression levels of related mRNAs in HepG2 and SK-Hep-1 cells. Note: (**A–D**) indicates the mRNA expression results of PPARα, CPT1B, CD36, SREBP1C, and FAFSN in HepG2 and SK-Hep-1 cells following 24 h and 48 h of exposure, respectively. "#" represents BPS compared to the control group. $p < 0.05$. n = 3.

3.7. Effects of BPS on the Expression Levels of the Lipid Synthesis Proteins SREBP1C and FASN in HepG2 Cells and SK-Hep-1 Cells

The protein expression levels of FASN and SREBP1C, which promote lipid synthesis, were found using Western blotting. After BPS treatment for 24 h, the protein expression levels of SREBP1C and FASN in the BPS group of HepG2 cells were markedly increased ($p < 0.05$) (Figure 8A,B). The expression of SREBP1C protein was markedly elevated ($p < 0.05$) in SK-Hep-1 cells (Figure 8E,F). There were no discernible alterations in HepG2 or SK-Hep-1 cells following 48 h of treatment (Figure 8C,D,G,H).

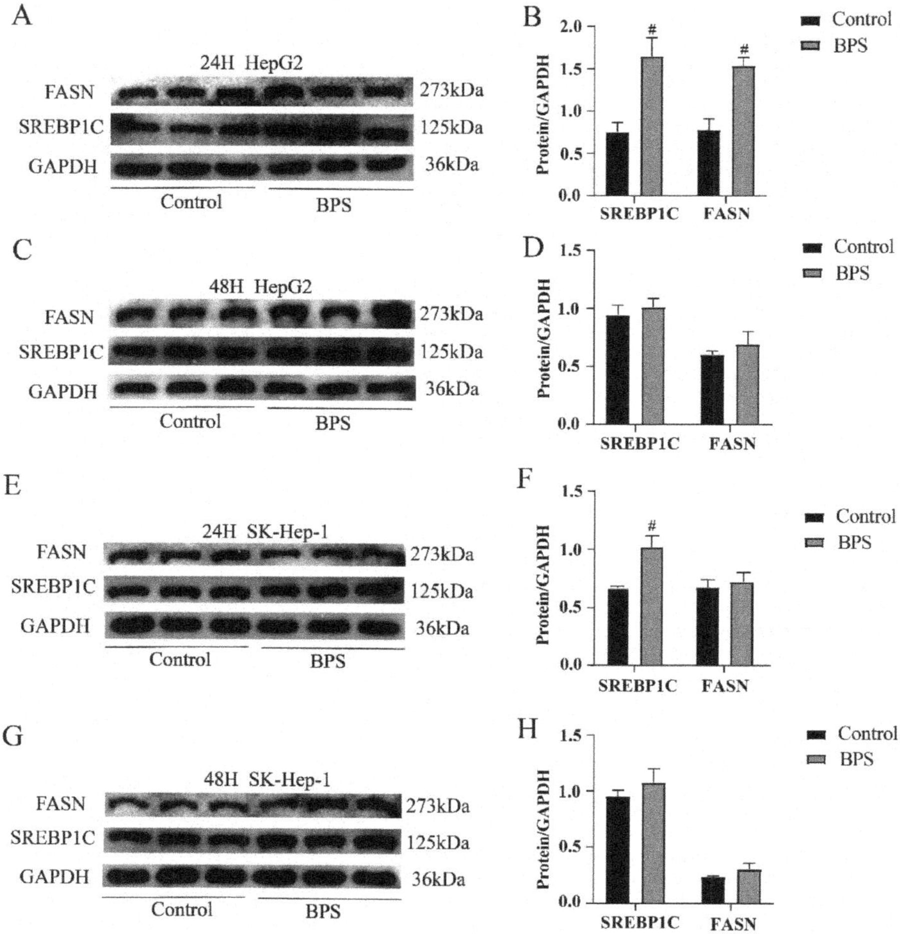

Figure 8. Effects of BPS on the expression levels of the lipid synthesis proteins SREBP1C and FASN in HepG2 and SK-Hep-1 cells. Note: (**A–H**) indicates the relative protein expression of SREBP1C and FASN in SK-Hep-1 and HepG2 cells after 24 h and 48 h of exposure, respectively. "#" represents BPS compared to the control group, $p < 0.05$. n = 3.

4. Discussion

Although BPS exerts endocrine-disrupting effects, the mechanisms underlying the metabolic disturbances triggered by BPS in hepatocytes remain unclear. Prolonged exposure to bisphenol compounds can increase cellular damage. When HepG2 cells were exposed to 0.625–10 μm BPS for 48 h, no or only slight cytotoxicity was produced, while after prolonged exposure, cytotoxicity was produced in a concentration-dependent manner [23]. The CCK-8 assay indicated that the viability of HepG2 and SK-Hep-1 cells gradually decreased after treatment with different concentrations (0, 50, 100, 150, 200, 250, 300, 350 μmol/L) of BPS for 24 or 48 h, indicating that BPS exerts a dose-dependent effect on cell damage. And increasing the concentration of the virus causes more obvious damage to cells. Studies have reported that oxidative stress leads to metabolic disorders and thus obesity [24] and that obesity can be alleviated by reducing and inhibiting liver oxidative stress and improving liver damage [25,26]. Obesity is often positively correlated with abnormal liver function. Zhang et al. [27] proposed that intracellular oxidative function is impaired in fatty liver lesions, and this can produce a large amount of ROS, leading to hepatocyte damage and the release of a large amount of ALT. Concurrently, AST levels increase with an increase in obesity [28], and antioxidant capacity also increases with an increase in TG and T-CHO levels [29]. Oxidative stress is both a precipitating factor and an endpoint of metabolic disorders [30,31]. Oral administration of BPS to mice at 5000 μg/kg/day or 50 mg/kg/day for 6–8 weeks resulted in liver damage, elevated ALT levels, and morphological changes to the liver [32,33]. In the present study, both the ROS content and MDA levels in HepG2 and SK-Hep-1 cells exposed to BPS for 24 h and 48 h were significantly increased, and the degree of oxidative stress in HepG2 cells was stronger after 48 h than 24 h of exposure to BPS, indicating that the cells not only developed oxidative stress, but also that the degree of oxidative stress might be enhanced by an increase in exposure time. The levels of ALT, T-CHO, and LDL-C in HepG2 and SK-Hep-1 cells treated with BPS for 24 h or 48 h significantly increased, including an increase in lipid droplets as assessed by Oil Red O staining, indicating that the cells were damaged to varying degrees after treatment with BPS for 24 h or 48 h. However, prolonged exposure to BPS increased lipid accumulation in HepG2 and SK-Hep-1 cells. In an analysis of a population-based study, elevated LDL-TG increased the risk of atherosclerosis, and it was therefore concluded that elevated LDL-TG could be used as a marker for atherosclerosis risk assessment [34]. Increased levels of ROS lead to oxidative stress in the vascular wall and support the oxidation of LDL, causing increased levels of ox-LDL, and when mitochondria are damaged by ROS accumulation, HDL and cholesterol metabolism will be defective [35]. This may be one of the reasons for increased levels of TG and T-CHO. Unexpectedly, after 24 h of BPS treatment, the TG content of SK-Hep-1 cells dropped, in contrast to HepG2 cells, and after 48 h, no discernible change was seen. According to previous studies, BPS increases leptin production in adipocytes [36] However, the TG content of SK-Hep-1 cells decreased after BPS treatment, and whether the pathway promoting fat metabolism was activated remains to be further explored. Notably, the CAT content in SK-Hep-1 cells decreased after 24 h and 48 h of BPS exposure, but the CAT content in HepG2 cells increased after 48 h of BPS exposure, indicating that BPS caused cell damage and oxidative stress in both SK-Hep-1 and HepG2 cells. However, HepG2 cells demonstrated that antioxidant capacity increased with increasing TG and T-CHO levels, which is in line with the findings of earlier research [29]. In the study of Mohan et al. [37], antioxidant defense mechanisms were activated in freshwater fish for resistance to BPS-induced oxidative stress after exposure to BPS, and anti-oxidative stress indices such as superoxide dismutase (SOD) and catalase were significantly elevated. In one study [38], bovine granulosa cells showed a significant increase in SOD1 levels after 12 h exposure to 50 μg/mL BPS, and an increase in SOD2 levels at 48 h exposure, even though there was no significant change in CAT levels. This reflects the fact that cells are also more resistant to oxidative stress in the presence of oxidative stress. SOD1 and SOD2, which also have anti-oxidative stress effects, were overexpressed at different times of staining, which may be a compensatory response of cells against oxidative stress. In the present study, CAT levels in HepG2 cells were increased at 48 h of staining, perhaps also as a compensatory effect.

Lipid accumulation is a result of increased lipid synthesis and decreased lipid metabolism [39]. Our group has previously demonstrated that BPS induces heightened hepatic lipid synthesis and reduced hepatic lipid metabolism in C57 mice [33]. To verify whether this phenomenon is also present in liver cells, we examined the levels of lipid metabolism-related mRNA expression of PPARα and CPT1B as well as the gene or protein expression of CD36, SREBP1C, and FASN, which are involved in fat synthesis. PPARα can promote lipid metabolism, and activated PPARα can reverse lipid accumulation in cells [40]. Agonists of PPARα can regulate various stages of lipid and lipoprotein metabolism through transcription factors with the effect of lowering TG levels [41]. CPT1B is involved in fatty acid β-oxidation and is directly regulated by PPARα [42]. In the current investigation, PPARα and CPT1B were significantly decreased in both cell lines after BPS exposure, indicating that intracellular lipid metabolism was weakened. It is possible that BPS indirectly regulates the expression of CPTIB by inhibiting the expression of PPARα, leading to a decrease in cellular metabolism and the occurrence of lipid aggregation. SREBP1C is a lipogenic transcription factor that regulates intracellular lipid accumulation and plays an important role in the regulation of lipid metabolism [43]. FASN overexpression promotes hepatic TG accumulation as a key regulator of lipid metabolism [44]. CD36 acts as a lipid sensor, promoting fatty acid uptake [45,46] and possibly inducing dysregulation of lipid protein levels [47]. The mRNA expression of PPARα in SK-Hep-1 cells decreased, the expression of CD36 increased significantly after 24 h of BPS exposure, and the expression of SREBP1C and FASN was significantly reduced. Following 48 h of exposure, there was a marked increase in the expression of SREBP1C and FASN. Because the lipid synthesis genes SREBP1C and FASN were altered in SK-Hep-1 cells after exposure to BPS, this resulted in altered levels of the effector indicators TG and T-CHO as well. The trends in the levels of TG and T-CHO were consistent with the trends in the mRNA expression of SREBP1C and FASN, suggesting that the production of TG and T-CHO may be induced by SREBP1C and FASN in SK-Hep-1 cells. After 24 h of treatment, HepG2 cells' expression levels of PPARα and CPT1B were markedly decreased. Although the expression level of CD36 was not significantly altered, the expression levels of SREBP1C and FASN were significantly increased, and this was consistent with the results of Western blotting. However, no significant changes in SREBP1C or FASN levels were observed after 48 h of BPS exposure. The results of qPCR and Western blotting indicated that the lipid metabolism of cells was inhibited and that lipid synthesis was promoted after BPS exposure. PPARα agonists are used in the clinic to reverse cholesterol transport and improve atherosclerotic lipoproteins [48], whereas activation of PPARα also ameliorates oxidative stress-induced organ damage [49]. The transcription factor, Krüppel-like factor 16, in the liver was found to target binding to PPARα to reduce oxidative stress in mice [50], and knockdown of PPARα causes lipid accumulation, whereas restoration of PPARα expression reduces mitochondrial oxidative stress [51]. In this study, inhibition of cellular PPARα expression by BPS resulted in enhanced oxidative stress, increased cholesterol transport, and increased levels of LDL-C, TG, and T-CHO. In summary, we hypothesize that BPS induces lipid metabolism disorders in HepG2 and SK-Hep-1 cells through oxidative stress by the following pathway: increased ROS and MDA content induces oxidative stress in cells, which directly or indirectly inhibits the expression of PPARα to regulate the expression of CPT1B, CD36, SREBPC, and FASN, and thus the cells undergo a disturbance in cholesterol metabolism, ultimately leading to cellular lipid accumulation. In this experiment, the mRNA or protein levels of SREBP1C and FASN related to lipid synthesis in HepG2 cells after 48 h of BPS exposure showed no discernible difference from those in the control group, and this may have been caused by the doubling of growth of HepG2 cells during culture in the presence of BPS without the exchange solution. It is also possible that the main pathway by which BPS causes lipid synthesis is the inhibition of PPARα expression, which reduces lipid metabolism and thus causes cellular lipid accumulation. In contrast, BPA, also an endocrine disruptor, increases SREBP1 mRNA expression to activate PPARγ which influences childhood obesity [52], and Di-2-ethylhexyl phthalate affects the normal metabolism of mouse liver through activation of LXR/SREBP1C and the PPARα signaling pathway [53]. This also illustrates the different mechanisms by which different chemicals affect different individuals.

In this study, although HepG2 and SK-Hep-1 cells are both human liver cancer cell lines, the biochemical indices and protein expression levels were not completely the same after BPS exposure, for example, after 48 h of BPS exposure, LDL-C levels were lower in SK-Hep-1 cells than in controls, and the difference between HepG2 cells and controls was not statistically significant, which further suggests that different individuals have different sensitivities to chemicals, which may undergo significant shifts over time, and may explain the differences between the two types of cells. This may result in different effects on different individuals in the population. Currently, the rate of obesity in the world is increasing, and BPS is widely used in various environmental media. Further studies are required to clarify the molecular mechanisms underlying the relationship among BPS, lipid accumulation, and obesity.

Author Contributions: Conceptualization, H.-C.Z.; methodology, K.-X.L. and Z.-Y.W.; validation, K.-X.L.; formal analysis, K.-X.L. and M.-L.Q.; resources, H.-C.Z.; data curation, K.-X.L.; writing—original draft preparation, K.-X.L.; writing—review and editing, H.-C.Z.; visualization, M.-L.Q. and K.-X.L.; supervision, H.-C.Z.; project administration, H.-C.Z.; funding acquisition, H.-C.Z. All authors have read and agreed to the published version of the manuscript.

Funding: This research was funded by the National Natural Science Foundation of China (NOs. 82160629, 82460653), the Science and Technology Department of Guangxi Zhuang Autonomous (NO. 2021JJA140831).

Institutional Review Board Statement: Not applicable.

Informed Consent Statement: Not applicable.

Data Availability Statement: The data that support the findings of this study are available from the corresponding author upon reasonable request.

Acknowledgments: The project was supported by grants from the National Natural Science Foundation of China (NO. 82160629, 82460653), the Science and Technology Department of Guangxi Zhuang Autonomous (NO. 2021JJA140831).

Conflicts of Interest: The authors declare that they have no known competing financial interests or personal relationships that could have appeared to influence the work reported in this paper.

References

1. Bousoumah, R.; Leso, V.; Iavicoli, I.; Huuskonen, P.; Viegas, S.; Porras, S.P.; Santonen, T.; Frery, N.; Robert, A.; Ndaw, S. Biomonitoring of occupational exposure to bisphenol A, bisphenol S and bisphenol F: A systematic review. *Sci. Total Environ.* **2021**, *783*, 146905. [CrossRef]
2. Pu, C.; Liu, Y.; Zhu, J.; Ma, J.; Cui, M.; Mehdi, O.M.; Wang, B.; Wang, A.; Zhang, C. Mechanisms insights into bisphenol S-induced oxidative stress, lipid metabolism disruption, and autophagy dysfunction in freshwater crayfish. *J. Hazard. Mater.* **2024**, *479*, 135704. [CrossRef] [PubMed]
3. An, H.; Yu, H.; Wei, Y.; Liu, F.; Ye, J. Disrupted metabolic pathways and potential human diseases induced by bisphenol S. *Environ. Toxicol. Pharmacol.* **2021**, *88*, 103751. [CrossRef] [PubMed]
4. Wang, H.; Gao, R.; Liang, W.; Wei, S.; Zhou, Y.; Zeng, F. Assessment of BPA and BPS exposure in the general population in Guangzhou, China-Estimation of daily intakes based on urinary metabolites. *Environ. Pollut.* **2022**, *315*, 120375. [CrossRef] [PubMed]
5. Ndaw, S.; Remy, A.; Denis, F.; Marsan, P.; Jargot, D.; Robert, A. Occupational exposure of cashiers to bisphenol S via thermal paper. *Toxicol. Lett.* **2018**, *298*, 106–111. [CrossRef]
6. Zhao, X.; Qiu, W.; Zheng, Y.; Xiong, J.; Gao, C.; Hu, S. Occurrence, distribution, bioaccumulation, and ecological risk of bisphenol analogues, parabens and their metabolites in the Pearl River Estuary, South China. *Ecotoxicol. Environ. Saf.* **2019**, *180*, 43–52. [CrossRef] [PubMed]
7. Danzl, E.; Sei, K.; Soda, S.; Ike, M.; Fujita, M. Biodegradation of bisphenol A, bisphenol F and bisphenol S in seawater. *Int. J. Environ. Res. Public Health* **2009**, *6*, 1472–1484. [CrossRef] [PubMed]
8. Kahn, L.G.; Philippat, C.; Nakayama, S.F.; Slama, R.; Trasande, L. Endocrine-disrupting chemicals: Implications for human health. *Lancet Diabetes Endocrinol.* **2020**, *8*, 703–718. [CrossRef] [PubMed]

9. Liu, B.; Lehmler, H.J.; Sun, Y.; Xu, G.; Liu, Y.; Zong, G.; Sun, Q.; Hu, F.B.; Wallace, R.B.; Bao, W. Bisphenol A substitutes and obesity in US adults: Analysis of a population-based, cross-sectional study. *Lancet Planet. Health* **2017**, *1*, e114–e122. [CrossRef] [PubMed]
10. Zhang, Y.; Dong, T.; Hu, W.; Wang, X.; Xu, B.; Lin, Z.; Hofer, T.; Stefanoff, P.; Chen, Y.; Wang, X.; et al. Association between exposure to a mixture of phenols, pesticides, and phthalates and obesity: Comparison of three statistical models. *Environ. Int.* **2019**, *123*, 325–336. [CrossRef]
11. Meng, Z.; Wang, D.; Yan, S.; Li, R.; Yan, J.; Teng, M.; Zhou, Z.; Zhu, W. Effects of perinatal exposure to BPA and its alternatives (BPS, BPF and BPAF) on hepatic lipid and glucose homeostasis in female mice adolescent offspring. *Chemosphere* **2018**, *212*, 297–306. [CrossRef]
12. Meng, Z.; Wang, D.; Liu, W.; Li, R.; Yan, S.; Jia, M.; Zhang, L.; Zhou, Z.; Zhu, W. Perinatal exposure to Bisphenol S (BPS) promotes obesity development by interfering with lipid and glucose metabolism in male mouse offspring. *Environ. Res.* **2019**, *173*, 189–198. [CrossRef] [PubMed]
13. Mornagui, B.; Rezg, R.; Repond, C.; Pellerin, L. Bisphenol S favors hepatic steatosis development via an upregulation of liver MCT1 expression and an impairment of the mitochondrial respiratory system. *J. Cell Physiol.* **2022**, *237*, 3057–3068. [CrossRef]
14. Gao, C.; He, H.; Qiu, W.; Zheng, Y.; Chen, Y.; Hu, S.; Zhao, X. Oxidative Stress, Endocrine Disturbance, and Immune Interference in Humans Showed Relationships to Serum Bisphenol Concentrations in a Dense Industrial Area. *Environ. Sci. Technol.* **2021**, *55*, 1953–1963. [CrossRef]
15. Singh, R.D.; Wager, J.L.; Scheidl, T.B.; Connors, L.T.; Easson, S.; Callaghan, M.A.; Alatorre-Hinojosa, S.; Swift, L.H.; Colarusso, P.; Jadli, A.; et al. Potentiation of Adipogenesis by Reactive Oxygen Species Is a Unifying Mechanism in the Proadipogenic Properties of Bisphenol A and Its New Structural Analogues. *Antioxid. Redox Signal* **2024**, *40*, 1–15. [CrossRef]
16. Chen, J.; Ding, X.; Wu, R.; Tong, B.; Zhao, L.; Lv, H.; Meng, X.; Liu, Y.; Ren, B.; Li, J.; et al. Novel Sesquiterpene Glycoside from Loquat Leaf Alleviates Type 2 Diabetes Mellitus Combined with Nonalcoholic Fatty Liver Disease by Improving Insulin Resistance, Oxidative Stress, Inflammation, and Gut Microbiota Composition. *J. Agric. Food Chem.* **2021**, *69*, 14176–14191. [CrossRef] [PubMed]
17. Evans, R.M.; Barish, G.D.; Wang, Y.X. PPARs and the complex journey to obesity. *Nat. Med.* **2004**, *10*, 355–361. [CrossRef] [PubMed]
18. Lee, Y.H.; Jang, H.J.; Kim, S.; Choi, S.S.; Khim, K.W.; Eom, H.J.; Hyun, J.; Shin, K.J.; Chae, Y.C.; Kim, H.; et al. Hepatic MIR20B promotes nonalcoholic fatty liver disease by suppressing PPARA. *Elife* **2021**, *10*, e70472. [CrossRef]
19. Qiu, W.; Yang, M.; Liu, J.; Xu, H.; Luo, S.; Wong, M.; Zheng, C. Bisphenol S-induced chronic inflammatory stress in liver via peroxisome proliferator-activated receptor gamma using fish in vivo and in vitro models. *Environ. Pollut.* **2019**, *246*, 963–971. [CrossRef] [PubMed]
20. Tao, Z.; Zhang, L.; Wu, T.; Fang, X.; Zhao, L. Echinacoside ameliorates alcohol-induced oxidative stress and hepatic steatosis by affecting SREBP1c/FASN pathway via PPARalpha. *Food Chem. Toxicol.* **2021**, *148*, 111956. [CrossRef] [PubMed]
21. Maćczak, A.; Cyrkler, M.; Bukowska, B.; Michałowicz, J. Bisphenol A, bisphenol S, bisphenol F and bisphenol AF induce different oxidative stress and damage in human red blood cells (in vitro study). *Toxicol. Vitr.* **2017**, *41*, 143–149. [CrossRef] [PubMed]
22. Kiseleva, O.I.; Kurbatov, I.Y.; Arzumanian, V.A.; Ilgisonis, E.V.; Vakhrushev, I.V.; Lupatov, A.Y.; Ponomarenko, E.A.; Poverennaya, E.V. Exploring Dynamic Metabolome of the HepG2 Cell Line: Rise and Fall. *Cells* **2022**, *11*, 3548. [CrossRef]
23. Yu, H.; Liu, Y. Impact of Extended and Combined Exposure of Bisphenol Compounds on Their Chromosome-Damaging Effect horizontal line Increased Potency and Shifted Mode of Action. *Environ. Sci. Technol.* **2023**, *57*, 498–508. [CrossRef] [PubMed]
24. Rani, V.; Deep, G.; Singh, R.K.; Palle, K.; Yadav, U.C. Oxidative stress and metabolic disorders: Pathogenesis and therapeutic strategies. *Life Sci.* **2016**, *148*, 183–193. [CrossRef] [PubMed]
25. Xue, R.; Wu, Q.; Guo, L.; Ye, D.; Cao, Q.; Zhang, M.; Xian, Y.; Chen, M.; Yan, K.; Zheng, J. Pyridostigmine attenuated high-fat-diet induced liver injury by the reduction of mitochondrial damage and oxidative stress via α7nAChR and M3AChR. *J. Biochem. Mol. Toxicol.* **2024**, *38*, e23671. [CrossRef] [PubMed]
26. Dhara, M.; Majumder, R.; Adhikari, L. Heliconia rostrata rhizomes mitigate chemical-induced liver injury by debilitating oxidative stress in HepG2 cells and rats. *J. Ethnopharmacol.* **2021**, *275*, 114113. [CrossRef] [PubMed]
27. Zhang, X.; Yang, J.; Guo, Y.; Ye, H.; Yu, C.; Xu, C.; Xu, L.; Wu, S.; Sun, W.; Wei, H.; et al. Functional proteomic analysis of nonalcoholic fatty liver disease in rat models: Enoyl-coenzyme a hydratase down-regulation exacerbates hepatic steatosis. *Hepatology* **2010**, *51*, 1190–1199. [CrossRef]
28. Huang, J.; Gao, T.; Zhang, H.; Wang, X. Association of obesity profiles and metabolic health status with liver injury among US adult population in NHANES 1999-2016. *Sci. Rep.* **2023**, *13*, 15958. [CrossRef]
29. Jakubiak, G.K.; Osadnik, K.; Lejawa, M.; Kasperczyk, S.; Osadnik, T.; Pawlas, N. Oxidative Stress in Association with Metabolic Health and Obesity in Young Adults. *Oxid. Med. Cell. Longev.* **2021**, *2021*, 9987352. [CrossRef]
30. Gianfrancesco, M.A.; Paquot, N.; Piette, J.; Legrand-Poels, S. Lipid bilayer stress in obesity-linked inflammatory and metabolic disorders. *Biochem. Pharmacol.* **2018**, *153*, 168–183. [CrossRef] [PubMed]

31. Lugo, R.; Avila-Nava, A.; Pech-Aguilar, A.G.; Medina-Vera, I.; Guevara-Cruz, M.; Gutiérrez Solis, A.L. Relationship between lipid accumulation product and oxidative biomarkers by gender in adults from Yucatan, Mexico. *Sci. Rep.* **2022**, *12*, 14338. [CrossRef]
32. Zhang, Z.; Lin, L.; Gai, Y.; Hong, Y.; Li, L.; Weng, L. Subchronic bisphenol S exposure affects liver function in mice involving oxidative damage. *Regul. Toxicol. Pharmacol.* **2018**, *92*, 138–144. [CrossRef] [PubMed]
33. Wu, Z.Y.; Luo, L.; Kan, Y.Q.; Qin, M.L.; Li, H.T.; He, Q.Z.; Zeng, H.C. Puerarin Prevents Bisphenol S Induced Lipid Accumulation by Reducing Liver Lipid Synthesis and Promoting Lipid Metabolism in C57BL/6J Mice. *Toxics* **2023**, *11*, 736. [CrossRef]
34. Balling, M.; Afzal, S.; Davey Smith, G.; Varbo, A.; Langsted, A.; Kamstrup, P.R.; Nordestgaard, B.G. Elevated LDL Triglycerides and Atherosclerotic Risk. *J. Am. Coll. Cardiol.* **2023**, *81*, 136–152. [CrossRef] [PubMed]
35. Masenga, S.K.; Kabwe, L.S.; Chakulya, M.; Kirabo, A. Mechanisms of Oxidative Stress in Metabolic Syndrome. *Int. J. Mol. Sci.* **2023**, *24*, 7898. [CrossRef]
36. Helies-Toussaint, C.; Peyre, L.; Costanzo, C.; Chagnon, M.C.; Rahmani, R. Is bisphenol S a safe substitute for bisphenol A in terms of metabolic function? An in vitro study. *Toxicol. Appl. Pharmacol.* **2014**, *280*, 224–235. [CrossRef]
37. Mohan, S.; Jacob, J.; Malini, N.A.; Prabhakar, R.; Kayalakkakathu, R.G. Biochemical responses antioxidant defense mechanisms in Channa Striatus exposed to Bisphenol, S.J. *Biochem. Mol. Toxicol.* **2024**, *38*, e23651. [CrossRef] [PubMed]
38. Sabry, R.; Nguyen, M.; Younes, S.; Favetta, L.A. BPA and its analogs increase oxidative stress levels in in vitro cultured granulosa cells by altering anti-oxidant enzymes expression. *Mol. Cell Endocrinol.* **2022**, *545*, 111574. [CrossRef]
39. Song, R.; Hu, M.; Qin, X.; Qiu, L.; Wang, P.; Zhang, X.; Liu, R.; Wang, X. The Roles of Lipid Metabolism in the Pathogenesis of Chronic Diseases in the Elderly. *Nutrients* **2023**, *15*, 3433. [CrossRef]
40. Wei, X.; Zhang, J.; Tang, M.; Wang, X.; Fan, N.; Peng, Y. Fat mass and obesity-associated protein promotes liver steatosis by targeting PPARalpha. *Lipids Health Dis.* **2022**, *21*, 29. [CrossRef]
41. Kumar, S.; Dhanwal, D.K. Central obesity & dyslipidemia in HIV patients on antiretroviral therapy. *Indian J. Med. Res.* **2018**, *148*, 366–368. [PubMed]
42. Zhao, Q.; Yang, R.; Wang, J.; Hu, D.D.; Li, F. PPARalpha activation protects against cholestatic liver injury. *Sci. Rep.* **2017**, *7*, 9967.
43. Lee, G.; Kim, Y.Y.; Jang, H.; Han, J.S.; Nahmgoong, H.; Park, Y.J.; Han, S.M.; Cho, C.; Lim, S.; Noh, J.R.; et al. SREBP1c-PARP1 axis tunes anti-senescence activity of adipocytes and ameliorates metabolic imbalance in obesity. *Cell Metab.* **2022**, *34*, 702–718. [CrossRef] [PubMed]
44. Liu, B.; Jiang, S.; Li, M.; Xiong, X.; Zhu, M.; Li, D.; Zhao, L.; Qian, L.; Zhai, L.; Li, J.; et al. Proteome-wide analysis of USP14 substrates revealed its role in hepatosteatosis via stabilization of FASN. *Nat. Commun.* **2018**, *9*, 4770. [CrossRef]
45. Hao, J.W.; Wang, J.; Guo, H.; Zhao, Y.Y.; Sun, H.H.; Li, Y.F.; Lai, X.Y.; Zhao, N.; Wang, X.; Xie, C.; et al. CD36 facilitates fatty acid uptake by dynamic palmitoylation-regulated endocytosis. *Nat. Commun.* **2020**, *11*, 4765. [CrossRef]
46. Zeng, H.; Qin, H.; Liao, M.; Zheng, E.; Luo, X.; Xiao, A.; Li, Y.; Chen, L.; Wei, L.; Zhao, L.; et al. CD36 promotes de novo lipogenesis in hepatocytes through INSIG2-dependent SREBP1 processing. *Mol. Metab.* **2022**, *57*, 101428. [CrossRef] [PubMed]
47. Nergiz-Unal, R.; Ulug, E.; Kisioglu, B.; Tamer, F; Bodur, M.; Yalcimin, H.; Yuruk, A.A. Hepatic cholesterol synthesis and lipoprotein levels impaired by dietary fructose and saturated fatty acids in mice: Insight on PCSK9 and CD36. *Nutrition* **2020**, *79–80*, 110954. [CrossRef] [PubMed]
48. Yanai, H.; Adachi, H.; Hakoshima, M.; Katsuyama, H. Molecular Biological and Clinical Understanding of the Statin Residual Cardiovascular Disease Risk and Peroxisome Proliferator-Activated Receptor Alpha Agonists and Ezetimibe for Its Treatment. *Int. J. Mol. Sci.* **2022**, *23*, 3418. [CrossRef] [PubMed]
49. Wen, C.; Yu, X.; Zhu, J.; Zeng, J.; Kuang, X.; Zhang, Y.; Tang, S.; Zhang, Q.; Yan, J.; Shen, H. Gastrodin ameliorates oxidative stress-induced RPE damage by facilitating autophagy and phagocytosis through PPARalpha-TFEB/CD36 signal pathway. *Free Radic. Biol. Med.* **2024**, *224*, 103–116. [CrossRef] [PubMed]
50. Sun, N.; Shen, C.; Zhang, L.; Wu, X.; Yu, Y.; Yang, X.; Yang, C.; Zhong, C.; Gao, Z.; Miao, W.; et al. Hepatic Kruppel-like factor 16 (KLF16) targets PPARalpha to improve steatohepatitis and insulin resistance. *Gut* **2021**, *70*, 2183–2195. [CrossRef]
51. Sun, J.; Bian, Y.; Ma, Y.; Ali, W.; Wang, T.; Yuan, Y.; Gu, J.; Bian, J.; Liu, Z.; Zou, H. Melatonin alleviates cadmium-induced nonalcoholic fatty liver disease in ducks by alleviating autophagic flow arrest via PPAR-alpha and reducing oxidative stress. *Poult. Sci.* **2023**, *102*, 102835. [CrossRef] [PubMed]
52. Hoepner, L.A. Bisphenol a: A narrative review of prenatal exposure effects on adipogenesis and childhood obesity via peroxisome proliferator-activated receptor gamma. *Environ. Res.* **2019**, *173*, 54–68. [CrossRef]
53. Liang, X.; Liang, J.; Zhang, S.; Yan, H.; Luan, T. Di-2-ethylhexyl phthalate disrupts hepatic lipid metabolism in obese mice by activating the LXR/SREBP-1c and PPAR-alpha signaling pathways. *Sci. Total Environ.* **2024**, *914*, 1699. [CrossRef]

Disclaimer/Publisher's Note: The statements, opinions and data contained in all publications are solely those of the individual author(s) and contributor(s) and not of MDPI and/or the editor(s). MDPI and/or the editor(s) disclaim responsibility for any injury to people or property resulting from any ideas, methods, instructions or products referred to in the content.

toxics MDPI

Article

Modulation of Paracetamol-Induced Hepatotoxicity by Acute and Chronic Ethanol Consumption in Mice: A Study Pilot

Allan Cristian Gonçalves [1], Maria Laura da Cruz Castro [1], Renata Rebeca Pereira [1], Natalia Pereira da Silva Araújo [1], Flávia Monteiro Ferreira [1], Pedro Alves Machado Júnior [2], Sirlaine Pio [3], Camilo Elber Vital [4], Frank Silva Bezerra [2], André Talvani [3], William de Castro Borges [4], Emerson Cruz de Oliveira [5] and Daniela Caldeira Costa [1,*]

1 Laboratory of Metabolic Biochemistry, Institute of Exact and Biological Sciences, UFOP, Ouro Preto 35402-136, MG, Brazil; allan.goncalves@aluno.ufop.edu.br (A.C.G.); alinemeireles0@yahoo.com.br (A.M.C.); maria.cruz@aluno.ufop.edu.br (M.L.d.C.C.); renatarp@ufop.edu.br (R.R.P.); nataliaop@gmail.com (N.P.d.S.A.); flavia.monteiro@aluno.ufop.edu.br (F.M.F.)
2 Laboratory of Experimental Pathophysiology, Institute of Exact and Biological Sciences, UFOP, Ouro Preto 35402-136, MG, Brazil; frank@ufop.edu.br (F.S.B.)
3 Laboratory of Immunobiology of Inflammation, Institute of Exact and Biological Sciences, UFOP, Ouro Preto 35400-000, MG, Brazil; sirlaine.silva@aluno.ufop.edu.br (S.P.); talvani@ufop.edu.br (A.T.)
4 Laboratory of Enzymology and Proteomics, Institute of Exact and Biological Sciences, UFOP, Ouro Preto 35402-136, MG, Brazil
5 Laboratory of Exercise of Physiology, School of Physical Education, UFOP, Ouro Preto 35400-000, MG, Brazil; emerson@ufop.edu.br
* Correspondence: daniela.costa@ufop.edu.br; Tel.: +55-(31)-3559-1761

Abstract: Paracetamol (APAP) overdose is the leading cause of drug-induced liver injury, leading to acute liver failure. However, the role of concurrent acute or chronic ethanol ingestion in this context requires further clarification. In this study, we investigated the effects of acute and chronic ethanol ingestion on APAP-induced hepatotoxicity. Male C57BL/6 mice were randomly allocated into four groups: control (C; water 2×/day for 7 days); APAP (single dose of APAP, 500 mg/kg); acute ethanol (AE; a single ethanol dose—10 mL/kg, and one hour later an overdose of APAP—500 mg/kg); chronic ethanol (CE; ethanol—10 mL/kg, 2×/day for 7 days; and on the last day, an overdose of APAP—500 mg/kg). The results showed that AE induced heightened liver damage, increased necrotic area, and elevated levels of ALT, AST, TBARS, and oxidized glutathione compared to the control group. The AE group exhibited diminished glutathione availability and elevated CYP2E1 levels compared to the other groups. CE maintained a hepatic profile similar to that of the control group in terms of necrosis index, ALT and AST levels, GSH/GSSG ratio, and CYP2E1 activity, along with the upregulation of gene expression of the glucuronidation enzyme compared to the APAP group. Proteomic analysis revealed that the AE protein profile closely resembled that of the APAP group, whereas the C and CE groups were clustered together. In conclusion, ethanol consumption differentially modulated APAP overdose-induced liver damage. Acute consumption exacerbated hepatotoxicity, similar to an APAP overdose alone, whereas chronic consumption appeared to mitigate this injury, at least within the parameters assessed in this study.

Keywords: paracetamol; acetaminophen; ethanol; alcohol; oxidative stress; hepatotoxicity; liver damage

1. Introduction

Paracetamol (N-acetyl-p-aminophenol, acetaminophen, APAP), available since the 1950s, has become one of the most widely used analgesics and antipyretics worldwide [1]. Although considered safe at therapeutic levels (4 g/day or less), when used in doses higher than therapeutic levels, it can cause serious liver damage, potentially progressing to acute liver failure (ALF) [2,3]. At therapeutic doses, most APAP is metabolized via the glucuronidation and sulfation pathways and subsequently excreted in the urine. The remaining APAP is converted into a potentially hepatotoxic metabolite, N-acetyl-p-benzoquinone imine (NAPQI), by cytochrome P450 enzymes, especially CYP2E1. The formed NAPQI is then reduced by glutathione to non-toxic, soluble mercapturic acid, which is also excreted in the urine. In cases of APAP overdose, the glucuronidation and sulfation pathways become saturated, and the cytochrome P450 pathway produces excessive NAPQI, leading to the depletion of glutathione reserves, causing liver toxicity mediated by the formation of free radicals [4,5]. The concomitant use of different drugs can lead to an adverse drug interaction resulting in a decrease in therapeutic efficacy or an increase in the rate of adverse effects. The consumption of ethanol, among other substances, is recognized as capable of causing such interactions by altering the pharmacodynamics or pharmacokinetics of medications when used simultaneously [6,7]. It is estimated that 2.3 billion people consume alcoholic beverages regularly (an average of 32.8 g of pure ethanol per day). Global per capita consumption increased between 1990 and 2017, and the World Health Organization (WHO) predicts an even greater increase by 2030. As the consumption of alcoholic beverages increases, there is a significant contribution to the increase in morbidity and mortality worldwide [8,9]. The liver metabolizes ethanol through three enzymatic pathways: alcohol dehydrogenase (ADH); cytochrome P450, in particular, by CYP2E1 (in this case, also called MEOS—microsomal ethanol oxidation system); and catalase (CAT). Class I alcohol dehydrogenase (ADH1) is considered the most important enzyme for ethanol metabolism. CYP2E1 and CAT are considered secondary pathways, while the other ADH classes (II, III, and IV) are considered less effective pathways [10]. Oxidative stress is believed to be an important factor in the development of alcoholic fatty liver lesions, and CYP2E1 activation is an important source of reactive oxygen species (ROS) in chronic alcoholic liver disease [11]. CYP2E1 is a microsomal enzyme that plays a crucial role in the metabolism of both ethanol and paracetamol. The interaction between these substances is known for its complexity, and the results of this interaction depend on certain factors, such as the dose administered and the duration of ethanol consumption [12]. Alcohol–drug interactions are common in individuals who regularly use paracetamol and/or are classified as frequent, heavy, or compulsive drinkers. In this context, although the medical community recognizes the interaction between paracetamol and ethanol, the underlying metabolic changes and short- and long-term toxic effects have not yet been completely understood [13]. Therefore, this study hypothesizes that acute and chronic ethanol consumption can modulate paracetamol-induced hepatotoxicity differently. Thus, the objective of this study was to evaluate metabolic outcomes in the liver of C57BL/6 mice through the combination of paracetamol overdose and acute and chronic ethanol consumption.

2. Materials and Methods

2.1. Animals and Ethical Care

To carry out this study, isogenic, adult male C57BL/6 mice were used, aged 8 to 12 weeks and weighing an average of 20 to 30 g. The animals were housed in polypropylene cages at the Animal Science Center of the Federal University of Ouro Preto (UFOP)—Brazil, with controlled temperature and humidity, subjected to 12-h light/dark cycles, access to water and food "ad libitum". The experimental procedures were approved by the UFOP Animal Ethics Committee (CEUA) under protocol number 2899150322.

2.2. Experimental Design

The APAP-induced hepatotoxicity model in C57BL/6 mice has been previously standardized in our laboratory [14–17]. Janssen brand liquid paracetamol (100 mg/mL, batch: AT5616) was used at a dose of 500 mg/kg. The ethanol dosage used for mice was based on the work of [18,19]. The animals received a 50% ethanol solution (10 mL/kg). Before administering the last dose of ethanol and paracetamol, the diet was removed, and the animals remained fasting for 6 h to ensure gastric emptying.

The sample size was calculated using G*Power software version 3.1.9.2, with a power of 0.90 and an alpha value of 0.05. For the present study, the animals were randomly distributed into a control group (C) (n = 12) that received, via orogastric gavage, water for 7 days; the paracetamol (APAP) group (n = 15) received a single dose of 500 mg/kg of paracetamol via orogastric gavage; acute ethanol group (AE) (n = 15) received a 50% ethanol solution (10 mL/kg) in a single dose via orogastric gavage and, one hour later, a single dose of 500 mg/kg of paracetamol was administered; chronic ethanol (CE) group (n = 15) received by orogastric gavage a 50% ethanol solution (10 mL/kg) twice a day for seven days and, one hour after the last dose of ethanol, the single dose of 500 mg/kg of paracetamol. To maintain the animals under the same experimental conditions (gavage stress and handling), the APAP and AE groups were also subjected to orogastric water gavage twice a day during the 7 days of the experiment. The calculation of the volume of liquid gavage (water, ethanol solution, or paracetamol) was carried out using the average weight of the animals placed in the same cage.

All animals were euthanized 12 h after administration of the paracetamol overdose. The animals were anesthetized by inhalation of isoflurane (Isoflurine, Cristália Ltd.a., São Paulo, Brazil, 1 mL/mL, lot: 21120059, 3–4% in air/O_2 mixture). Then, exsanguination and collection of the animal's blood and liver were carried out (Figure 1).

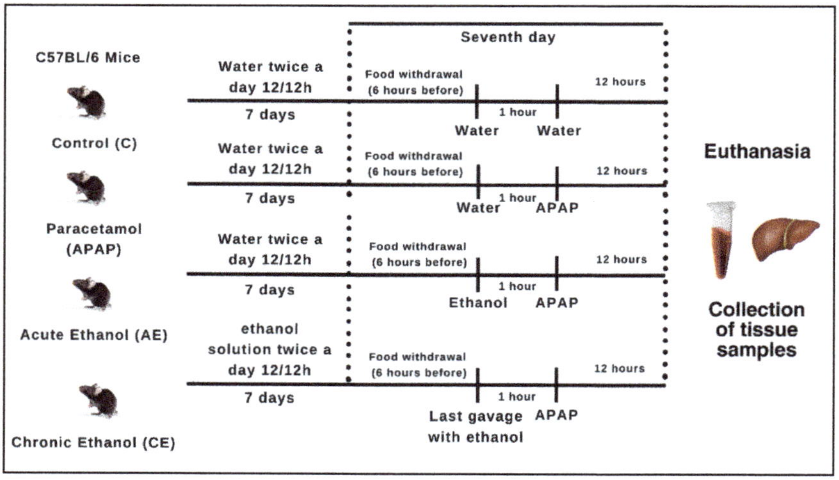

Figure 1. Experimental design. Source: Illustration created by the author himself through the website canva.com.

2.3. *Serum Inflammatory Mediators*

The concentration of inflammatory cytokines was determined in serum using commercial kits (PeproTech®, Rocky Hill, NJ, USA). The immunoabsorption assay was performed according to the manufacturer's instructions using the kits described below: Murine IL-10 (catalog #900-K153) and Murine TNF-α (catalog #900-K54). Absorption readings were taken at 405 nm, allowing for wavelength correction, with adjustment to 630 nm.

2.4. *Histological and Morphometric Analysis*

Histopathological analyses of the liver parenchyma were carried out quantitatively and semi-quantitatively using morphometry and digital densitometry techniques through image scanning. The slides containing the liver sections were stained with hematoxylin-eosin and digitized with a 40× objective using a PRIMO STAR optical microscope coupled to an AXIOCAM 102 COLOR camera using ZEN© Blue edition Software (version 3.3). Based on a normality test, 20 fields per animal were defined for each analysis. After obtaining the images with the 40× objective, we used the Image Pro Plus© software—version 4.5.0.29 (Media cybernetics) for all analyses carried out. Histopathological analyses were carried out by a pathologist with experience in the field. The inflammatory nuclei present in the liver tissue were analyzed quantitatively by isolating the inflammatory nuclei through the application of contrast, saturation, dilation/erosion, and measurement of the nuclei's area and automatic counting by the software Binucleated hepatocytes were counted manually in each image, taking as the criteria for binucleation the absence of space between the hepatocyte nuclei. The area of necrosis was assessed in all the images by manually measuring the extent of the necrotic area based on the morphology of the lesion, expressed in μm^2/area. The presence of hepatic steatosis was assessed semi-quantitatively by applying a grid made up of 100 squares in which each square represented 1% of the area, and then evaluated according to a scoring system: (0) absent; (1) steatosis present between approximately 1–9%; (2) steatosis present between approximately 10–33%; (3) steatosis present between approximately 34–66%; (4) steatosis present between approximately 67–100% of the total tissue area [20,21].

2.5. *Assessment of Liver Injury Biomarkers*

2.5.1. Measurement of ALT and AST Levels

To evaluate the activity of the hepatic enzymes alanine aminotransferase (ALT) and aspartate aminotransferase (AST), serum samples were used, and the analysis was carried out using commercial kits from the LABTEST® laboratory (Lagoa Santa—Minas Gerais, Brazil), according to the protocols available by the manufacturer.

2.5.2. Quantification of Thiobarbituric Acid Reactive Substances (TBARS)

To perform the TBARS dosage, 125 µL of trichloroacetic acid (TCA), 125 µL of thiobarbituric acid (TBA), and 62.5 µL of butylated hydroxytoluene (BHT) were added, according to a previously standardized protocol [14,15]. The reading was carried out on a plate reader with a wavelength of 535 nm. The straight-line equation was generated to calculate the concentration of the samples. The value obtained from the equation was divided by the protein content determined using the Lowry method [22].

2.5.3. Carbonylated Protein

The quantification of carbonylated proteins was performed using a UV spectrophotometer at a wavelength of 370 nm, and the procedure was carried out by adding 10% TCA reagents, 2,4-dinitrophenylhydrazine (DNPH), ethanol/acetate, and SDS, followed by centrifugation and incubation at room temperature, protected from light, according to the protocol standardized by [14,15]. The results were expressed as nmol of incorporated DNPH/mL.

2.5.4. Matrix Metalloproteinase 9 (MMP9) Activity

Matrix metalloproteinase 9 activity was quantified by zymography assay. Liver samples were homogenized using RIPA buffer (pH 8.0), which contained 150 mM NaCl, 1% IGEPAL® CA-630 (Sigma-Aldrich® Co., St. Louis, MO, USA), 0.5% sodium deoxycholate, 0.1% SDS, and 50 mM Tris, and then centrifuged at 10,000× *g* for 10 min at 4 °C. Samples were prepared and inserted into polyacrylamide gels containing 8% gelatin (2 mg/mL). After running, the gels were washed in 2.5% Triton mM CaCl2 and 0.05% NaN3 (pH 7.5). The gels were stained using 0.05% Coomassie Brilliant blue G-250 for 3 h and then decolorized in 4% methanol with 3% acetic acid solution. Gelatinase activity was visualized as discolored bands against a blue background, indicating areas of proteolysis. The marked bands were quantified using Image J software version 1.32j (National Institutes of Health, Bethesda, MD, USA), where the optical density of each band was detected.

2.6. *Assessment of the Antioxidant Profile*

2.6.1. Superoxide Dismutase (SOD) Activity

In the method used, the SOD enzyme competes with the superoxide radical, formed by the auto-oxidation of pyrogallol, responsible for the reduction of 3-[4,5-dimethylthiazol-2,5-diphenyltetrazolium] (MTT) to formazan crystals. Briefly, the plate was incubated in an oven at 37 °C for 5 min. The reaction was then stopped by adding 150 μL of dimethyl sulfoxide (DMSO), and the absorbance was measured at 570 nm using a plate reader.

2.6.2. Catalase (CAT)

Liver homogenate samples were diluted in H_2O_2 (10 mM), and every 30 s, a spectrophotometer reading was taken at 240 nm to determine the absorbance of the samples until 2 min had been completed. For the blank, distilled water was used. Catalase activity was calculated using delta absorbance over 2 min. (final absorbance − initial absorbance/2) and the molar extinction coefficient of H_2O_2 (ε = 39.4 $L/mol^{-1}/cm^{-1}$). Therefore, 1 U of catalase was equivalent to the hydrolysis of 1 μmol of H_2O_2.

2.6.3. Total Glutathione (GSHt) and Oxidized (GSSG) and Reduced (GSH) Fractions

The intracellular content of total glutathione (GSHt) and glutathione disulfide (GSSG) in the liver was determined using 5.5′dithio-bis (2-nitrobenzoic acid) (DTNB) and GSSG reductase (25). This assay employs a kinetic method based on the reduction of DTNB to TNB (5-thio-2-nitrobenzoic acid), which can be detected on a spectrophotometer at 412 nm.

For GSHt measurement, 10 μL of the supernatant was placed in a 96-well microplate. Then, 150 μL of the working mixture [95 mM phosphate buffer (pH 7.0), 0.95 mM EDTA, 48 μM NADPH, 0.031 mg/mL DTNB, 0.115 units/mL glutathione reductase were added. and 0.24% sulfosalicylic acid]. The samples were then incubated for 5 min at room temperature. The next step was to add 50 μL of NADPH (0.16 mg/mL). Absorbance readings were taken every minute for 5 min at 412 nm in an ELISA reader.

The procedure used to measure GSSG was the same as that adopted for total glutathione. However, the sample underwent a derivatization step by adding 2 μL of 2-vinyl pyridine. Derivatized samples were used in the assay following the same procedure described above. Absorbances were measured in serial dilutions of standard solutions of reduced and oxidized glutathione to generate calibration curves. The straight line equation was used to determine the concentrations in moles of total and oxidized glutathione per mL of sample. Reduced glutathione was obtained by subtracting the oxidized glutathione value from the total glutathione value.

2.6.4. Quantification of Cytochrome P450 2E1 (CYP2E1)

The cytochrome P450 isoform 2E1 (CYP2E1) was quantified in the liver homogenate using the immunoenzymatic ELISA kit for mouse samples from the company ABclonal™ [Mouse Cytochrome P450 2E1 (CYP2E1) ELISA Kit]. CYP2E1-specific antibody was pre-coated on the microplate. Samples and standards were pipetted into the wells, and the CYP2E1 present bound to the immobilized antibody. Unbound substances were washed, and an antibody conjugate specific for CYP2E1 was added to the wells and bound to the CYP2E1 capture antibody combination in the sample. After a wash to remove any unbound antibody–enzyme combination, the conjugate was added to the wells. After the incubation and washing steps, a substrate solution was added to the wells. Absorbance was measured at 450 nm.

2.6.5. Gene Expression Analysis by qRT-PCR

To analyze the expression of the genes under study, the quantitative post-reverse transcription polymerase chain reaction (qRT-PCR) technique was used. The concentration (measured at 260 nm) and purity (indicated by the 260/280 nm ratio) of total RNA were assessed using the NanoDrop ND1000 spectrophotometer (Nano Drop Technologies, Wilmington, DE, USA). The reactions were conducted in 96-well plates, with each well containing

1 µL of cDNA (diluted 5× in water), 0.5 µL of each primer (forward and reverse, 10 µM), and 5 µL of SYBR® Green PCR Master Mix (Applied Biosystems®) and 3 µL of DNAse-free water, totaling a final volume of 10 µL. The assays were performed in technical triplicate for all genes evaluated, with the reference gene (GAPDH) present in all plates. The qRT-PCR reaction was conducted according to the programming contained in the ABI 7300 Applied Biosystems® device. The specificity of the products obtained was confirmed by analyzing the dissociation curves of the amplified products at the end of each reaction. Expression level analyses were carried out using the relative gene expression quantification method (comparative Cq or ΔCq), which allows evaluation of the expression level of a specific gene between different samples. In this way, the expression of the target genes was normalized by the levels of the reference gene (GAPDH), and the results obtained through the difference between the expression of the target genes (ADH, CYP2E1, UGT1A1, and UGT2A1) and the expression of the gene of GAPDH reference. The sequence of the primers used was (1) ADH: F′ TAATGCCTCGGGGGACTTTG, R′ GAGAAGGTGCTGGTGCTGAT; (2) CYP2E1: F′ TTTCCCTAAGTATCCTCCGTGAC, R′ TCGTAATCGAAGCGTTTGTTG; (3) UGT1A1: F′ CTGGGAGGCTGTTAGTGTTCC, R′ GAGGCTTCAGGTGCTATGAC; (4) UGT2A1: F′ CTCATCTGGCCCATGGAAGG, R′ GGCCACAAGGACAGTCACAT; (5) GAPDH: F′ ATGTGTCCGTCGTGGATCTG, R′ GTAGCCCAAGATGCCCTTCA.

2.6.6. Proteomic Analysis

Protein concentration was determined using the BCA protein assay kit (Thermo Scientific, Cramlington, UK). Fifty micrograms of protein were used for digestion. Samples were diluted in ammonium bicarbonate (AmBic, 25 mM) containing RapiGest (Waters Corporation, Milford, MA, USA) (0.06% final concentration), homogenized and incubated in a thermoblock at 80 °C for 10 min. Ten microliters of a dithiothreitol solution (DTT, Vetec, code: 13-1318-0001) were added, undergoing further homogenization and incubation for 10 min at 60 °C. The proteins were alkylated with the addition of 10 µL of an iodoacetamide solution (GE Healthcare UK Limited, code: RPM6302V) (33 mg/mL), homogenized again, and incubated for 45 min protected from light. Trypsin was added in a 50:1 ratio (protein: trypsin) followed by homogenization and incubated overnight (12 h). Next, 2 µL of peptides were separated using an UltiMate® 3000 nanoUHPLC 3000 system (Dionex®), which was configured with an Acclaim PepMap100 C18 Nano-Trap capture column (75 µm i.d. × 2 cm, 3 µm, 100 Å; Thermo Scientific®) and an Easy Column C18 capillary column (75 µm i.d. × 10 cm, 3 µm, 120 Å; Thermo Scientific®) conditioned at 40 °C, at a flow rate of 300 nL/min. The peptides were previously washed with 2% acetonitrile and 0.05% trifluoroacetic acid for 5 min, then separated at 40 °C using a nonlinear solvent gradient A (0.1% formic acid) and B (80% acetonitrile/0.1% formic acid). Spectrum scans were acquired on the Q-Exactive™ mass spectrometry instrument (Thermo Scientific) coupled to the nano UHPLC system containing a nanoelectrospray ion source. The instrument operated at 3.5 kV, positive mode, resolution of 70,000 in the range 300–2000 m/z, maximum injection time of 120 ms, and automatic gain control (AGC) of 1 × 106 ions. Up to 12 most intense precursor ions with charge state ≥ 2 were isolated in a 2 m/z window and fragmented via high-energy collisional dissociation—HCD (30 V collision energy). MS/MS spectra were acquired at 35,000 resolution with a maximum injection time of 150 ms and AGC of 5 × 105 ions. Dynamic exclusion was set to 40 s. The .raw files obtained from the Q-Exactive instrument were searched in a database using Peaks Studio software, version 8.5. Protein identification was performed against a mus musculus database obtained from UniProt containing 55305 protein sequences. Relative protein quantification was performed and statistically tested using ANOVA, which was performed automatically by the software. Only proteins with a p-value ≤ 0.05 were considered differentially abundant between samples. The IDs of the researched proteins were used to search for the corresponding genes and the species, defined as *mus musculus*, in the database KEGG (Kyoto Encyclopedia of Genes and Genomes; http://bioinformatics.sdstate.edu/go/, accessed on 23 May 2024).

2.6.7. Statistical Analyzes

Statistical analyses were performed using GraphPad Prism9® software (GraphPad Software Inc., Solana Beach, CA, USA). Data normality was assessed using the Kolmogorov–Smirnov test. For data with a normal distribution, one-way ANOVA (analysis of variance) followed by the Bonferroni post-test was performed, and results were represented as the mean ± standard error of the mean. For data not following a normal distribution, the Kruskal–Wallis test followed by Dunn's post-test was conducted, and results were represented as a median with an interquartile range. Differences were considered significant when $p < 0.05$.

3. Results

3.1. Assessment of Serum Inflammatory Profile

The serum inflammatory profile was assessed by measuring the levels of TNF-α and IL-10. Figure 2A shows that the APAP group had higher levels of TNF-α compared to the control group ($p < 0.0001$) and the AE ($p = 0.0034$) and CE ($p = 0.0037$) groups. The AE ($p = 0.0013$) and CE ($p = 0.0047$) groups were superior to the control group but equal to each other. A similar pattern was observed for IL-10 (Figure 2B), with the APAP group exhibiting higher values than the control group ($p < 0.0001$) and the AE ($p < 0.0001$) and CE ($p = 0.0001$). The AE ($p = 0.0029$) and CE ($p = 0.0132$) groups exhibited higher levels compared to the control group but did not differ from each other.

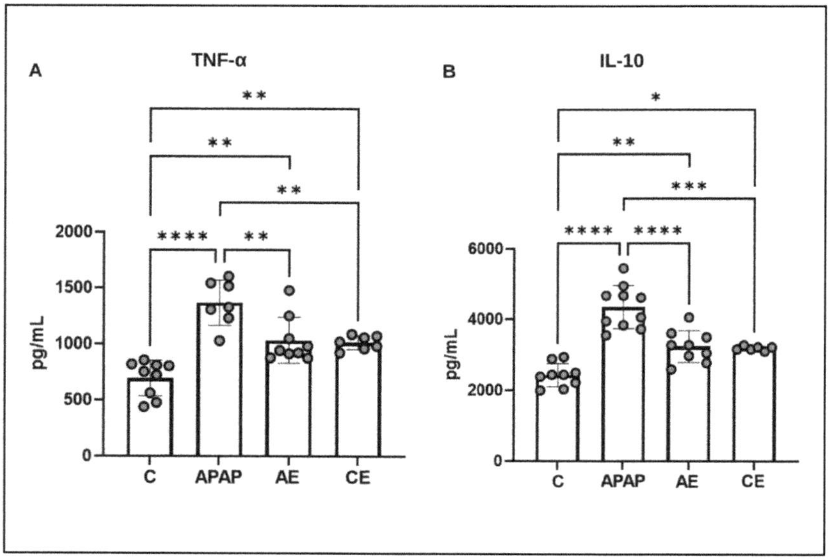

Figure 2. Assessment of the serum inflammatory profile using TNF-α (**A**) and IL-10 (**B**) measurements. Statistical analysis was performed using the one-way ANOVA test and Bonferroni post-test. TNF-α: Tumor necrosis factor alpha; IL-10: Interleukin 10. (*) represents a significant difference between groups. **** ($p < 0.0001$); *** ($p < 0.001$); ** ($p < 0.01$), and * ($p < 0.05$).

3.2. Histological and Morphometric Analysis

Representative images of the liver tissue are shown in Figure 3A–D at 40× magnification, highlighting the histopathological aspects of the liver parenchyma, and Figure 3E–H at 20× magnification, showing general pathological changes. The morphometric analyses conducted on the liver parenchyma of control animals (C) showed a preserved parenchyma without significant pathological aspects (Figure 3A,E). The other experimental groups presented: the presence of foci of inflammation in the APAP and AE groups (Figure 3B,C,F,G), a general increase in inflammatory nuclei, hydropic and fatty degeneration (Figure 3D), sinusoidal dilation, ischemic-type necrosis, with prevalent areas in zones 3 and 2, further away from the afferent blood supply, in addition to regenerative processes such as hepatocyte binucleation and karyomegaly.

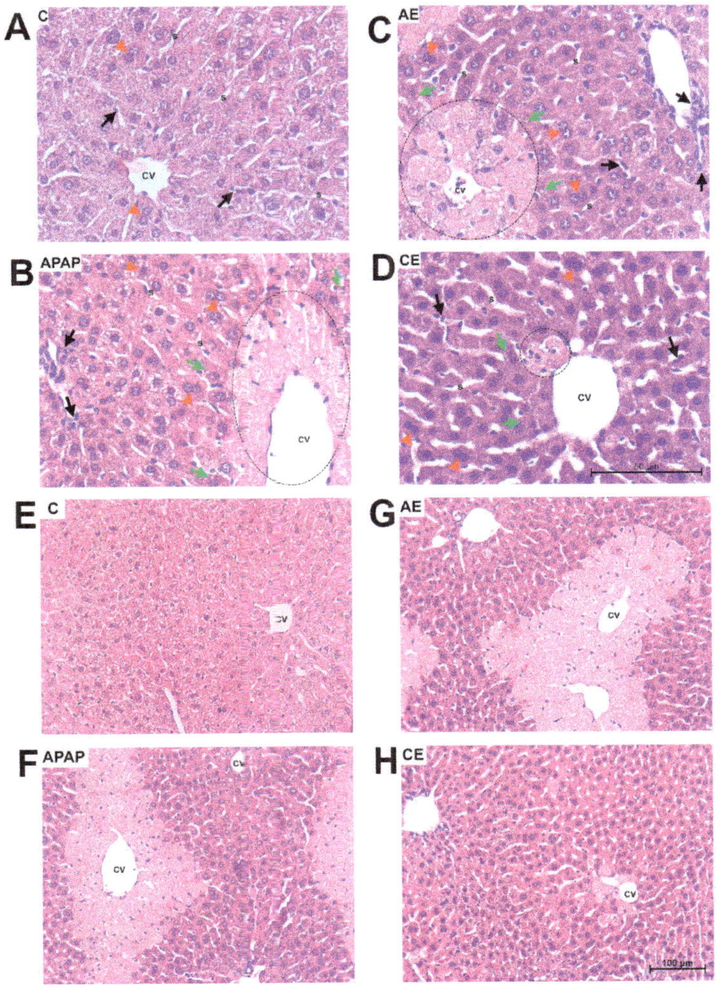

Figure 3. Histopathological aspects of the liver parenchyma. Photomicrographs of liver sections stained with hematoxylin and eosin. Bar = 50 µm, 400× magnification (**A–D**) and Bar = 100 µm, 200× magnification (**E–H**). (**A**,**E**) Representative image of the control group (**C**). (**B**,**F**) Representative image of the lesions found in the group treated with paracetamol (APAP). (**C**,**G**) Representative image of the group treated with acute ethanol (AE). (**D**,**H**) Representative image of the group treated with chronic ethanol (CE). In (**A**,**E**) preserved liver parenchyma, the presence of inflammatory cells in a normal pattern (black arrow), preserved sinusoidal capillaries (S), and few binucleated hepatocytes (red triangle). (**B**,**C**) Fatty degeneration (green arrow), binucleated hepatocytes (red triangle), area of extensive necrosis (dotted circle), and inflammatory infiltrates (black arrow). (**D**) Fatty degeneration (green arrow), binucleated hepatocytes (red triangle), and area of necrosis to a lesser extent (dotted circle), central vein (CV).

The inflammatory nucleus count was higher in the APAP and AE groups compared to the control group and CE group. APAP was higher than the control group ($p < 0.0001$) and CE ($p = 0.0002$). AE was greater than the control ($p = 0.0006$) and CE ($p = 0.0095$) (Figure 4A). Intoxication with paracetamol (APAP) and its association with an acute dose of ethanol (AE) promoted hepatocellular hypoxia. The APAP ($p = 0.0033$) and AE ($p = 0.0456$) groups showed a greater extent of the necrosis area compared to the control group, with no statistical difference between APAP and AE ($p > 0.05$). The APAP group presented a larger area of necrosis when compared to CE ($p = 0.0073$). The CE group was statistically equal to the AE and C groups ($p > 0.05$) (Figure 4B). Regarding the count of binucleated hepatocytes, the APAP and AE groups were statistically equal ($p > 0.05$). APAP was higher than the control group ($p < 0.0001$) and CE ($p = 0.0117$). AE was greater than the control ($p = 0.0005$) and equal to CE (Figure 4C). Fatty degeneration or steatosis was evident in a higher percentage in the APAP ($p = 0.0309$) and AE ($p = 0.0152$) groups compared to the control group. The CE group was not different from the control and, likewise, it was not different from the other groups (Figure 4D).

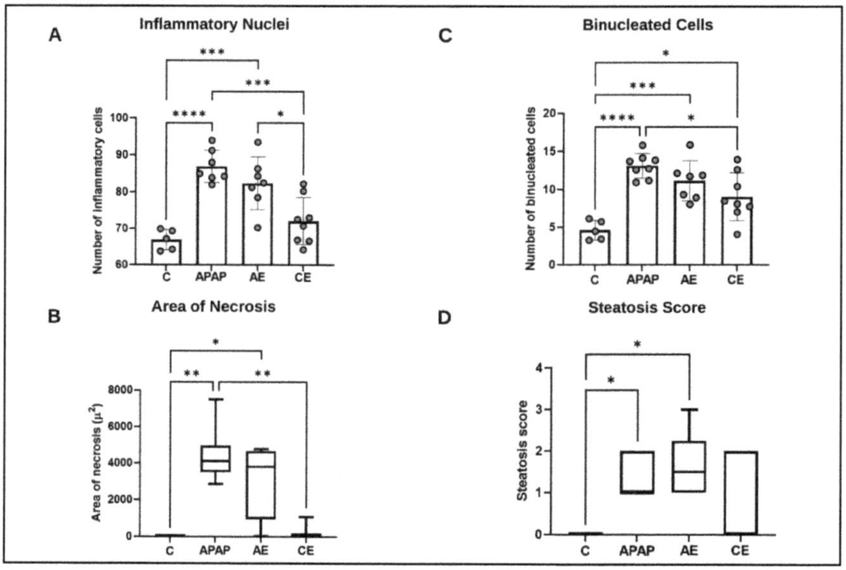

Figure 4. Morphometric and semiquantitative analyses of the liver in relation to inflammatory nuclei (**A**), binucleated cells (**B**), area of necrosis (**C**), and steatosis score (Panel **D**). (**C**) Control group; (*APAP*) paracetamol group; (AE) acute ethanol group; (CE) chronic ethanol group. For results, number of inflammatory nuclei, number of binucleated cells, and area of necrosis, data were expressed as mean ± standard deviation of the mean and were analyzed by (one-way ANOVA) followed by the Bonferroni post-test. For the non-parametric results of necrosis area and steatosis score, data were expressed as the median and interquartile range (25th–75th percentile) and analyzed using the Kruskal–Wallis test followed by Dunn's post hoc test. (*) represents a significant difference between groups. **** ($p < 0.0001$); *** ($p < 0.001$); ** ($p < 0.01$), and * ($p < 0.05$).

3.3. *Assessment of Liver Injury Markers*

Regarding ALT activity (Figure 5A), there was a significant increase in the APAP ($p < 0.0001$) and AE ($p < 0.0001$) groups compared to the control group and the CE group ($p < 0.0001$ for both). The APAP and AE groups did not differ significantly. There was no difference between the CE group and the control group for this parameter. For AST activity (Figure 5B), there was greater activity in the APAP ($p = 0.0017$) and AE ($p = 0.0472$) groups compared to the control group. Similarly, the APAP ($p = 0.0014$) and AE ($p = 0.0442$) groups were higher than the CE group. The APAP and AE groups did not differ significantly from each other for this parameter, nor did the CE group differ from the control group.

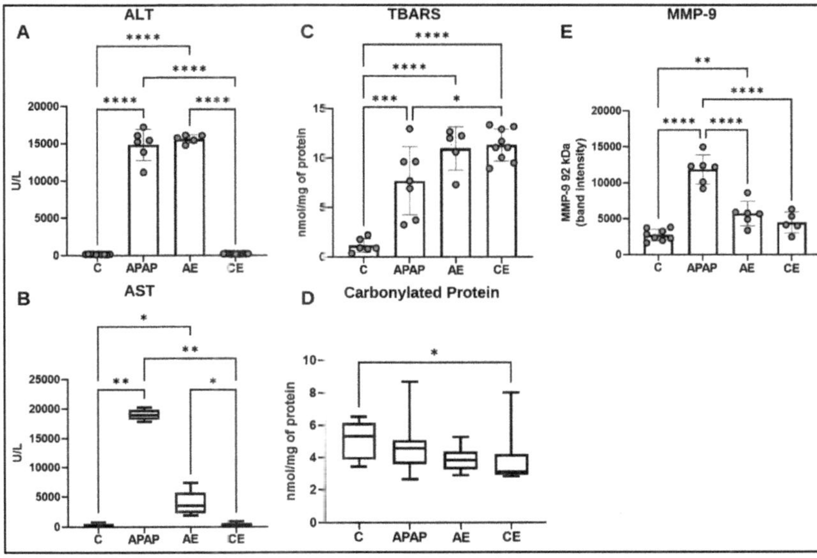

Figure 5. Assessment of markers of liver damage by evaluating the activities of ALT (**A**), AST (**B**), the concentration of TBARS (**C**), carbonylated protein (**D**), and the activity of MMP-9 (**E**). Statistical analysis for ALT, TBARS, and MMP-9 was performed using the one-way ANOVA test and Bonferroni post-test. For the statistical analysis of AST and carbonylated protein data, the Kruskal-Wallis test was applied, followed by the Dunns post-test. ALT: Alanine aminotransferase; AST: Aspartate aminotransferase; TBARS: Substances reactive to thiobarbituric acid; MMP-9: Matrix metalloproteinase—9. (*) represents a significant difference between groups. **** ($p < 0.0001$); *** ($p < 0.001$); ** ($p < 0.01$) and * ($p < 0.05$).

Regarding TBARS, there was an increase in the APAP ($p = 0.0001$), AE, and CE ($p < 0.0001$ for both) groups compared to the control group. The AE and CE groups were not significantly different from each other; however, the CE group ($p = 0.0226$) was statistically higher than the APAP group. There was no significant difference between the APAP and AE groups (Figure 5C). As for carbonyl protein, the CE group ($p = 0.0457$) showed a significant reduction compared to the control group (Figure 5D). There was no statistical difference between the experimental groups for this parameter, nor was there any difference between the APAP and AE groups compared to the control group.

Regarding MMP-9 activity, the APAP group ($p < 0.0001$) showed the highest results compared to the control group and the AE and CE groups ($p < 0.0001$ for both). The AE group ($p = 0.0093$) showed a significant difference from the control group, which was not observed for the CE group (Figure 5E).

3.4. Assessment of the Hepatic Antioxidant Profile

Total glutathione levels (Figure 6A) in the AE group exhibited the lowest values compared to the control ($p < 0.0001$), APAP ($p = 0.0023$), and CE ($p = 0.0003$) groups. The control, APAP, and CE groups were not significantly different from each other. Regarding the GSH/GSSG ratio (Figure 6B), the lowest values were observed for the AE and APAP groups ($p < 0.0001$ for both) compared to the control group. The APAP ($p = 0.0009$) and AE ($p = 0.0002$) groups were also smaller than CE. When evaluating the levels of reduced glutathione (Figure 6C), once again, the scenario presents itself with the lowest values for the AE group ($p < 0.0001$) compared to the control group. The AE group also has lower values than the APAP ($p = 0.0038$) and CE ($p = 0.0001$) groups. Finally, the results for oxidized glutathione (Figure 6D) show that the APAP group presented the highest levels for this parameter, being significantly higher than the control and CE groups ($p < 0.0001$ for both); however, it was no different from the AE group. The AE group, in turn, was higher than the control group ($p < 0.0001$) and CE ($p = 0.0004$).

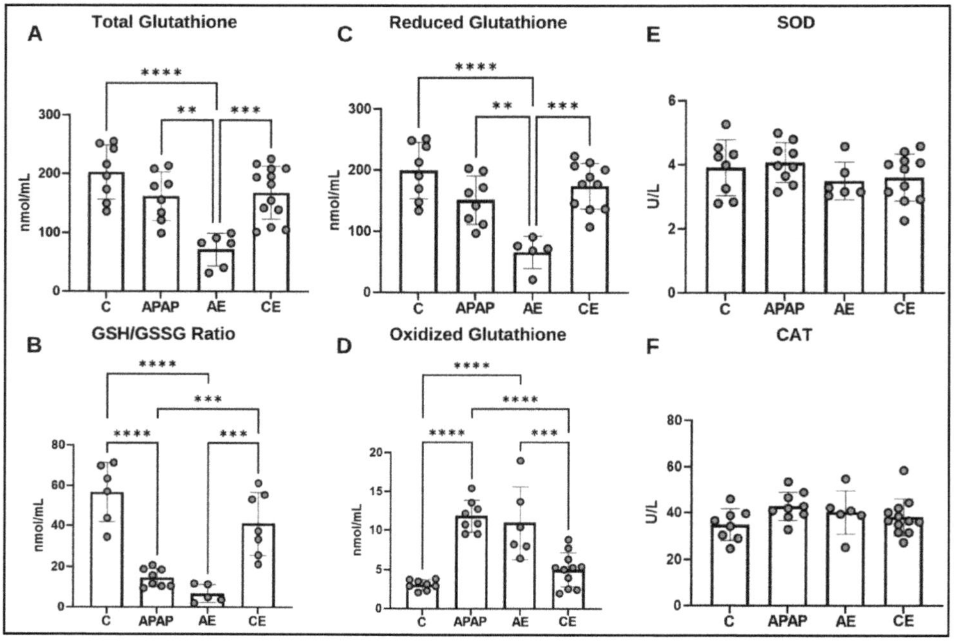

Figure 6. Assessment of the hepatic antioxidant profile by evaluating the levels of total glutathione (**A**), GSH/GSSG ratio (**B**), oxidized glutathione (**C**), reduced glutathione (**D**), SOD (**E**), and CAT (**F**). Statistical analysis was performed using the one-way ANOVA test and Bonferroni post-test. GSH: Reduced glutathione; GSSG: Oxidized glutathione; SOD: Superoxide dismutase; CAT: Catalase. (*) represents a significant difference between groups. **** ($p < 0.0001$); *** ($p < 0.001$), and ** ($p < 0.01$).

Regarding the activity of the antioxidant enzymes SOD (Figure 6E) and CAT (Figure 6F), no significant differences were observed between the groups.

3.5. Assessment of CYP2E1 Levels and Expression of Genes Related to APAP and Ethanol Metabolism

CYP2E1 is a microsomal enzyme active in both APAP and ethanol metabolism. When quantifying this enzyme (Figure 7A), it was found that the highest concentration values were found in the AE group, which was significantly higher in the control group ($p = 0.0064$), APAP ($p = 0.0550$) and CE ($p = 0.0749$). There was no significant difference in CYP2E1 gene expression between the experimental groups (Figure 7B).

ADH is an important enzyme in ethanol metabolism. Regarding gene expression for this enzyme, the CE group exhibited the highest values compared to the control group ($p = 0.0004$) and compared to the APAP and AE groups ($p < 0.0001$) (Figure 7C).

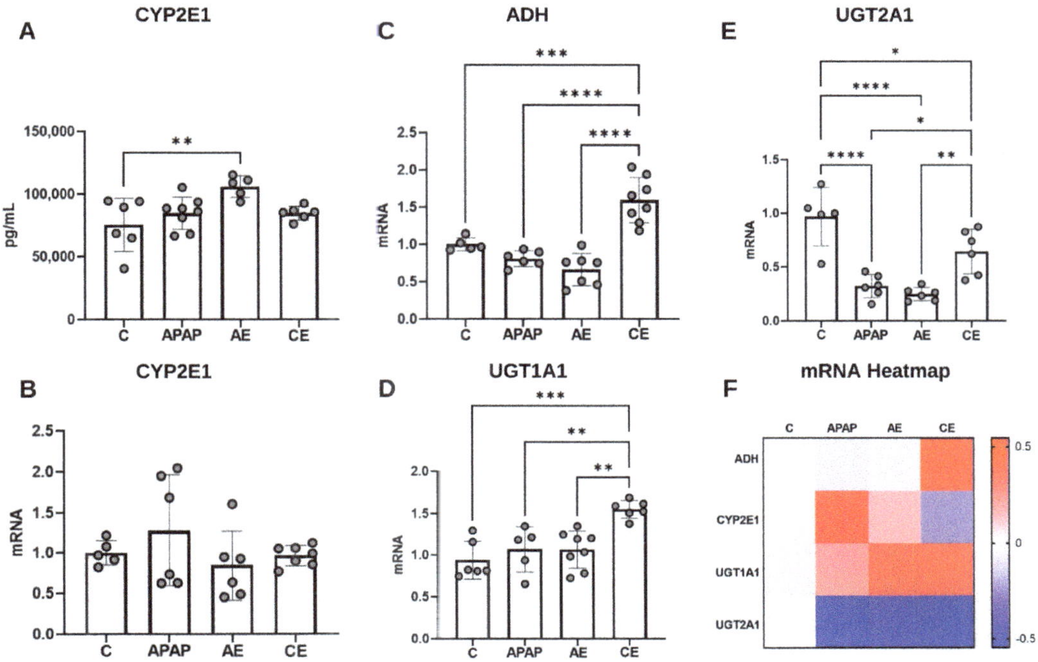

Figure 7. Assessment of hepatic CYP2E1 concentration (**A**), CYP2E1 gene expression (**B**), ADH (**C**), UGT1A1 (**D**), UGT2A1 (**E**) and gene expression heatmap (**F**). Statistical analysis for CYP2E1 concentration and expression of CYP2E1, ADH, and UGT2A1 genes was performed using the one-way ANOVA test and Bonferroni post-test. For statistical analysis of UGT1A1 gene expression data, the Kruskal–Wallis test was applied, followed by Dunn's post-test. CYP2E1: cytochrome P450 2E1; ADH: Alcohol dehydrogenase; UGT1A1: Glucuronosyltransferase Family 1 Member A1; UGT2A1: Glucuronosyltransferase Family 2 Member A1. (*) represents a significant difference between groups. **** ($p < 0.0001$); *** ($p < 0.001$); ** ($p < 0.01$), and * ($p < 0.05$).

Regarding the expression of UGT1A1 (Figure 7D), the greatest difference was observed between the CE group ($p = 0.0045$) and the control group. The CE group also differed significantly from the APAP ($p = 0.0071$) and AE ($p = 0.0024$) groups. Finally, for UGT2A1 (Figure 7E), the APAP and AE groups presented the lowest values. These groups do not present statistical differences between them; however, they are significantly lower than the values of the control group ($p < 0001$ for both). The APAP group has lower results than the CE group ($p = 0.0238$), as well as the AE group ($p = 0.0048$). It can be considered that the CE group has intermediate values, lower than the control group ($p = 0.0313$) and, as already described, higher than the other experimental groups.

Figure 7F displays the heatmap graph referring to the qualitative analysis of the modulation of gene expression related to APAP/ethanol metabolizing enzymes. It is noted that in the APAP, AE, and CE groups, there is upregulation of the UGT1A1 gene and downregulation of the UGT2A1 gene. In the APAP and AE groups, upregulation of CYP2E1 was observed, while in the CE group, upregulation of the ADH gene was observed.

3.6. The Hepatic Proteome Is Altered During Acute and Chronic Alcohol Consumption and Acetaminophen Overdose

The scope of the proteome observed through spectral data obtained from the soluble fraction of the liver proteome was compared with the databases available for *mus musculus* animals at UniProt. Thus, it was possible to identify 937 distinct groups of proteins. Thus, it was possible to identify 937 distinct groups of proteins. Among the groups identified, 588 (62.75%) are present in all treatments. It was found that in the four experimental groups, there were groups of proteins that were expressed exclusively in each group (Supplementary Material—Figure S1). The dynamic range of identified proteins covered five orders of magnitude of difference between the highest and lowest abundance constituents in the liver, as assessed by the area under the curve. Around 200 proteins cover more than 90% of the accumulated area; among these, only 15 proteins correspond to more than 50% of the total ionic signal (Supplementary Material—Figure S2A,B). The 15 most abundant proteins are presented in decreasing order of abundance in Table S1 (Supplementary Materials—Table S1).

The analysis of proteomic data obtained from the soluble fraction of the liver proteome confirmed the presence of the proteins of interest that were quantified and evaluated through biochemical analyses in the present study. From the KEGG database, it was found that the genes for these proteins are involved in several drug and xenobiotic metabolism pathways via the cytochrome P450 pathway and glutathione metabolism, both involved in the metabolism and detoxification of paracetamol and ethanol (Supplementary Material—Figure S3).

Principal component analysis (PCA) demonstrated that the different experimental groups produced isolation or groupings of protein constituents according to the treatment used. The PCA graph revealed, according to the data from the label-free quantitative analysis, that the samples from the AE group were more closely related to those from the APAP group. Groups C and CE appear close to each other and further apart from groups APAP and AE. This analysis demonstrated that an acute dose of ethanol presents a profile of protein constituents closer to the acetaminophen overdose group (Figure 8), confirming the profile of the biochemical and morphometric analyses.

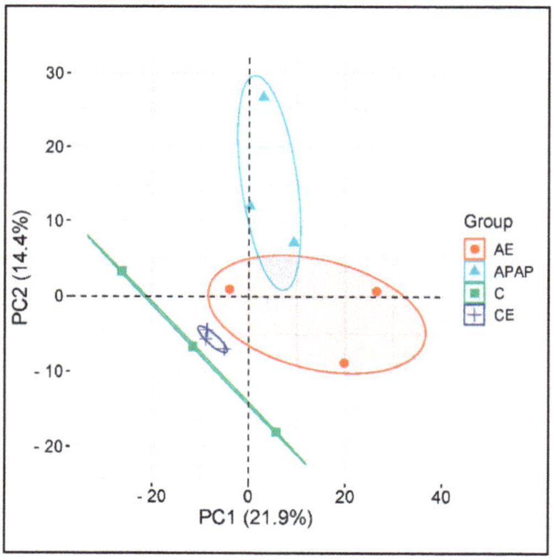

Figure 8. Principal components analysis (PCA). Axes demonstrate principal component 1 and principal component 2, showing 21.9% and 14.4% of the total variance, respectively.

The heatmap graph shows that among the most differentially abundant proteins, treatments with paracetamol and its association with an acute dose or chronic use of ethanol promoted positive regulation in several proteins. This result is likely associated with a compensatory mechanism aimed at maintaining cellular functions under the stress induced by the drugs (Figure 9A). Figure 9B shows the classification of proteins analyzed in the heatmap according to their biological function.

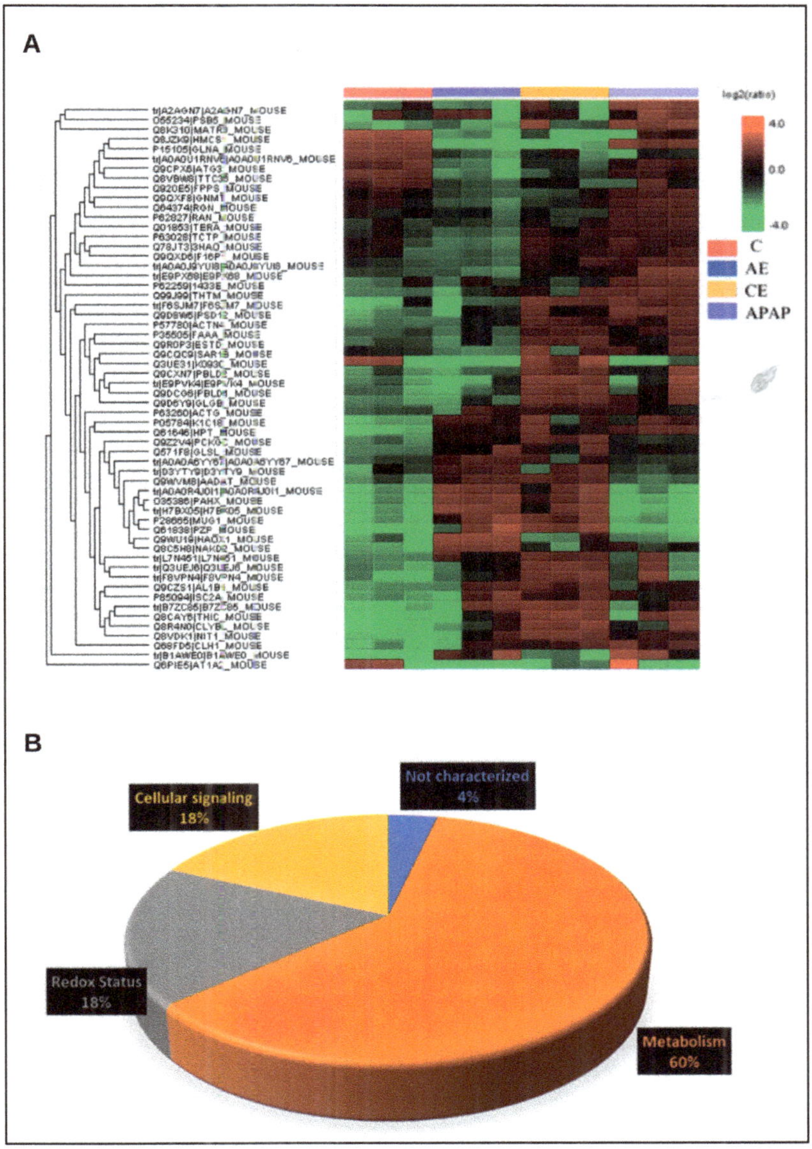

Figure 9. Heatmap of differentially abundant hepatic proteins when comparing different treatments. Red coloring indicates positive regulation, while green coloring indicates negative regulation (**A**) and classification of proteins according to their biological function (**B**).

4. Discussion

The risk of APAP toxicity associated with alcohol consumption has been recognized since the 1980s; however, the mechanisms underlying liver injury are still not completely understood [23,24].

Our study was based on the premise that ethanol metabolism plays a critical role in modulating the extent of liver damage induced by paracetamol overdose. Consequently, the primary objective was to investigate the effects of co-exposure to ethanol and paracetamol. The 1-h interval between administrations was strategically chosen to maximize the interaction between the two compounds. This design allowed for the evaluation of co-exposure effects in both acute and chronic contexts, simulating clinical scenarios such as occasional alcohol consumption followed by analgesic use or repeated ethanol exposure accompanied by paracetamol intake.

Our results indicated that acute ethanol consumption maintained a hepatic profile similar to that of the group intoxicated with APAP. Although we observed a reduction in GSH levels beyond what was observed in the APAP group and an increase in CYP2E1 levels, the other parameters evaluated remained similar to those in the APAP group. This suggested that acute ethanol consumption does not worsen the hepatic response to APAP overdose. Chronic ethanol consumption improved the liver response to APAP. This was demonstrated by the reduction in inflammatory nuclei, area of necrosis, MMP-9, carbonylated protein, ALT, and AST, in addition to the increase in the GSH/GSSG ratio and gene expression of the enzymes UGT1A1 and UGT2A1, which are responsible for the non-toxic metabolism of APAP. Thus, it is suggested that, despite the observed increase in TBARS levels, chronic ethanol consumption minimizes APAP-induced hepatotoxicity. However, it is important to note that these results were observed after seven days of ethanol consumption; therefore, we cannot extrapolate these results to longer consumption.

During liver injury, exaggerated production of inflammatory cytokines can trigger a systemic inflammatory response syndrome. In this scenario, the analysis of serum cytokines is essential to understand and evaluate drug-induced liver failure [25]. TNF is a pleiotropic cytokine that can contribute to the induction of apoptosis and activation of endothelial cells and platelets, in addition to increased vascular permeability and activation of soluble mediators. The increase in TNF during the course of APAP-induced acute liver failure appears to be a crucial event in determining its outcome [26]. In our study, the APAP group exhibited the highest TNF values. Even with a lower dosage of APAP (300 mg/kg), it is possible to observe an increase in the levels of pro-inflammatory cytokines (TNF, IL-1β, and IL-6) 12 h after its administration [27]. Our results showed that the AE and CE groups had higher levels of TNF compared to the control group, although they were lower than the values in the APAP group. Chronic and acute ethanol consumption can increase TNF-production. This increase is attributed to an increase in the intestinal permeability caused by ethanol, which can lead to endotoxemia. Endotoxemia, in turn, results in the increased production of lipopolysaccharide, which activates Kupffer cells and ultimately leads to the generation of pro-inflammatory cytokines [28]. However, the deleterious effects of pro-inflammatory cytokines can be counterbalanced by the upregulation of immunoregulatory cytokines such as IL-10. IL-10 is an anti-inflammatory cytokine that is markedly released in cases of hepatotoxicity induced by both APAP and ethanol. IL-10 is capable of negatively regulating the synthesis of pro-inflammatory cytokines such as TNF [29]. Similar to the TNF results, higher levels of IL-10 were observed in the APAP group compared to the control group and the other experimental groups (AE and CE). However, the latter presented values that were lower than those observed in the APAP group but still higher than those in the control group. Even with a lower dose of APAP (300 mg/kg), a previous study [29] showed an increase in the serum concentration of IL-10, which peaked 24 h after drug administration. In another study, animals that received an ethanol dose of 5 g/kg three times at 12 h intervals also exhibited an increase in serum concentrations of IL-10 [30]. In contrast [31], using an ethanol dose of 7 g/kg in C57BL/6 mice, no changes were observed in TNF or IL-10 4 h after euthanasia. According to [31], in addition to the dose and the time of exposure, the serum concentrations of these cytokines can also be influenced by the strain of animals used. Therefore, C57BL/6 mice are less susceptible to changes in the systemic inflammatory response in models of excessive ethanol consumption.

After analyzing systemic TNF and IL-10 levels, we next evaluated histopathological changes in the liver. Morphometric analyses showed that treatment with APAP alone and in combination with an acute dose of ethanol (group AE) promoted hepatocellular hypoxia, a larger area of necrosis, and hepatic steatosis compared to groups C and CE. Similarly, both the APAP and AE groups exhibited higher counts of binucleated hepatocytes, which is evidence of tissue regeneration. A 300 mg/kg dose of APAP can promote necrosis and centrilobular liver degeneration [32]. Thus, the observed liver damage indicated a typical and consistent pattern caused by paracetamol overdose, which was maintained by acute ethanol consumption. The results of the histopathological analyses in the APAP group were consistent with those of previous studies conducted by our research group [14–17]. The literature suggests that when a combination of APAP (200 mg/kg) and ethanol [23] is used, following a protocol in which ethanol is administered via a liquid diet containing 5% ethanol (5% *v*/*v*) for 10 days, followed by ethanol gavage adjusted to the weight of the animals on the eleventh day (a longer period than that used in our study), the development of micro- and macroscopic hepatic steatosis was observed, in addition to hepatocellular ballooning. This indicated that ethanol administration aggravated APAP-induced liver injury.

Administration of 400 mg/kg of APAP is considered sufficient to cause significant liver toxicity within 6–24 h [33]. Even at a lower dose (300 mg/kg) than that used in our study, high plasma levels of ALT and AST were observed at different time points (3, 6, and 12 h) [32]. In previous studies (15–17), we administered a toxic dose of 500 mg/kg and performed euthanasia 12 h after drug administration, which revealed increased serum ALT and AST levels. An increase in ALT and AST activities was observed in C57BL/6 mice at a dose of 500 mg/kg, even 24 h after administration of the toxic dose [34]. Taken together, the results obtained from the different studies fall within the time window in which the ability of APAP to promote liver toxicity was observed (6–24 h). Consistent with these findings, in the present study, the APAP group showed higher ALT and AST levels. The AE group also showed higher serum activity of these enzymes compared to group C and similar to the APAP group, which was not observed in the CE group. Our data indicated that the combination of APAP overdose and acute ethanol administration promoted a greater degree of liver damage than chronic ethanol administration.

According to the literature, in the case of an APAP overdose, NAPQI can react even more with cellular proteins, increasing the formation of free radicals and lipid peroxidation and potentially worsening oxidative damage [35]. Similar to APAP, ethanol metabolism results in an increased production of free radicals, which play a crucial role in the development of liver damage caused by this substance. CYP2E1 is one of the three main enzymes involved in ethanol metabolism and is capable of converting it into more reactive products and increasing the generation of ROS [36,37]. Both acute and chronic ethanol administration can increase ROS production and lipid peroxidation in animal models and humans. Studies in which ethanol was administered via orogastric gavage showed that ethanol-induced liver injury was associated with increased lipid peroxidation and carbonyl protein formation and decreased hepatic antioxidant defense [18,28]. In both cases, free radical formation played an important role in inducing lipid, DNA, and protein damage [35,36]. Even in animals treated with ethanol ingested orally through a liquid diet (containing 36% of the calories from ethanol) for six weeks, the concentration of TBARS increased significantly, indicating oxidative damage to cellular lipids [37]. When evaluating the effects of acute ethanol administration (5 g/kg administered three times separated by 12 h), an almost nine-fold increase in hepatic TBARS content was observed in ethanol-treated animals compared to that in the control group [38], in which the concentration of TBARS was twice as high in animals chronically treated with ethanol via a liquid diet (Lieber–DeCarli). In our study, we observed an increase in lipid peroxidation as indicated by the TBARS levels in groups AE and CE, which were higher than those in groups C and APAP. Mice of the C57Bl/6J lineage were administered two doses of ethanol (6 g/kg) by orogastric gavage with an interval of 12 h between them [39]. As observed in the AE and CE groups, the cited study found an increase in the production of free radicals and lipid peroxidation through TBARS measurements. According to the authors, because the liver is the main site of ethanol metabolism, a reduction in hepatic proteasome activity by ethanol may have resulted in the formation of adducts or oxidative modifications of the proteasome subunit proteins when reacting with ethanol-derived acetaldehyde and/or secondary products (ROS and lipid peroxides) derived from ethanol oxidation.

The increase in TBARS levels in the APAP group was consistent with results obtained in previous studies conducted by our research group using the same APAP administration protocol [14,16]. These data demonstrated that the combination of APAP and ethanol intensified hepatic lipid peroxidation. Hepatic carbonylated proteins are considered important markers of APAP-induced oxidative stress [40]. In a previous study, no significant differences were found in this parameter between animals treated with ethanol and those in the control group [38]. However, regarding carbonylated proteins, we found that the APAP and AE groups showed no difference compared with the control group, and there was a reduction in this parameter in the CE group. Because protein carbonyls are markers of protein oxidation by ROS, the fact that the CE group presented the lowest values does not necessarily represent an inconsistency; rather, there was less protein damage caused by oxidative stress, which is also typical in cases of APAP overdose. This result does not necessarily represent a protective effect of ethanol and might be an adaptative mechanism of the organ to the oxidative insult caused by prolonged ethanol intake. However, given that the APAP and AE groups were not statistically different from the control group, we understand that the protein carbonylated assay protocol used in our study was probably less sensitive in assessing hepatic oxidative damage than the TBARS measurement.

MMP-9, also known as type IV collagenase (gelatinase B), belongs to a family of matrix zinc-dependent proteinases (MMPs), almost all of which play an important role in liver regeneration and in controlling the number of proteins in the extracellular matrix. They are also involved in other biological processes, such as fibrosis, cirrhosis, and carcinogenesis [41]. In our study, increased MMP-9 activity was observed in the APAP and AE groups. In another study, an increase in MMP-9 activity was observed 6 h after the administration of an APAP dose of 600 mg/kg [42]. These data suggest that an increase in MMP-9 activity resulting from APAP overdose is associated with liver injury. Sinusoidal endothelial cells (ESCs) are direct targets of APAP hepatotoxicity, as evidenced by the formation of clefts in the endothelium of centrilobular sinusoids formed by the destruction and/or coalescence of fenestrae. The formation of larger clefts in the sinusoidal endothelial cells results in increased infiltration of red blood cells into the extrasinusoidal space, causing additional hypoxic damage to the liver [43,44]. These events precede any evidence of histological or chemical injury. These cracks are larger and more frequent in animals treated with ethanol, acutely or chronically, after receiving a toxic dose of APAP. The inhibition of MMP-2 and MMP-9 can minimize endothelial injury and red blood cell infiltration, as they affect the ESC cytoskeleton, which, in turn, reduces cleft formation [43]. The increase in MMP-9 levels during APAP intoxication, as well as its association with acute ethanol administration, may be associated with hepatocellular damage and microcirculatory dysfunction, resulting in significant hepatocellular hypoxia, in line with the histological data from our study.

APAP toxicity is primarily associated with excessive production of NAPQI. Hepatic cytochrome P450 enzymes, particularly CYP2E1, play fundamental roles in the oxidative activation of APAP. In cases of APAP overdose, large amounts of NAPQI are generated and subsequently conjugated with glutathione (GSH), which can neutralize it [45]. The CYP2E1 pathway can also produce ROS, mainly superoxide anions and hydrogen peroxide, in alcohol-induced liver injury [46]. Both these mechanisms lead to mitochondrial dysfunction, resulting in increased ROS production, decreased ATP production, and compromised cellular antioxidant profiles [47]. Regarding the antioxidant profile, the AE group exhibited the lowest total glutathione values as well as the lowest GSH/GSSG ratio. The ICR mice were treated with APAP (400 mg/kg) or ethanol (4 g/kg) [48]. According to the authors, the administration of ethanol itself did not change the hepatic GSH and GSSG content; however, in animals that received combined APAP and ethanol, the GSH content decreased, although not significantly. However, both the APAP and ethanol dosages used by these authors were lower than those used in our study, and the animal strains used were different. In animals chronically treated with ethanol (5% v/v) and receiving an acute dose of APAP

(200 mg/kg), the total glutathione values were the lowest among all groups studied. Finally, we found that both the AE and APAP groups presented the highest levels of oxidized glutathione. These findings suggested that the combination of acutely administered APAP and ethanol leads to a greater depletion of glutathione reserves, potentially resulting in increased liver damage due to the formation of protein adducts and underlying oxidative stress, ultimately leading to cellular collapse and necrosis.

Enzymes such as CYP2E1, alcohol dehydrogenase (ADH), and catalase (CAT) are involved in the oxidative pathway of hepatic metabolism. The microsomal respiratory chain and the CYP2E1-dependent microsomal monooxygenase system are the main sources of ROS during ethanol ingestion. When addressing the ability to produce diverse hepatotoxic substrates related to APAP and ethanol metabolism, CYP2E1 is of particular interest [49]. In the present study, group AE exhibited the highest levels of CYP2E1 compared to group C. However, when evaluating gene expression for the same parameter, we found no difference between the experimental groups. Taken together, these results suggested a temporal differentiation in the regulation of gene expression and protein levels. Thus, it is possible to infer that an increase in CYP2E1 gene expression in the AE group may have occurred more quickly, not allowing the detection of significant differences within 12 h, whereas only CYP2E1 protein levels were shown to increase after APAP overdose in the same time interval.

Chronic alcoholics are at greater risk of developing APAP-induced liver injury owing to the induction of CYP2E1 in the MEOS, which is also responsible for the production of NAPQI from APAP metabolism. Thus, it is assumed that high CYP2E1 activity results in greater conversion of APAP to NAPQI, thereby increasing APAP-induced liver toxicity [50,51]. Large-scale clinical studies on APAP poisoning have not observed a negative change in the prognosis due to prior ethanol ingestion [52]. However, when analyzing studies on APAP toxicity in combination with chronic ethanol use, it is necessary to consider factors that may significantly interfere with the observed results. For example, in rats, fasting increases APAP hepatotoxicity by depressing the glucuronide and sulfate conjugation pathways, resulting in a significantly increased formation of the toxic metabolite NAPQI. This effect has been reported in humans [53,54]. Furthermore, malnutrition reduces hepatic glutathione levels, limiting the ability to metabolize reactive metabolites and worsening intoxication owing to the deficiency of phase II metabolizing enzymes [53]. In our study, the animals received food ad libitum to avoid interference with results related to their nutritional status. In addition, the animals were subjected to a short fasting period of 6 h before APAP administration to ensure gastric emptying and minimize possible interference in drug absorption. Animal models have demonstrated that ethanol acts as a competitive inhibitor of APAP metabolism mediated by cytochrome P450. However, evidence of the inhibition of APAP metabolism and reduction in APAP toxicity due to the concomitant use of ethanol in humans is limited [52,55]. This mechanism has been used to justify the hypothesis that an acute dose of ethanol has protective effects.

Acute ethanol ingestion inhibits the microsomal oxidation of paracetamol by CYP2E1 and alters the redox state, resulting in the reduced synthesis of NAPQI. However, only a few clinical studies have reported the protective effects of acute ethanol ingestion in humans. [56], it was pointed out that a low proportion of patients who consumed ethanol during acute APAP ingestion developed subsequent hepatotoxicity. According to the authors, factors such as the ingestion of smaller amounts of APAP and early arrival at the hospital for treatment may have influenced the results. In a multivariate analysis that considered the declared dosage of APAP ingested by the patient and the interval between ingestion and hospital admission, acute ethanol consumption had no independent effect on the risk of hepatotoxicity. Finally, the authors suggested that there may be a dose threshold for the possible protective effects of acute ethanol consumption against APAP hepatotoxicity. According to [57], the most important factors determining the development of hepatotoxicity are the relative doses and timing of ethanol and APAP ingestion. This is because CYP2E1 is inhibited in the presence of ethanol [52]. A study [58] found that the hepatic ethanol content was significantly modulated by ethanol ingestion. These authors observed that in a group of active drinkers, the hepatic level of CYP2E1 was, on average, twice as high as that in individuals with moderate abstinence (5–10 days). Furthermore, after the cessation of ethanol consumption, the level of CYP2E1 decreased rapidly and appeared to return to lower levels after five days. Hepatic CYP2E1 levels can be increased up to eight-fold by ethanol in rodents, and its activity is increased in association with the consumption of alcoholic beverages in humans [59].

Alcohol dehydrogenase (ADH) catalyzes the conversion of ethanol to acetaldehyde, which is then rapidly converted to acetate by aldehyde dehydrogenase (ALDH). ADH is activated at low ethanol concentrations. However, ethanol oxidation is limited by the amount of ADH present in the liver. This is a saturable pathway; therefore, ADH is unable to sufficiently oxidize all the ethanol present. When the metabolic capacity via ADH is exceeded, ethanol metabolism via the CYP2E1, CYP1A2, and CYP3A4 pathways is predominant [60,61]. In the present study, it was observed that the CE group presented the highest ADH expression values compared to the other groups.

UDP-glucuronosyltransferases (UGTs), which catalyze the glucuronidation of compounds by transferring glucuronic acid from its co-substrate (UDP-glucuronic acid) to other compounds, are of great relevance in phase II metabolic reactions because of their ability to increase hydrophilicity, enabling the excretion of these substances through bile and urine [62,63]. Regarding the expression of UGTs, we found that, in the case of UGT1A1, the CE group presented significantly higher values than the other groups. A study conducted in C57BL/6 mice found that chronic alcohol intake caused an increase in plasma bilirubin levels and induced an increase in the expression of UGT1A1 mRNA and protein, which mediated the detoxification of bilirubin into less toxic substrates for biliary and urinary excretion [64], thus corroborating the data observed here. The enzyme UGT2A1, also involved in the glucuronidation of xenobiotics, although belonging to the same family as UGT1A1, was downregulated in all treatments compared to the control group. However, it is worth noting that the expression of UGT2A1 was also increased in the CE group compared to that in the APAP group, further suggesting that APAP was metabolized in the CE group through a non-toxic route. The increase in the expression of both isoforms in the CE group compared to the APAP group may contribute to the clearance of toxic metabolites. This, in turn, contributed to the reestablishment of the GSH/GSSG ratio observed in the CE group.

Using spectral data of the soluble fraction of the liver proteome, we identified 937 distinct protein groups among the experimental groups. Proteins were uniquely identified in each study group. Another research group observed that in C57BL/6 mice (susceptible to APAP poisoning) treated with APAP (300 mg/kg), a series of proteins were highly expressed compared to SJL lineage mice (resistant to APAP poisoning) undergoing the same treatment. This difference was attributed to the greater susceptibility of the C57BL/6 lineage to APAP-induced liver injury, which caused the selective loss of hepatic proteins, especially mitochondrial proteins, because of APAP overdose [65]. In our study, the CE group showed the highest number of proteins that could not be detected in the other experimental groups. Prolonged ethanol use in C57BL/6 mice can cause significant changes in hepatic proteins related to phosphorylation, including a range of proteins involved in cell death signaling [66]. We found that treatment with APAP, as well as treatments associated with acute or chronic EtOH consumption, promoted positive regulation of a series of proteins mainly related to metabolism, redox status, and cell signaling. This result is likely associated with a compensatory mechanism to maintain cellular functions in response to the stress induced by APAP and/or ethanol overdose.

The liver is an organ that functions as a critical center for numerous physiological processes essential for the maintenance of life. Drug-induced liver injury is an important cause of liver disease. Alcohol–drug interactions have a potential aggravating effect on drug-induced hepatotoxicity. In the present study, the combination of APAP and an acute dose of ethanol resulted in hepatotoxicity similar to that observed in the APAP group.

In contrast, chronic ethanol consumption attenuated paracetamol-induced hepatotoxicity. These findings highlight the complexity of the interactions between ethanol and paracetamol in the context of hepatotoxicity and indicate that further studies are needed to elucidate adaptive response mechanisms during chronic ethanol consumption.

5. Conclusions

Ethanol consumption modulates liver damage caused by paracetamol overdose differently. While acute ethanol consumption maintains a liver injury profile similar to the hepatotoxicity profile caused by APAP overdose, chronic ethanol consumption appears to reduce this injury, at least at the dose and time evaluated in this study.

Supplementary Materials: The following supporting information can be downloaded at: https://www.mdpi.com/article/10.3390/toxics12120857/s1, Figure S1: Venn diagram showing the overlapped identified protein groups between treatments. Figure S2: Compositional analysis of liver proteome in the mice. (A) The dynamic range of identified proteins encompassed five orders of magnitude difference between the most and least abundant liver constituent, as judged by Area Under Curve (AUC). (B) The cumulative abundance plot revealed 15 molecules contributing to 54% of the total ion signal. Figure S3: Protein genes are evaluated by biochemical analyses according to the KEGG database and categorized according to the metabolic pathways in which they act. Table S1: Main differentially most abundant proteins.

Author Contributions: Conceptualization, D.C.C. and A.C.G.; formal analysis, D.C.C., A.C.G., E.C.d.O., P.A.M.J., F.S.B., A.T. and W.d.C.B.; investigation, A.M.C., M.L.d.C.C., R.R.P., N.P.d.S.A., F.M.F., S.P. and C.E.V.; resources, D.C.C.; data curation, D.C.C. and A.C.G.; writing—original draft preparation, A.C.G.; writing—review and editing, D.C.C. and E.C.d.O.; supervision, D.C.C.; project administration, D.C.C.; funding acquisition, D.C.C. All authors have read and agreed to the published version of the manuscript.

Funding: This research and the APC were funded by the Minas Gerais Research Support Foundation (FAPEMIG), grant number APQ-00782-22, APQ-02511-22 and APQ-01703-24.

Institutional Review Board Statement: The animal study protocol was approved by the Ethics Committee for the Use of Animals (CEUA) of the Federal University of Ouro Preto (UFOP) under protocol number 2899150322.

Informed Consent Statement: Not applicable.

Data Availability Statement: The original contributions presented in this study are included in the article; further inquiries can be directed to the corresponding author/s.

Acknowledgments: The authors are grateful for the support of the Federal University of Ouro Preto (UFOP). D.C.C., F.S.B., W.d.C.B. and A.T. thank CNPq for the productivity fellowship. The authors are grateful for the Laboratório Multiusuário de Proteômica e Biomoléculas (LMU-ProtBio), from Núcleo de Pesquisas em Ciências Biológicas, Universidade Federal de Ouro Preto, MG, Brazil for providing the required equipments and technical expertise for sample processing and analyses.

Conflicts of Interest: The authors declare no conflicts of interest.

References

1. Rotundo, L.; Pyrsopoulos, N. Liver injury induced by paracetamol and challenges associated with intentional and unintentional use. *World J. Hepatol.* **2020**, *12*, 125–136. [CrossRef] [PubMed]
2. Ramachandran, A.; Jaeschke, H. Acetaminophen Hepatotoxicity. *Semin Liver Dis.* **2019**, *39*, 221–234. [CrossRef] [PubMed]
3. Tittarelli, R.; Pellegrini, M.; Scarpellini, M.G.; Marinelli, E.; Bruti, V.; Di Luca, N.M.; Busardò, F.P.; Zaami, S. Hepatotoxicity of paracetamol and related fatalities. *Eur. Rev. Med. Pharmacol. Sci.* **2017**, *21* (Suppl. 1), 95–101. [PubMed]
4. Lv, L.; Ren, S.; Jiang, H.; Yan, R.; Chen, W.; Yan, E.; Dong, J.; Shao, L.; Yu, Y. The oral administration of *Lacticaseibacillus casei* Shirota alleviates acetaminophen-induced liver injury through accelerated acetaminophen metabolism via the liver-gut axis in mice. *mSphere* **2024**, *9*, e0067223. [CrossRef]
5. Bryan, A.; Pingali, P.; Faber, A.; Landry, J.; Akakpo, J.Y.; Jaeschke, H.; Li, H.; Lee, W.S.; May, L.; Patel, B.; et al. High dose acetaminophen with concurrent CYP2E1 inhibition has profound anti-cancer activity without liver toxicity. *J. Pharmacol. Exp. Ther.* **2024**, *388*, 209–217. [CrossRef]

6. Maideen, N.M.P. Drug Interactions of Acetaminophen (Paracetamol) involving CYP and UGT Enzymes. *Eur. J. Med.* **2019**, *7*, 30–34. [CrossRef]
7. Breslow, R.A.; Dong, C.; White, A. Prevalence of Alcohol-Interactive Prescription Medication Use Among Current Drinkers: United States, 1999 to 2010. *Alcohol Clin. Exp. Res.* **2015**, *39*, 371–379. [CrossRef]
8. Huang, D.Q.; Mathurin, P.; Cortez-Pinto, H.; Loomba, R. Global epidemiology of alcohol-associated cirrhosis and HCC: Trends, projections and risk factors. *Nat. Rev. Gastroenterol. Hepatol.* **2023**, *20*, 37–49. [CrossRef]
9. Hyun, J.; Han, J.; Lee, C.; Yoon, M.; Jung, Y. Pathophysiological Aspects of Alcohol Metabolism in the Liver. *Int. J. Mol. Sci.* **2021**, *22*, 5717. [CrossRef]
10. Contreras-Zentella, M.L.; Villalobos-García, D.; Hernández-Muñoz, R. Ethanol Metabolism in the Liver, the Induction of Oxidant Stress, and the Antioxidant Defense System. *Antioxidants.* **2022**, *11*, 1258. [CrossRef]
11. Iturrospe, E.; da Silva, K.M.; Robeyns, R.; van de Lavoir, M.; Boeckmans, J.; Vanhaecke, T.; van Nuijs, A.L.; Covaci, A. Metabolic Signature of Ethanol-Induced Hepatotoxicity in HepaRG Cells by Liquid Chromatography–Mass Spectrometry-Based Untargeted Metabolomics. *J. Proteome Res.* **2022**, *21*, 1153–1166. [CrossRef] [PubMed]
12. Kumar, S.; Singla, B.; Singh, A.K.; Thomas-Gooch, S.M.; Zhi, K.; Singh, U.P. Hepatic, Extrahepatic and Extracellular Vesicle Cytochrome P450 2E1 in Alcohol and Acetaminophen-Mediated Adverse Interactions and Potential Treatment Options. *Cells* **2022**, *11*, 2620. [CrossRef] [PubMed]
13. Jaber, M.A.; Ghanim, B.Y.; Al-Natour, M.; Arqoub, D.A.; Abdallah, Q.; Abdelrazig, S.; Alkrad, J.A.; Kim, D.H.; Qinna, N.A. Potential biomarkers and metabolomics of acetaminophen-induced liver injury during alcohol consumption: A preclinical investigation on C57/BL6 mice. *Toxicol. Appl. Pharmacol.* **2023**, *465*, 116451. [CrossRef]
14. Coelho, A.M.; Queiroz, I.F.; Lima, W.G.; Talvani, A.; Perucci, L.O.; de Souza, M.O.; Costa, D.C. Temporal analysis of paracetamol-induced hepatotoxicity. *Drug Chem. Toxicol.* **2023**, *46*, 472–481. [CrossRef]
15. Coelho, A.M.; Queiroz, I.F.; Perucci, L.O.; de Souza, M.O.; Lima, W.G.; Talvani, A.; Costa, D.C. Piperine as Therapeutic Agent in Paracetamol-Induced Hepatotoxicity in Mice. *Pharmaceutics* **2022**, *14*, 1800. [CrossRef]
16. Bandeira, A.C.B.; da Silva, R.C.; Rossoni, J.V.; Figueiredo, V.P.; Talvani, A.; Cangussú, S.D.; Bezerra, F.S.; Costa, D.C. Lycopene pretreatment improves hepatotoxicity induced by acetaminophen in C57BL/6 mice. *Bioorganic Med. Chem.* **2017**, *25*, 1057–1065. [CrossRef]
17. Bandeira, A.C.B.; da Silva, T.P.; de Araujo, G.R.; Araujo, C.M.; da Silva, R.C.; Lima, W.G.; Bezerra, F.S.; Costa, D.C. Lycopene inhibits reactive oxygen species production in SK-Hep-1 cells and attenuates acetaminophen-induced liver injury in C57BL/6 mice. *Chem. Biol. Interact.* **2017**, *263*, 7–17. [CrossRef]
18. Koneru, M.; Sahu, B.D.; Kumar, J.M.; Kuncha, M.; Kadari, A.; Kilari, E.K.; Sistla, R. Fisetin protects liver from binge alcohol-induced toxicity by mechanisms including inhibition of matrix metalloproteinases (MMPs) and oxidative stress. *J. Funct. Foods* **2016**, *22*, 588–601. [CrossRef]
19. Khan, I.; Bhardwaj, M.; Shukla, S.; Min, S.-H.; Choi, D.K.; Bajpai, V.K.; Huh, Y.S.; Kang, S.C. Carvacrol inhibits cytochrome P450 and protects against binge alcohol-induced liver toxicity. *Food Chem. Toxicol.* **2019**, *131*, 110582. [CrossRef]
20. Rocha, D.F.A.; Machado-Junior, P.A.; Souza, A.B.F.; Castro, T.D.F.; Costa, G.D.P.; Talvani, A.; Bezerra, F.S.; Cangussú, S.D. Lycopene Ameliorates Liver Inflammation and Redox Status in Mice Exposed to Long-Term Cigarette Smoke. *BioMed Res. Int.* **2021**, *2021*, 7101313. [CrossRef]
21. Machado-Junior, P.A.; Araújo, N.P.S.; Souza, A.B.F.; Castro, T.F.; Oliveira, M.; Costa, G.P.; Matos, N.A.; Vieira, P.M.A.; Talvani, A.; Bezerra, F.S.; et al. Protective Effects of Quercetin on Livers from Mice Exposed to Long-Term Cigarette Smoke. *BioMed Res. Int.* **2020**, *2020*, 2196207. [CrossRef] [PubMed]
22. Lowry, O.H.; Rosebrough, N.J.; Farr, A.L.; Randall, R.J. Protein measurement with the Folin phenol reagent. *J. Biol. Chem.* **1951**, *193*, 265–275. [CrossRef] [PubMed]
23. Hu, S.; Yao, Y.; Wei, Z.Y.; Wang, S.X.; Wu, Y.C.; Hu, Y.; Yang, C.C.; Min, J.L.; Li, L.Y.; Zhou, H.; et al. Deletion of p38γ attenuates ethanol consumption- and acetaminophen-induced liver injury in mice through promoting Dlg1. *Acta Pharmacol. Sin.* **2022**, *43*, 1733–1748. [CrossRef]
24. Kim, S.H.; Choi, H.J.; Seo, H.; Kwon, D.; Yun, J.; Jung, Y.-S. Downregulation of Glutathione-Mediated Detoxification Capacity by Binge Drinking Aggravates Acetaminophen-Induced Liver Injury through IRE1α ER Stress Signaling. *Antioxidants* **2021**, *10*, 1949. [CrossRef]
25. Yang, K.; Huang, Z.; Wang, S.; Zhao, Z.; Yi, P.; Chen, Y.; Xiao, M.; Quan, J.; Hu, X. The Hepatic Nerves Regulated Inflammatory Effect in the Process of Liver Injury: Is Nerve the Key Treating Target for Liver Inflammation? *Inflammation* **2023**, *46*, 1602–1611. [CrossRef]
26. de Freitas Souza, B.S.; Nascimento, R.C.; de Oliveira, S.A.; Vasconcelos, J.F.; Kaneto, C.M.; de Carvalho, L.F.P.P.; Ribeiro-dos-Santos, R.; Soares, M.B.P.; de Freitas, L.A.R. Transplantation of bone marrow cells decreases tumor necrosis factor-α production and blood–brain barrier permeability and improves survival in a mouse model of acetaminophen-induced acute liver disease. *Cytotherapy* **2012**, *14*, 1011–1021. [CrossRef]
27. Shen, X.L.; Guo, Y.N.; Lu, M.H.; Ding, K.N.; Liang, S.S.; Mou, R.W.; Yuan, S.; He, Y.M.; Tang, L.P. Acetaminophen-induced hepatotoxicity predominantly via inhibiting Nrf2 antioxidative pathway and activating TLR4-NF-κB-MAPK inflammatory response in mice. *Ecotoxicol. Environ. Saf.* **2023**, *252*, 114590. [CrossRef]

28. Cederbaum, A.I. CYP2E1- and TNFalpha/LPS-Induced Oxidative Stress and MAPK Signaling Pathways in Alcoholic Liver Disease. *Curr. Pathobiol. Rep.* **2015**, *3*, 263–272. [CrossRef]
29. Bourdi, M.; Eiras, D.P.; Holt, M.P.; Webster, M.R.; Reilly, T.P.; Welch, K.D.; Pohl, L.R. Role of IL-6 in an IL-10 and IL-4 Double Knockout Mouse Model Uniquely Susceptible to Acetaminophen-Induced Liver Injury. *Chem. Res. Toxicol.* **2007**, *20*, 208–216. [CrossRef]
30. Yan, S.; Yin, M. Protective and Alleviative Effects from 4 Cysteine-Containing Compounds on Ethanol-Induced Acute Liver Injury through Suppression of Oxidation and Inflammation. *J. Food Sci.* **2007**, *72*, S511–S515. [CrossRef]
31. Bavia, L. The influence of genetic background of C57Bl/6 and A/J mice on the development of acute inflammatory response induced by alcohol. *Rev. Soc. Bras. Ciências Animais Laboratório* **2013**, *2*, 124–135. [CrossRef]
32. Li, C.; Ming, Y.; Hong, W.; Tang, Y.; Lei, X.; Li, X.; Mao, Y. Comparison of hepatic transcriptome profiling between acute liver injury and acute liver failure induced by acetaminophen in mice. *Toxicol. Lett.* **2018**, *283*, 69–76. [CrossRef] [PubMed]
33. Maes, M.; Vinken, M.; Jaeschke, H. Experimental models of hepatotoxicity related to acute liver failure. *Toxicol. Appl. Pharmacol.* **2016**, *290*, 86–97. [CrossRef] [PubMed]
34. Bavia, L. A/J mice are more susceptible than C57BL/6 to acetaminophen-induced hepatotoxicity. *J. Pharmacol. Toxicol. Methods* **2021**, *108*, 106960. [CrossRef]
35. Wang, X.; Wu, Q.; Liu, A.; Anadón, A.; Rodríguez, J.L.; Martínez-Larrañaga, M.R.; Yuan, Z.; Martínez, M.A. Paracetamol: Overdose-induced oxidative stress toxicity, metabolism, and protective effects of various compounds in vivo and in vitro. *Drug Metab. Rev.* **2017**, *49*, 395–437. [CrossRef]
36. Herath, K.H.I.N.M.; Bing, S.J.; Cho, J.; Kim, A.; Kim, G.; Kim, J.S.; Kim, J.B.; Doh, Y.H.; Jee, Y. Sasa quelpaertensis leaves ameliorate alcohol-induced liver injury by attenuating oxidative stress in HepG2 cells and mice. *Acta Histochem.* **2018**, *120*, 477–489. [CrossRef]
37. Noh, J.R.; Kim, Y.H.; Gang, G.T.; Hwang, J.H.; Lee, H.S.; Ly, S.Y.; Oh, W.K.; Song, K.S.; Lee, C.H. Hepatoprotective effects of chestnut (*Castanea crenata*) inner shell extract against chronic ethanol-induced oxidative stress in C57BL/6 mice. *Food Chem. Toxicol.* **2011**, *49*, 1537–1543. [CrossRef]
38. Smathers, R.L.; Galligan, J.J.; Shearn, C.T.; Fritz, K.S.; Mercer, K.; Ronis, M.; Orlicky, D.J.; Davidson, N.O.; Petersen, D.R. Susceptibility of L-FABP$^{-/-}$ mice to oxidative stress in early-stage alcoholic liver. *J. Lipid Res.* **2013**, *54*, 1335–1345. [CrossRef]
39. Arumugam, M.K.; Chava, S.; Perumal, S.K.; Paal, M.C.; Rasineni, K.; Ganesan, M.; Donohue, T.M.; Osna, N.A.; Kharbanda, K.K. Acute ethanol-induced liver injury is prevented by betaine administration. *Front. Physiol.* **2022**, *13*, 940148. [CrossRef]
40. Dobariya, P.; Xie, W.; Rao, S.P.; Xie, J.; Seelig, D.M.; Vince, R.; Lee, M.K.; More, S.S. Deletion of Glyoxalase 1 Exacerbates Acetaminophen-Induced Hepatotoxicity in Mice. *Antioxidants* **2024**, *13*, 648. [CrossRef]
41. Lebedeva, E.I.; Babenka, A.S.; Shchastniy, A.T. MMP-9 mRNA Expression and Bridging Fibrosis Progression in Toxic Liver Injury. *Acta Naturae* **2023**, *15*, 50–58. [CrossRef] [PubMed]
42. Ito, Y.; Abril, E.R.; Bethea, N.W.; McCuskey, R.S. Inhibition of Matrix Metalloproteinases Minimizes Hepatic Microvascular Injury in Response to Acetaminophen in Mice. *Toxicol. Sci.* **2005**, *83*, 190–196. [CrossRef] [PubMed]
43. McCuskey, R.S. Sinusoidal endothelial cells as an early target for hepatic toxicants. *Clin. Hemorheol. Microcirc.* **2006**, *34*, 5–10. [PubMed]
44. Ito, Y.; Abril, E.R.; Bethea, N.W.; Mccuskey, R.S. Ethanol Binging Enhances Hepatic Microvascular Responses to Acetaminophen in Mice. *Microcirculation* **2004**, *11*, 625–632. [CrossRef]
45. Xiao, Q.; Zhao, Y.; Ma, L.; Piao, R. Orientin reverses acetaminophen-induced acute liver failure by inhibiting oxidative stress and mitochondrial dysfunction. *J. Pharmacol. Sci.* **2022**, *149*, 11–19. [CrossRef]
46. Du, K.; Ramachandran, A.; Jaeschke, H. Oxidative stress during acetaminophen hepatotoxicity: Sources, pathophysiological role and therapeutic potential. *Redox Biol.* **2016**, *10*, 148–156. [CrossRef]
47. Dogaru, G.; Bulboaca, A.E.; Gheban, D.; Boarescu, P.M.; Rus, V.; Festila, D.; Sitar-Taut, A.-V.; Stanescu, I. Effect of Liposomal Curcumin on Acetaminophen Hepatotoxicity by Down-regulation of Oxidative Stress and Matrix Metalloproteinases. *In Vivo* **2020**, *34*, 569–582. [CrossRef]
48. Lee, S.-M.; Cho, T.-S.; Kim, D.-J.; Cha, Y.-N. Protective effect of ethanol against acetaminophen-induced hepatotoxicity in mice: Role of role of NADH: Quinone reductase. *Biochem. Pharmacol.* **1999**, *58*, 1547–1555. [CrossRef]
49. Sandoval, C.; Mella, L.; Godoy, K.; Adeli, K.; Farías, J. β-Carotene Increases Activity of Cytochrome P450 2E1 during Ethanol Consumption. *Antioxidants* **2022**, *11*, 1033. [CrossRef]
50. Draganov, P.; Durrence, H.; Cox, C.; Reuben, A. Alcohol-acetaminophen syndrome. *Postgrad. Med.* **2000**, *107*, 189–195. [CrossRef]
51. Walker, R.M.; McElligott, T.F.; Power, E.M.; Massey, T.E.; Racz, W.J. Increased acetaminophen-induced hepatotoxicity after chronic ethanol consumption in mice. *Toxicology* **1983**, *28*, 193–206. [CrossRef] [PubMed]
52. Schmidt, L.E.; Dalhoff, K.; Poulsen, H.E. Acute versus chronic alcohol consumption in acetaminophen-induced hepatotoxicity. *Hepatology* **2002**, *35*, 876–882. [CrossRef] [PubMed]
53. Bray, G.P.; Mowat, C.; Muir, D.F.; Tredger, J.M.; Williams, R. The Effect of Chronic Alcohol Intake on Prognosis and Outcome in Paracetamol Overdose. *Hum. Exp. Toxicol.* **1991**, *10*, 435–438. [CrossRef]
54. Prescott, L.F. Paracetamol, alcohol and the liver. *Br. J. Clin. Pharmacol.* **2000**, *49*, 291–301. [CrossRef]
55. McGill, M.R.; Jaeschke, H. Metabolism and Disposition of Acetaminophen: Recent Advances in Relation to Hepatotoxicity and Diagnosis. *Pharm. Res.* **2013**, *30*, 2174–2187. [CrossRef]

56. Waring, W.S.; Stephen, A.F.; Malkowska, A.M.; Robinson, O.D. Acute Ethanol Coingestion Confers a Lower Risk of Hepatotoxicity after Deliberate Acetaminophen Overdose. *Acad. Emerg. Med.* **2008**, *15*, 54–58. [CrossRef]
57. Bromer, M.Q.; Black, M. Acetaminophen hepatotoxicity. *Clin. Liver Dis.* **2003**, *7*, 351–367. [CrossRef]
58. Perrot, N.; Nalpas, B.; Yang, C.S.; Beaune, P.H. Modulation of cytochrome P450 isozymes in human liver, by ethanol and drug intake. *Eur. J. Clin. Investig.* **1989**, *19*, 549–555. [CrossRef]
59. Liangpunsakul, S.; Kolwankar, D.; Pinto, A.; Gorski, J.C.; Hall, S.D.; Chalasani, N. Activity of CYP2E1 and CYP3A enzymes in adults with moderate alcohol consumption: A comparison with nonalcoholics. *Hepatology* **2005**, *41*, 1144–1150. [CrossRef]
60. Wang, X.; Yang, Y.; Chen, Y.; Duan, Y.; Han, J.; Yang, X. MEK1/2 inhibitors induce class I alcohol dehydrogenase (ADH1) expression by regulating farnesoid X receptor in hepatic cell lines and C57BL/6J mouse. *Mol. Biol. Rep.* **2022**, *49*, 5843–5852. [CrossRef]
61. Hedgpeth, B.; Missall, R.; Bambaci, A.; Smolen, M.; Yavuz, S.; Cottrell, J.; Chu, T.; Chang, S.L. A Review of Bioinformatics Tools to Understand Acetaminophen-Alcohol Interaction. *Medicines* **2019**, *6*, 79. [CrossRef] [PubMed]
62. Kutsuno, Y.; Itoh, T.; Tukey, R.H.; Fujiwara, R. Glucuronidation of Drugs and Drug-Induced Toxicity in Humanized *UDP-Glucuronosyltransferase 1* Mice. *Drug Metab. Dispos.* **2014**, *42*, 1146–1152. [CrossRef] [PubMed]
63. Shiratani, H.; Katoh, M.; Nakajima, M.; Yokoi, T. Species Differences in UDP-Glucuronosyltransferase Activities in Mice and Rats. *Drug Metab. Dispos.* **2008**, *36*, 1745–1752. [CrossRef]
64. Wang, X.; Zheng, L.; Wu, J.; Tang, B.; Zhang, M.; Zhu, D.; Lin, X. Constitutive androstane receptor activation promotes bilirubin clearance in a murine model of alcoholic liver disease. *Mol. Med. Rep.* **2017**, *15*, 3459–3466. [CrossRef]
65. Welch, K.D.; Wen, B.; Goodlett, D.R.; Yi, E.C.; Lee, H.; Reilly, T.P.; Nelson, S.D.; Pohl, L.R. Proteomic Identification of Potential Susceptibility Factors in Drug-Induced Liver Disease. *Chem. Res. Toxicol.* **2005**, *18*, 924–933. [CrossRef]
66. Singh, V.; Huang, E.; Pathak, V.; Willard, B.B.; Allende, D.S.; Nagy, L.E. Phosphoproteomics identifies pathways underlying the role of receptor-interaction protein kinase 3 in alcohol-associated liver disease and uncovers apoptosis signal-regulating kinase 1 as a target. *Hepatol. Commun.* **2022**, *6*, 2022–2041. [CrossRef]

Disclaimer/Publisher's Note: The statements, opinions and data contained in all publications are solely those of the individual author(s) and contributor(s) and not of MDPI and/or the editor(s). MDPI and/or the editor(s) disclaim responsibility for any injury to people or property resulting from any ideas, methods, instructions or products referred to in the content.

toxics

MDPI

Article

The Acute Toxicity and Cardiotoxic Effects of Protocatechuic Aldehyde on Juvenile Zebrafish

Jiufeng Yin [1,†], Hui Wang [1,†], Feng Zhao [2], Dan Liang [1], Wenqing Yang [1,3,*] and Dan Zhang [2,3,*]

1 Institute for Chinese Medicine Innovation, Shandong University of Traditional Chinese Medicine, Jinan 250300, China; yjf17854598221@163.com (J.Y.); m15192536410@163.com (H.W.); liangd980@163.com (D.L.)
2 Laboratory Centre, Shandong University of Traditional Chinese Medicine, Jinan 250300, China; 60019116@sdutcm.edu.cn
3 Department of Classical Theory of Chinese Medicine, Key Laboratory of the Ministry of Education, Jinan 250355, China
* Correspondence: wenqing-yang@hotmail.com (W.Y.); zhangdansdtcm@aliyun.com (D.Z.)
† These authors contributed equally to this work.

Abstract: Protocatechuic aldehyde (PCA) is a natural phenolic acid compound with pharmacological effects such as anti-oxidative stress, antibacterial, anti-apoptotic, anti-inflammatory, anti-platelet aggregation, and anti-tumor. Despite the favorable therapeutic effects of PCA, it is imperative to recognize that adverse drug reactions can arise even with satisfactory quality assurance measures and during standard clinical application and dosing. Additionally, the acute toxicity and cardiotoxic sequelae of PCA are frequently under reported in the available documentation. To investigate the acute toxicity and cardiotoxic effects of PCA, the present study comprehensively assessed the acute toxicity and cardiotoxic effects of PCA by administering different concentrations of PCA and by monitoring the phenotypic changes in zebrafish, using AB wild-type *Tg(cmlc2:EGFP)* zebrafish as the experimental model organism. Meanwhile, the target genes of PCA that may cause cardiotoxicity were predicted and validated using a network pharmacology approach. Our findings indicated that PCA exhibited severe acute toxicity and cardiotoxic effects in zebrafish at 70 μg/mL and 80 μg/mL. Furthermore, PIK3CA, PARP1, and GSK3β may be involved in the mechanism of action of the cardiotoxicity-inducing effects of this compound. The present investigation has afforded a deeper insight into the acute toxicity and cardiotoxic impacts of PCA on zebrafish and has established a significant theoretical foundation for the evaluation of toxicity in pharmaceuticals incorporating PCA.

Keywords: zebrafish; PCA; acute toxicity; cardiotoxic

1. Introduction

PCA is widely found in the roots of Salvia miltiorrhiza as well as in the leaves of the ophiopogon and hollyhock. It is a natural phenolic acid compound found in Salvia miltiorrhiza and other traditional Chinese medicinal herbs, and consists of a benzene ring and an acrolein moiety. Three hydroxyl groups are distributed on the benzene ring and the acrolein group is attached to the benzene ring, and this structure makes PCA hydrophilic and active [1,2]. Studies have shown that PCA possesses a variety of pharmacological activities such as antioxidant, antibacterial, anti-apoptotic, anti-inflammatory, anti-platelet aggregation, and anti-tumor, as well as many other pharmacological activities [3–7]. Currently, Cao found [8] that in rat animal experiments, PCA can be converted to protocatechuic acid in vivo, and the subsequent generation of vanillyl-CoA PCA has been a popular conjugate that inhibits the binding of long-chain fatty acids to CoA and reduces the AcCoA/CoA value [9–12].

In acute myocardial ischemia, the metabolism of PCA is slowed down, and the metabolism of protocatechuic acid and vanillic acid is slowed down in vivo, resulting in cardiotoxicity caused by accumulation [13]. This provides a rationale for the cardiotoxicity of the animal model in recent years for evaluating pharmaceutical effectiveness and safety. The zebrafish is a non-mammalian vertebrate known for its rapid development, tiny embryos and individuals, translucent body, high spawning rates, and rapid reproduction. The benefits of using zebrafish for experiments include reduced costs, shorter cycle times, and fewer ethical restrictions. It usually takes only about 3 days from the subject's exposure to zebrafish to the completion of the evaluation experiment [14]. Furthermore, this study used transgenic fluorescently tagged zebrafish to reveal the labeled position under the corresponding excitation light and quantitatively analyze the area of cardiac fluorescence imaging. The zebrafish heart's response to exogenous drugs is highly similar to that of human hearts [15]. This helps observe damage to organ shape and target the PCA medication.

PCA's cardiotoxic effects in zebrafish have not been documented in any national or international publication. We selected zebrafish as a new model organism for this study and administered different concentrations of the drug to zebrafish larvae to thoroughly assess the potential acute toxicity and cardiotoxicity of PCA exposure. This allowed us to provide important theoretical references for the evaluation of the toxicity of PCA drugs.

2. Materials and Methods

2.1. Instrumentation

A zebrafish aquaculture system (Beijing Aisheng Technology Co., Ltd., Beijing, China), Leica M205FA stereo fluorescence microscope (Leica Microsystems, Wetzlar, Germany), Zeiss LSM880 + Fast Airyscan Laser Confocal Microscope (with Live Cell Workstation), Leica RM2255 Paraffin Slicer, water bath LWB-24, pathological tissue processing staining system (YB-6LF, YR-19, ZT-12M), Gradient PCR Instrument T100, LongGene Real-Time Fluorescence PCR Instrument Q200B, Zebrafish Behavior Analyzer (ZebraLab), and ViewPoint Microscope ZEB6202 were used.

2.2. Medicines and Reagents

Procatechaldehyde (batch No. S30202-5g), xylene (batch No. W14278), hematoxylin anhydrous ethanol solution (batch No. R20587), and neutral gum (batch No. S30509) were acquired from Yuanye Biotechnology Co. (Shanghai, China). Tricine MS-222 (batch No. M14788) was bought from Jinan Anxia Biotechnology Co. Ltd, AbMole (Jinan, China). Fish fixative sodium carboxy methyl cellulose (CMC-Na, lot 419281) was bought from Sigma-Aldrich, St. Louis, MO, USA. Paraformaldehyde (batch No. CR2209049) was bought from Sevier (Wuhan, China). Biotechnology Co. 2xSYBR Green qPCR Mix (with ROX) (batch No. C13720975) was acquired from Ciscojet Biotechnology Co. A SPARKscript II RT Plus Kit (with a gDNA eraser) (batch No. AG0304-B) was bought from Cisco Jie Biotechnology Co. (San Jose, CA, USA).

2.3. Animals

AB wild-type zebrafish *Tg(cmlc2:EGFP)* were acquired courtesy of Zebrafish Laboratory, New Animal Centre, Shandong University of Traditional Chinese Medicine, China. In a zebrafish culture system, every adult male and female zebrafish were kept apart and maintained at 28 °C, pH 7.2 $\pm$ 0.2, with a photoperiod of 14 h/10 h (light/dark) and twice-daily feedings of penaeid shrimp.

3. Methodology

3.1. Breeding and Culture of Zebrafish

Zebrafish reach sexual maturity at three months of age. Four to six pairs of mature fish were chosen from the tanks and put in a spawning device one night beforehand. The male and female fish were arranged in a 1:1 ratio, with an insert plate between them. To select high-quality embryos for zebrafish spawning, the lights were turned on and the transparent inserts were taken out the next morning.

3.2. Zebrafish Drug Delivery Solution Preparation

For this experiment, the PCA concentration gradient group (50 µg/mL, 60 µg/mL, 70 µg/mL, and 80 µg/mL) was chosen. One milligram of PCA was precisely weighed, put in a 1.5 mL EP tube, and dissolved in one milliliter of purified water to create a master batch with a drug mass concentration of one mg/mL. Next, 100 µL, 120 µL, 140 µL, and 160 µL of the masterbatch were taken from each tube and added to another 15 mL EP tube. Finally, 1900 µL, 1800 µL, 1600 µL, and 1400 µL of the masterbatch were added to the zebrafish embryo culture and diluted with water to the equivalent drug mass concentration of 50 µg/mL, 60 µg/mL, 70 µg/mL, and 80 µg/mL. The dispensed solution was diluted with water to an equivalent drug mass concentration of 50 µg/mL, 60 µg/mL, 70 µg/mL, and 80 µg/mL for further experimental drug delivery. The drug mass concentration drug delivery system was then formulated in each well of the total fish culture water of 2 mL in a 24-well plate. One liter of clean water included 0.633 g of KCl, 2.452 g of $CaCl_2$, 14.658 g of NaCl, and 4.06 g of $MgSO_4 \cdot 7H_2O$ for zebrafish embryo culture. The anesthetic was a 0.4mg/mL tricaine solution prepared in purified water.

3.3. Grouping Interventions for Zebrafish

Five groups of experimental zebrafish per Section 2.3 were created: control and 50 µg/mL, 60 µg/mL, 70 µg/mL, and 80 µg/mL drug concentration groups for PCA. The drug concentration groups of 50 µg/mL, 60 µg/mL, 70 µg/mL, and 80 µg/mL PCA were immersed in drug preparation concentrations based on the experimental requirements, as determined by the method of Section 3.2. Meanwhile, the control group was maintained in zebrafish culture water without any intervention.

3.4. Zebrafish with Acute Exposure to PCA Exhibit Teratogenic Toxicity and Epimorphological Alterations

Normal zebrafish embryos were chosen under a somatic microscope upon spawning and placed onto 24-well plates, with ten embryos per well. The subjects had exposure to three duplicate wells in each of the following groups: the control group, the PCA concentration gradient group (50 µg/L, 60 µg/L, 70 µg/L, and 80 µg/mL), and soak-in drugs. To enable the embryos to continue developing, each well was filled to a total amount of 2 mL of embryo culture water, sealed, and kept in a fish room with a thermostat set at 28 °C. Per FET guidelines [16] and OECD guidelines [17], all developmental endpoints were identified. Every 24 h, the exposure solution was replaced at 24 hpf (hours after the hour after fertilization), 48 hpf, 72 hpf, and 96 hpf, respectively. The mortality of each group was recorded for four days in a row. Thirty zebrafish were fixed under a somatotopic microscope in 0.3% methylcellulose solution after being anesthetized with 0.4 mg/mL of tricaine as needed for observation. The zebrafish were then positioned sideways on slides with their eyes facing opposite directions to observe the embryos with aberrant development at various times. Every 24 h, hatchability and mortality were carefully tallied. At 96 h, the malformation rate was computed.

3.5. Acute Exposure to PCA's Effects on Zebrafish Larvae's Behavioral Alterations

Similar to the grouping under Section 3.3, zebrafish embryos subjected to a gradient concentration of 120 hpf PCA were placed in a Zebrabox, a Zebrafish ViewPoint Behaviore Analyzer, with one larval fish per well, on a 96-well plate. As soon as the analytical setup was complete, the behaviors of the zebrafish were investigated.

3.6. Acute Exposure to PCA and Its Impact on the Zebrafish Heart's Sinus Venosus–Arteriolar Bulb (SV-BA) Distance

Zebrafish with 96hpf *Tg(cmlc2:EGFP)* were chosen and followed Section 3.3. Under a stereo microscope, thirty zebrafish were fixed in 0.3% methylcellulose solution after being anesthetized with 0.4 mg/mL tricaine. The fish were then placed sideways on slides across from their eyes, and the heart's fluorescence was recorded and captured on camera. Confocal imaging analysis measured the area of PCA on the fluorescent heart, measured the distance between the sinus venous (SV) and the bulb of the artery (BA) to quantify the cardiac tube ring, and photographed the zebrafish fluorescent heart under excitation light [18].

3.7. Morphological Alterations in the Heart of Zebrafish Exposed to PCA

In vivo imaging of the heart of zebrafish at the macroscopic and histological levels was observed under excitation light using the 96 hpf *Tg(cmlc2:EGFP)* zebrafish line of EGFP-labeled cardiomyocytes, as described in Section 3.3 Calculation of the effect of PCA on the fluorescence morphology area of the zebrafish heart at gradient concentrations and confocal imaging was carried out to analyze differences in cardiac morphology. The study used confocal imaging to examine variations in heart morphology.

3.8. Acute Exposure to PCA: Effects on the Heart Function of Zebrafish

The AB zebrafish were chosen and arranged in Section 3.3. Following a 96 h drug administration period, 30 zebrafish were anesthetized with 0.4 mg/mL tricaine, fixed in 0.3% methylcellulose solution under a somatotrope, and arranged sideways on slides with their eyes facing opposite directions. Heart rates were then counted every 20 s using the ViewPoint system's photos and videos, which allow for the visual analysis of animal behavior. Zebrafish embryo heart rates were recorded at 20 s intervals in pictures and movies. To evaluate PCA-induced cardiotoxicity, the pericardial area was measured and drawn to determine the degree of pericardial edema [19].

3.9. The Impact of Brief Exposure to PCA on the Zebrafish Heart's Histological Composition

After fixation with a gradient of ethanol, alcohol benzene, and xylene in an embedding machine in paraffin embedding, 4 μm sections were cut, deparaffinized to water, rinsed in pure water, and stained with hematoxylin–eosin (HE). The 96 hpf AB wild-type zebrafish, which are the same as the Section 3.3 grouping drug modeling for 96 h, were taken in the appropriate amount of 0.4 mg/mL tricaine anesthesia. Sections were cleaned, sealed with neutral gum, dried by air, and then put in gradient ethanol xylene and dehydrated until transparent before being photographed.

3.10. Prediction and Enrichment Analysis of Target Genes for PCA-Induced Cardiotoxicity

Using the SwissTarget website prediction (https://swisstargetprediction.ch, accessed on 1 January 2024) for PCA, possible target genes for the agent's action were found. You may discover targets of cardiotoxic effects by searching for the word "cardiotoxicity" at https://www.genecards.org/Sitesearch, accessed on 1 January 2024. The 84 proteins that were obtained from SwissTarget and Gene Cards were entered into the String database (https://cn.string-db.org, accessed on 1 January 2024) to identify the corresponding zebrafish target genes. Utilizing the Microbiotics Online Analysis Network (https://www.bioinformatics.com.cn, accessed on 1 January 2024), the target genes identified by screening were imported. Figure 1 depicts the network pharmacological flow. The GO functional classification and KEGG enrichment analysis were performed based on the gene identifications for MF (molecular function), BP (biological process), and CC (cellular components). PIK3CA, PARP1, and GSK3β were identified as the main target genes of PCA cardiotoxicity using network pharmacogenomics. By using RT-PCR, this identity was verified. Using 96 hpf AB wild-type zebrafish (the same as Section 3.3), which were split into groups and immersed in the drug for 96 h, each group's 50 zebrafish underwent two rounds of rinsing in pure water to remove any leftover water. The fish tissue was then extracted in its entirety to prepare the total RNA and transferred to 1.5 mL of non-enzymatic sterilization of EP tubes, and reverse transcription was carried out according to the instructions provided by the RNA Reverse Transcription Kit. The cDNA was reverse transcribed following the directions included with the RNA Reverse Transcription Kit, using β-actin as an internal reference throughout the PCR process. Reaction conditions: 95 °C for 3 min; 94 °C for 10 s; 65 °C for 30 s; 40 cycles. The $2^{-\Delta\Delta Ct}$ method was used to ascertain the mRNA's relative expression. The primer sequences are shown in Table 1.

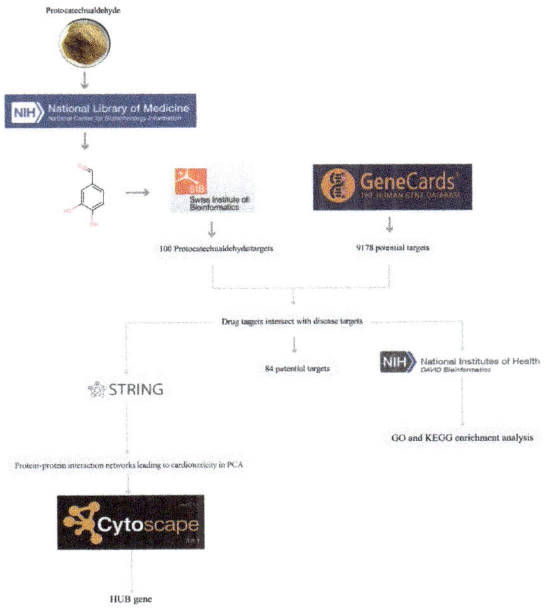

Figure 1. Schematic diagram of the network pharmacology process.

Table 1. Primer sequences (5′–3′).

β-Actin	**F: AGAGCTATGAGCTGCCTGACG**	**R: CCGCAAGATTCCATACCCA**
Pik3ca	F: GATCGCCGAAGCCATCAGGAAG	R: GTCACAGCCGCAGACCTTCAG
Parp1	F: CATTTGGGTCCCTGAAGCCT	R: ACCCAGTCTTTGCGATCAGG
Gsk3β	F: AACTCTGCGACTTTGGCAGT	R:CGGTGGCTCCAAAGATGAGT

3.11. Statistical Analysis

All experiments were carried out at least three times, and all data are presented as mean ± S.D. Statistical significance and correlation between the groups were performed by SPSS 25.0 software (SPSS, Inc., Chicago, IL, USA). All data were analyzed with one-way analysis of variance (ANOVA) followed by Duncan's multiple range tests. Values of $p < 0.05$ were considered statistically significant.

4. Results

4.1. Examination of the Morphological Alterations and Teratogenic Effects of Acute Exposure to PCA in Zebrafish

PCA gradient concentrations of 50 µg/mL, 60 µg/mL, 70 µg/mL, and 80 µg/mL were selected for observation and photographed at 24 hpf, 48 hpf, 72 hpf, and 96 hpf, respectively (Figure 2a–c). The figure shows that the zebrafish in the 60 µg/mL exposure group exhibited noticeable deformities at 72 h. Zebrafish showed spine curvature as the length of exposure to PCA increased. Zebrafish in the 60 µg/mL exposure group also showed swim bladder closure, loss, and pericardial edema in addition to yolk cysts. At 96 h, the zebrafish in the 80 µg/mL exposure group had the most prominent exhibition of the previously indicated phenomena, and their mortality rate significantly increased as the exposure concentration increased. This suggests that acute exposure to PCA affects zebrafish larval development in a concentration-dependent manner.

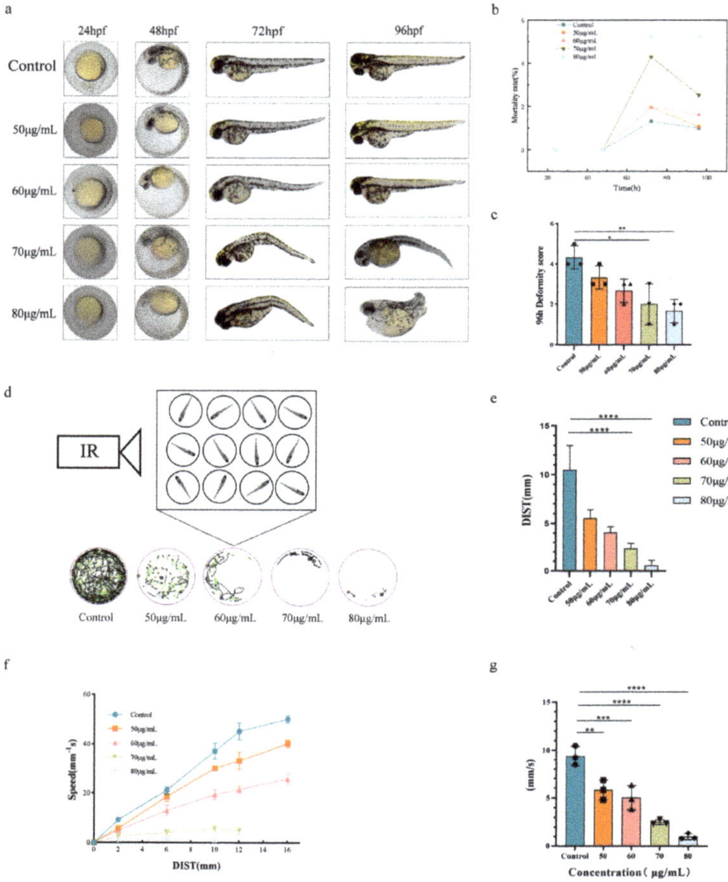

Figure 2. Acute toxic effects of PCA in zebrafish. (**a**) Single fish images of zebrafish larvae exposed to PCA gradient concentrations at 24 hpf, 48 hpf, 72 hpf, and 96 hpf (**b**) Mortality of zebrafish larvae exposed to PCA gradient concentrations at 96 hpf. (**c**) Deformity score of zebrafish larvae exposed to PCA gradient concentrations at 96 hpf. (**d**) Schematic diagram of the behavioral trajectory recordings of 120 hpf zebrafish at a gradient concentration of PCA under Zebrabox. (**e**) Statistical graph of distance analysis of the behavioral trajectory of 120 hpf zebrafish at a gradient concentration of PCA. (**f**) Statistical graph of the speed analysis of the behavioral trajectory of 120 hpf zebrafish at a gradient concentration of PCA. (**g**) Statistical graph of speed–distance analysis of the behavioral trajectory of 120 hpf zebrafish at a gradient concentration of PCA. Comparison with the blank control group: * $p < 0.05$; ** $p < 0.01$; *** $p < 0.001$; **** $p < 0.001$ (n = 30). The circles, squares, triangles, inverted triangles, and diamonds in the diagram represent the data in the histogram. Concentrations of PCA are expressed in μg/mL.

4.2. An Examination of the Behavior of Zebrafish Larvae Exposed to PCA Acutely

Using a video monitoring and behavioral analysis system, the activity process of zebrafish exposed to different doses of PCA was recorded in this work. Before filming, the fish were allowed ten minutes to become used to their new environment. Behavioral data including speed, distance traveled, and duration of activity were then extracted from the video recordings. The overall decrease in the three previously indicated behavioral traits of the juvenile fish in the exposure group of 70 μg/mL is shown in Figure 2d–g. Conversely, in zebrafish at 120 hpf, the 80 μg/mL exposure group suppressed the mean rate and distance traveled and significantly reduced activity time and distance traveled. Therefore, PCA significantly reduced the zebrafish larvae's ability to move their locomotor system at dosages of 70 μg/mL and 80 μg/mL. Meanwhile, PCA led to behavioral limitations in zebrafish, indicating the occurrence of some neurotoxicity.

4.3. Evaluation of the Acute Exposure of Zebrafish Larvae Heart SV-BA Distance to PCA

Zebrafish cardiac SV-BA distance may be used to gauge the extent of heart injury. A decrease in the heart stroke volume, per pulse output, ejection fraction, and short axis shortening rate, is linked to an increase in this distance [20]. Thus, the SV-BA distance was the main indication used in this experiment to evaluate the toxicity of PCA to zebrafish. The effects of gradient PCA concentrations at 50 μg/mL, 60 μg/mL, 70 μg/mL, and 80 μg/mL on morphological changes in the *Tg(cmlc2:EGFP)* heart after 96 h were seen using a confocal imaging system. As compared to the control group, Figure 3a,b shows that the 80 μg/mL exposed group saw an increase in pericardial enlargement and SV-BA distance ($p < 0.01$). There was a discernible decrease in cardiac output and output per beat, along with a significant delay in the zebrafish yolk sac's absorption, in the 70 μg/mL and 80 μg/mL exposure groups. It has been shown that the drug PCA may induce severe cardiotoxicity in zebrafish larvae at doses of 70 μg/mL and 80 μg/mL.

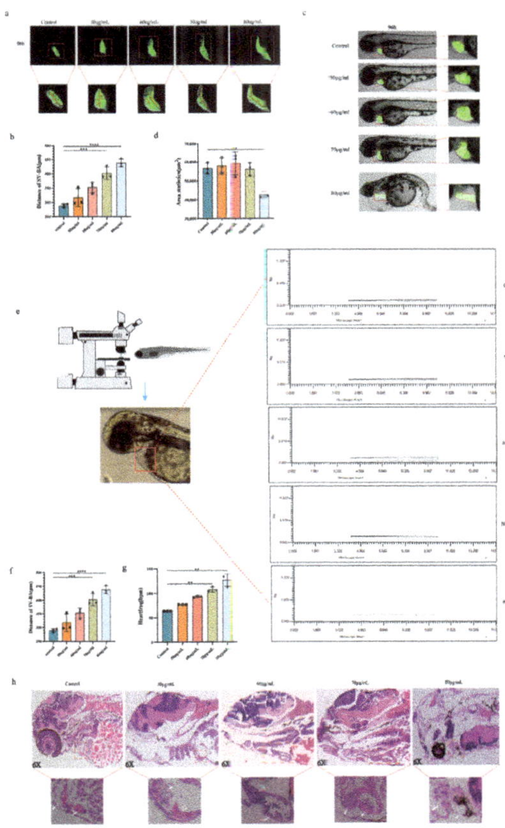

Figure 3. Cardiotoxicity effects of PCA in *Tg(cmlc2:EGFP)* zebrafish. (**a**) Confocal imaging of *Tg(cmlc2: EGFP)*: The control group and PCA gradient concentration group zebrafish larvae SV-BA distances in

bright and fluorescent fields of view. (**b**) Statistical analysis graph (SV-BA distance). (**c**) Morphology of zebrafish larvae heart in bright and fluorescent fields of view in the confocal imaging: the control group and PCA gradient concentration group of *Tg(cmlc2:EGFP)*. (**d**) Graph of statistical analysis of the fluorescence area of the heart. (**e**) Schematic diagram of zebrafish heartbeat frequency observed under the ViewPoint system. (**f**) Statistical graph of the heartbeat frequency (HZ). (**g**) Statistical graph of the heartbeat frequency (bpm). (**h**) Effect of PCA gradient concentration on the histopathological structure of the heart of zebrafish larvae. White arrows represent V-A: ventricle–atrium. Note: comparison with blank control group: ** $p < 0.01$; *** $p < 0.001$; **** $p < 0.001$(n = 30). The circles, squares, triangles, inverted triangles, and diamonds in the diagram represent the data in the histogram.

4.4. Examination of the Morphological Alterations in the Heart of Zebrafish Exposed to PCA

Zebrafish cardiotoxicity from PCA may be seen right away in the atypical changes in their cardiac anatomy. Therefore, after 96 h, experiments were conducted using confocal imaging equipment to determine the effects of gradient concentrations of PCA of 50 μg/mL, 60 μg/mL, 70 μg/mL, and 80 μg/mL on the changes in heart shape of *Tg(cmlc2: EGFP)*. Figure 3c,d show that the zebrafish heart shape was not altered substantially in the 50 μg/mL and 60 μg/mL exposure groups compared to the control group. On the other hand, the zebrafish heart morphology in the 70 μg/mL exposure group exhibited longitudinal malformation, whereas the heart ventricle in the 80 μg/mL exposure group had distinct alterations, such as pericardial edema and longitudinal deformity of the atria and ventricles. According to these results, cardiac damage in PCA was seen at concentration of 70 μg/mL and 80 μg/mL. This implies that cardiac damage occurred at 70 μg/mL and 80 μg/mL of PCA.

4.5. Evaluation of Zebrafish Heart Function after Acute PCA Exposure

An excessive heart rate causes the coronary artery flow to decrease and the myocardial diastolic period to shorten, results in inadequate filling, and even causes the compensatory significance to disappear because of the decrease in output per minute. Blood enters the zebrafish heart via the venous sinus and leaves the ventricle through the arterial bulb. Since the zebrafish heart rate reflects the heart's pumping function [21], it is employed as a supplemental indicator to assess the zebrafish heart function. The effects of gradient concentrations of PCA at 50 μg/mL, 60 μg/mL, 70 μg/mL, and 80 μg/mL on changes in zebrafish larval heart function at 96 hpf were identified using the Zebrafish ViewPoint system. As shown in Figure 3e, a deeper black line denotes a regular and powerful heartbeat, whereas a lighter black line with short intervals suggests a rapid, feeble, and irregular heartbeat. As shown in Figure 3f,g, compared to the control group, the heartbeat frequencies of the exposed groups at 70 μg/mL and 80 μg/mL were weak, rapid, irregular, and dysfunctional. The phenotypic traits were also more prominent in the 80 μg/mL exposed group. At concentrations of 70 μg/mL and 80 μg/mL, PCA was shown to affect zebrafish heart function, leading to abnormalities in heart rate and rhythm, cardiac insufficiency, and a reduction in the pumping capacity.

4.6. Analysis of the Histopathological Slice of the Heart of a Zebrafish Exposed to PCA

After 96 h, HE staining was used to investigate the effects of gradient concentrations of PCA (50 μg/mL, 60 μg/mL, 70 μg/mL, and 80 μg/mL) on histopathological alterations in the heart of zebrafish larvae. As per Figure 3h, there was no discernible difference between the 50 μg/mL and 60 μg/mL exposure groups and the control group in the histopathological sections of the heart. Conversely, the zebrafish heart tissues subjected to 70 μg/mL and 80 μg/mL had pronounced intercellular vacuoles, damaged nuclei, inflammatory infiltration, and hazy cell-to-cell borders, indicating serious structural abnormalities and impairments in the heart cellular structure.

4.7. *Cardiotoxic Target Gene Prediction and Enrichment Analysis Triggered by Acute PCA Exposure*

4.7.1. Potential Targets for PCA-Induced Cardiotoxicity

The SwissTarget database was used to determine the 100 active component targets of PCA. The active ingredient targets were retrieved from the SwissTarget database, and 100 drug targets were acquired after duplicates were removed. As shown in Figure 4a, 9179 cardiotoxic illness targets were retrieved using GeneCards, and 84 common targets were produced by crossing drug targets with disease targets. These common targets are probable targets of cardiotoxicity induced by PCA.

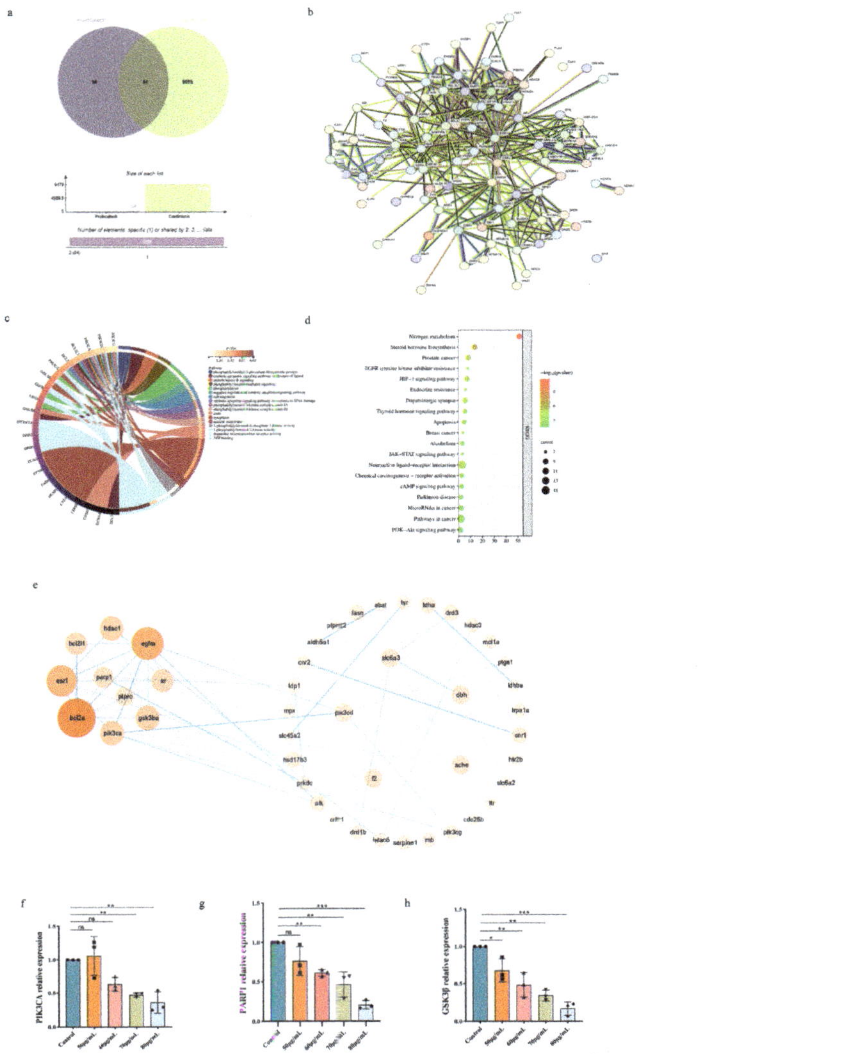

Figure 4. Network pharmacology chart. (**a**) Wayne diagram of cardiotoxicity and PCA intersection genes. (**b**) PPI network diagram. (**c**) GO analysis chart. (**d**) KEGG analysis chart. (**e**) Cytoscape HUB gene map. (**f–h**) Effect of PCA on PIK3CA, PARP1, and GSK3β mRNA expression of key target genes of zebrafish cardiotoxicity. Note: comparison with blank control group: * $p < 0.05$; ** $p < 0.01$; *** $p < 0.001$ (n = 50). The circles, squares, triangles, inverted triangles, and diamonds in the diagram represent the data in the histogram.

4.7.2. Networks of Protein Interactions

Figure 4b shows the PPI network of possible targets of cardiotoxicity induced by PCA dispersions by (https://string-db.org/, accessed on 1 January 2024). The top 10 target genes of PIK3CA, PARP1, HDAC1, GSK3β, EGFRA, ESR1, BAL211, BCL2A, AR, and PTPRC were selected based on the degree of significance targeting values by using Cytoscape 3.9.1 software, as shown in Figure 4e.

4.7.3. GO and KEGG Pathway Enrichment Analysis Results

To investigate the potential cardiotoxicity mechanisms of PCA, we used network pharmacology to predict the target genes that PCA might act on and performed KEGG and GO functional enrichment analyses of these target genes. As shown in Table 2, the target genes were found to be enriched in multiple pathways, including "phosphorylation, phosphatidyli-n-ositol-3-phosphatebiosynthesis, phosphatidylinositol-mediated, signaling, cytoplasmic, axonal, phosphatidylinositol-3-kinase, complexclasslA, ATPbinding, 1-phosphatidylinositol-4-ph-osp-hate, 1-phosphatidylinositol-3-kinase, or phosphate action". Entries were filtered by $p \leq 0.05$ and plotted as an enrichment analysis circle diagram in Figure 4c. We found that PCA may act on zebrafish cardiotoxicity through biological processes. The results of KEGG analysis showed that these biological processes mainly include "ErbB signaling pathway, apoptosis and inositol phosphate metabolism" (Table 3, Figure 4d). Combining the results of the enrichment analyses, we found that the mechanism of action of PCA-induced cardiotoxicity in zebrafish may be related to the core targets of PIK3CA, PARP 1, HDAC 1, GSK3β, EGFRA, ESR 1, BAL211, BCL 2A, AR, and PTPRC. Based on the existing reports, we selected three key target genes (PIK3CA, PARP1, and GSK3β), which are closely related to cardiotoxicity, from which we performed mRNA validation.

Table 2. GO enrichment analysis including molecular function (MF), cellular composition (CC), and biological process (BP).

GO Term	Subgroup	Count
Phosphatidylinositol-3-phosphate biosynthetic process	Biological Processes	3
Extrinsic apoptotic signaling pathway in the absence of ligand	Biological Processes	3
Protein kinase B signaling	Biological Processes	3
Phosphatidylinositol-mediated signaling	Biological Processes	3
Phosphorylation	Biological Processes	5
Negative regulation of intrinsic apoptotic signaling pathway	Biological Processes	2
Cell migration	Biological Processes	3
Intrinsic apoptotic signaling pathway in response to DNA damage	Biological Processes	2
Phosphatidylinositol 3-kinase complex, class lA	Cellular Components	2
Phosphatidylinositol3-kinase complex, class lB	Cellular Components	2
axon	Cellular Components	3
Cytoplasm	Cellular Components	10
Nuclear membrane	Cellular Components	2
1-Phosphatidylinositol-4-phosphate 3-kinase activity	Molecular Functions	3
1-Phosphatidylinositol-3-kinase activity	Molecular Functions	3
Dopamine neurotransmitter receptor activity	Molecular Functions	2
ATP binding	Molecular Functions	7

Table 3. Analysis of KEGG enrichment.

Number	Pathway	Enrichment	*p*-Value	Count
zab00140	ErbB signaling pathway	26.31292517	0.000364195	4
zab04210	Apoptosis	10.96371882	0.000778384	5
zab04140	Inositol phosphate metabolism	8.05028305	0.002457148	5
zab04012	FoxO signaling pathway	12.44530245	0.003254212	4
zab04510	Autophagy-animal	6.692967885	0.004793276	5
zab04068	Insulin signaling pathway	8.372294372	0.009852925	4

Table 3. *Cont.*

Number	Pathway	Enrichment	p-Value	Count
zab04910	Herpes simplex virus 1 infection	7.804681195	0.011931379	4
zab01100	Salmonella infection	2.030969565	0.017097321	11
zab05168	Human cytomegalovirus infection	6.771708683	0.017480242	4
zab00562	Metabolic pathways	10.62637363	0.028938037	3

4.7.4. Acute Exposure to PCA's Effects on the mRNA Expression of the Main Target Genes for Cardiotoxicity in Zebrafish

We exposed zebrafish larvae to gradient concentrations of PCA (50 μg/mL, 60 μg/mL, 70 μg/mL, and 80 μg/mL) for 96 h. RT-PCR validation revealed a decreasing trend in the expression of PIK3CA, PARP1, and GSK3β in the gradient concentrations of PCA with the increase in drug concentration. As shown in Figure 4f, compared with the control, at PCA concentrations of 50 μg/mL and 60 μg/mL, there was no significant change in the mRNA expression of the PIk3CA gene. However, at 60 μg/mL and 70 μg/mL, the expression of the gene PIk3CA showed a decreasing trend compared with the control. There was no significant change in the mRNA expression of the PARP1 gene at 50 μg/mL PCA concentration compared with the control group, but the expression showed a decreasing trend at 60 μg/mL, 70 μg/mL, and 80 μg/mL, as shown in Figure 4g. As shown in Figure 4h, the mRNA expression of gene GSK3β decreased with the increase in PCA concentration, and the difference was statistically significant. This suggests that PCA may cause cardiotoxicity by inducing the expression of PIK3CA, PARP1, and GSK3β, especially the GSK3β gene; however, further systematic validation is needed to illustrate this.

5. Discussion

PCA has a wide range of pharmacological activities, and its pharmacological effects have been mainly focused on cardioprotective effects [22]. Several studies have reported that acute/chronic exposure to PCA may lead to toxic effects. In the present study, we used zebrafish as a sensitive and susceptible biological model for evaluating the toxicity of PCA drugs. Acute toxicity in zebrafish embryos is commonly manifested as behavioral changes such as the closure of the swim bladder, yolk cysts, loss of swim bladder, bending of the zebrafish trunk, and abnormal motor trajectories, suggesting the manifestation of neurotoxicity [23,24]. Pericardial edema and abnormal ring formation are frequently observed in zebrafish embryos as morphological changes of cardiac defects [25,26], and these changes can be reported on the basis of quantification of the pericardial area and SV-BA distance [27,28]. In addition, the most common dysfunction of the zebrafish cardiovascular system is abnormal heart rhythms, including tachycardia, bradycardia, atrioventricular block, premature beats, or fibrillation [29]. Miao Wenyu [30] showed that the Pearson correlation coefficient between zebrafish embryonic LC50 values and rodent LD50 values was 0.9271, showing a very strong positive correlation, and a one-way regression was fitted to the equation y = 0.4525x. Combined with previous studies [22], the LD50 of PCA in rodents was 1627 ± 115 mg/kg. The LD50 equation was used to calculate the LD50 of PCA on zebrafish as 57.297 ± 5.02 μg/mL. In addition, in an attempt to further investigate the degree of toxicity of PCA to zebrafish at the lethal concentration, we combined the pre-test with a simultaneous selection of concentrations exceeding the upper limit of the PCA (LD50) concentration to observe the maximal toxicity of PCA to zebrafish. On this basis, the doses of 50 μg/mL, 60 μg/mL, 70 μg/mL, and 80 μg/mL were selected for the phenotypic observation of 96 hpf zebrafish. At these dose-induced doses, we observed severe acute toxic injury and cardiac morphological changes in zebrafish, including pericardial edema, structural deformities, altered cardiac function, and pathological structural damage. Based on this, in the present study, we observed the acute toxicity of wild-type zebrafish by counting the acute toxicity after the administration of a gradient concentration of PCA, including observation of the overall morphological deformity changes, and monitoring the behavioral ability and cardiotoxicity by observing the cardiotoxicity in *Tg(cmlc2: EGFP)* zebrafish, including the area of cardiac fluorescence, cardiac function, and cardiac pathology slides for comprehensive evaluation of the intensity of the acute and cardiotoxicity of the gradient concentration of PCA. It was found that the concentration of PCA at 70 μg/mL resulted in irregular growth patterns, restricted behavioral function, led to cardiac malformation, and caused abnormal cardiac function in zebrafish, and this abnormality increased with the increase in exposure concentration. In order to investigate the locomotor behavior of zebrafish under acute exposure to PCA, an autonomous locomotion experiment was conducted in this study, and the results showed that zebrafish larvae exposed to PCA at the concentrations of 70 μg/mL and 80 μg/mL showed a significant decrease in the distance and speed of locomotion. These abnormal behaviors indicated that the exposure to PCA at 70 μg/mL and 80 μg/mL resulted in acute toxicity and abnormal behavioral functions in zebrafish. Based on this, the present study was the first to comprehensively and systematically evaluate the effects of PCA on acute toxicity and cardiotoxicity and to preliminarily elucidate the mechanism of action of PCA-induced cardiotoxicity using a combination of phenotypic observation, network pharmacology, and experimental validation using zebrafish of the AB and *Tg(cmlc2:EGFP)* strains. It provides an important theoretical reference for the evaluation of the drug toxicity of PCA.

In the follow-up experiments, combined with enrichment analysis, three key genes, PIK3CA, PARP1, and GSK3β, were selected. Among the key target genes, we enriched the KEGG pathway and further analyzed it by combining it with the existing literature. The PI3K-AKT signaling pathway in the signaling pathway enrichment results has been proven to be related to a variety of cardiovascular diseases [31–34]. The phosphatidylinositol-45-bisphosphate 3-kinase catalytic subunit alpha PIK3CA gene consists of multiple exons and is expressed in a variety of tissues and organs, and is widely involved in cell proliferation, survival, and cell cycle regulation, as well as other cellular functional activities [35]. Studies have shown that PIK3CA can activate PI3K, mediate the phosphorylation of Akt, and then regulate mTOR and GSK3β, which are involved in the regulation of cell proliferation, differentiation, and apoptosis [36–38]. PIK3CA is a key initiator of the PI3K-AKT signaling pathway, which has an important role in regulating biological signaling and pathway activation. He Yazhou [39] found that miR-320a could promote myocardial fibrosis through its target gene PIK3CA in protein interaction analysis of PI3K-AKT pathway target genes. PARP-1 (poly-ADP-ribose polymerase-1) is an important member of the PARP family whose main role is DNA damage repair and regulation of apoptosis [40]. Some studies have found that single nucleotide polymorphism changes in PARP-1 are associated with genetic susceptibility to many diseases [41]. Rumei Men [42] found that metoprolol reduces cardiomyocyte apoptosis and thus ameliorates MI/R injury mainly by inhibiting PARP-1 protein expression levels. GSK3β (glycogen synthase kinase 3β) is a class of highly structurally conserved serothreonine protein kinases that are prevalent in organisms and eukaryotes and play an important role in the regulation of cellular functions, such as cellular structure regulation, intracellular signaling, cell division, apoptosis, microtubule movement, and determination of the fate of cells in the process of embryonic development [43–47]. In recent years, many studies have confirmed that GSK3β is an important factor in the regulation of apoptosis [48]. Some studies have confirmed that the PI3K/AKT/GSK3β pathway promotes fibrosis in myocardial tissues, and its upregulation damages cardiomyocytes and participates in the pathogenesis of acute myocardial infarction [49–51]. Huang Jing [52] found that downregulation of miR-208 could inhibit PI3K/AKt/GSK3β signaling pathway-related proteins, which in turn inhibited cardiomyocyte apoptosis, alleviated the body's inflammatory response, protected the body's cardiomyocytes, and ultimately slowed down the degree of cardiac muscle damage. Combined with the above studies, it is hypothesized that the three key target genes, PIK3CA, PARP1, and GSK3β, are all associated with cardiomyocyte apoptosis. Apoptosis is a form of programmed cell death regulated by the exogenous death receptor pathway and the endogenous mitochondrial pathway, and it is essential for the normal development of the cardiovascular system in zebrafish [53]. However, the relevance of PIK3CA, PARP1, and GSK3β to PCA and their regulatory mechanisms to induce cardiotoxicity in PCA have rarely been reported [54,55]. Therefore, we performed RT-PCR to validate the expression of PIK3CA, PARP1, and GSK3β and found that the expression of PIK3CA, PARP1, and GSK3β decreased in a concentration-dependent manner with the PCA concentration gradient. It can be preliminarily speculated that the mechanism of PCA-induced cardiotoxicity may be related to the apoptosis of cardiomyocytes caused by the three core target genes, PIK3CA, PARP1, and GSK3β. This still needs further investigation and research.

In this experiment, we found that PCA produced severe acute toxicity and cardiotoxic effects in zebrafish at concentrations of 70 μg/mL and 80 μg/mL. In addition, PIK3CA, PARP1, and GSK3β may be involved in the mechanism of action of this compound to induce cardiotoxic effects In addition, more biological model experiments are needed to help avoid the toxic side effects and improve the safety of drug use.

6. Conclusions

For the first time, we observed the acute toxicity and cardiotoxic effects of PCA in wild-type and transgenic zebrafish models and initially explored the mechanism of toxicity of PCA, with the aim of better understanding the potential toxicity of PCA in order to achieve the purpose of reducing the adverse effects of PCA and enhancing the medicinal value of PCA, to provide strong evidence for accelerating the development of new highly efficient and low-toxicity drugs containing PCA, and also to provide a valuable theoretical framework for assessing the toxicity of PCA containing drugs. This study provides strong evidence for accelerating the development of new efficient and low-toxicity drugs for PCA and provides a valuable theoretical framework for assessing the toxicity of PCA-containing drugs.

Author Contributions: J.Y. and H.W. carried out the conceptualization, data curation, methodology, and original draft of the study; F.Z. carried out the formal analysis, investigation, methodology, and most of the literature review; D.L. participated in the data curation and formal analysis; and W.Y. and D.Z. participated in the funding acquisition, supervision, visualization, and review and editing of the text. All authors have read and agreed to the published version of the manuscript.

Funding: This work was supported by the National Natural Science Foundation of China (NSFC) (No. 82174337), the Outstanding Youth Innovation Team of Shandong Institutions of Higher Learning (2022KJ257), the Shandong Traditional Chinese Medicine Science and Technology Project (Z-2022045), and the Natural Science Foundation of Shandong Province (ZR2023MH160).

Institutional Review Board Statement A license for the use of laboratory animals was obtained from the Shandong University of Traditional Chinese Medicine (i.e., document SYXK(lu)2022 0009, approved on 8 May 2022). As we conducted embryonic and juvenile experiments earlier than 7 dpf, which did not involve adult zebrafish, and we did not perform damaging surgeries or treatments on the juveniles, a separate ethical certificate was not required.

Informed Consent Statement: Not applicate.

Data Availability Statement: The raw data supporting the conclusions of this article will be made available by the authors upon request.

Acknowledgments: The authors special acknowledge Associate Wenqing Yang and Dan Zhang, from the University of Shandong Traditional Chinese Medicine, who helped in editing the article. The authors would also like to thank the Medical Research Platform and the Zebrafish Laboratory of the Animal Centre of Shandong University of Traditional Chinese Medicine for their technical support, especially Feng Zhao. Information was obtained from a variety of sources, and the views and conclusions of this study do not necessarily represent those of other organizations or institutions.

Conflicts of Interest: The authors declare no conflicts of interest.

References

1. Zhang, C.; Guo, L.; Wang, J. Progress of pharmacological studies on protocatechuic aldehyde. *Chin. J. Exp. Formulas* **2013**, *19*, 338–342.
2. Ji, G.L.; Zhou, W.; Ba, R.R.; Lin, C.H.; Liu, Y.L. Determination of six phenolic acid components in Danshen formula granules by double-labeled multi-assay method. *J. Pharm. Anal.* **2023**, *43*, 1326–1333. [CrossRef]
3. Krzysztoforska, K.; Mirowska-Guzel, D.; Widy-Tyszkiewicz, E. Pharmacological effects of protocatechuic acid and its therapeutic potential in neurodegenerative diseases: Review on the basis of in vitro and in vivo studies in rodents and humans. *Nutr. Neurosci.* **2019**, *22*, 72–82. [CrossRef] [PubMed]
4. Xing, Y.L.; Zhou, Z.; Agula; Zhong, Z.Y.; Ma, Y.J.; Zhao, Y.L.; Xiao, X.H.; Wang, S.Q. Protocatechuic aldehyde inhibits lipopolysaccharide-induced human umbilical vein endothelial cell apoptosis via regulation of caspase-3. *Phytother. Res.* **2012**, *26*, 1334–1341. [CrossRef]
5. Fang, X.; Liu, Y.; Lu, J.; Hong, H.; Yuan, J.; Zhang, Y.; Wang, P.; Liu, P.; Ye, J. Protocatechuic aldehyde protects against isoproterenol-induced cardiac hypertrophy via inhibition of the JAK2/STAT3 signaling pathway. *Naunyn-Schmiedeberg's Arch. Pharmacol.* **2018**, *391*, 1373–1385. [CrossRef]
6. Wan, Y.J.; Guo, Q.; Liu, D.; Jiang, Y.; Zeng, K.W.; Tu, P.F. Protocatechualdehyde reduces myocardial fibrosis by directly targeting conformational dynamics of collagen. *Eur. J. Pharmacol.* **2019**, *855*, 183–191. [CrossRef]
7. Yang, S.Y.; Xiao, Y.; An, C.; Qiu, C.L.; Li, J.A.; Chu, J.X. Neuroprotective mechanism of protocatechuic aldehyde. *Chin. Herbal. Med.* **2024**, *55*, 2463–2471.
8. Cao, Y.G.; Zhang, L.; Ma, C.; Chang, B.B.; Chen, Y.C.; Tang, Y.Q.; Liu, X.D.; Liu, X.Q. Metabolism of protocatechuic acid influences fatty acid oxidation in rat heart: New anti-angina mechanism implication. *Biochem. Pharmacol.* **2009**, *77*, 1096–1104. [CrossRef]
9. Zhou, J.; Zhang, J.; Cao, Y.; Chen, Y.; Yu, D.; Liu, X. Effect of acute myocardial ischemia on methylation metabolism of danshenin in rats. *J. China Pharm. Univ.* **2009**, *40*, 72–76.
10. Zhu, B.T. Catechol-O-Methyltransferase (COMT)-mediated methylation metabolism of endogenous bioactive catechols and modulation by endobiotics and xenobiotics: Importance in pathophysiology and pathogenesis. *Curr. Drug Metab* **2002**, *3*, 321–349. [CrossRef]
11. Xu, M.; Zhang, Z.; Fu, G.; Sun, S.; Sun, J.; Yang, M.; Liu, A.; Han, J.; Guo, D. Liquid chromatography-tandem mass spectrometry analysis of protocatechuic aldehyde and its phase I and II metabolites in rat. *J. Chromatogr. B Anal. Technol. Biomed. Life Sci.* **2007**, *856*, 100–107. [CrossRef] [PubMed]
12. Cao, W.; Cao, Y.; Zhang, L.; Chang, Z.; Tang, Y.; Liu, X. Effects of acute myocardial ischemia on the pharmacokinetics of protocatechuic acid in rats. *J. China Pharm. Univ.* **2010**, *41*, 156–159.
13. Gao, L.; Wu, W.F.; Dong, L.; Ren, G.L.; Li, H.D.; Yang, Q.; Li, X.F.; Xu, T.; Li, Z.; Wu, B.M.; et al. Protocatechuic Aldehyde Attenuates Cisplatin-Induced Acute Kidney Injury by Suppressing Nox-Mediated Oxidative Stress and Renal Inflammation. *Front. Pharmacol.* **2016**, *7*, 479. [CrossRef]
14. MacRae, C.A.; Peterson, R.T. Zebrafish as tools for drug discovery. *Nat. Rev. Drug Discov.* **2015**, *14*, 721–731. [CrossRef] [PubMed]
15. OECD. *Validation Report (Phase 2) for the Zebrafish Embryo Toxicity Test I*; OECD Series on Testing and Assessment 179; The OECD Observer; Organisation for Economic Co-Operation and Development: Paris, France, 2012; Volume 25.
16. OECD. *Test No. 236: Fish Embryo Acute Toxicity (FET) Test*; OECD: Paris, France, 2013.
17. Huang, M.; Jiao, J.; Wang, J.; Xia, Z.; Zhang, Y. Exposure to acrylamide induces cardiac developmental toxicity in zebrafish during cardiogenesis. *Environ. Pollut.* **2018**, *234*, 656–666. [CrossRef] [PubMed]
18. Liu, H.; Chu, T.; Chen, L.; Gui, W.; Zhu, G. In vivo cardiovascular toxicity induced by acetochlor in zebrafish larvae. *Chemosphere* **2017**, *181*, 600–608. [CrossRef]
19. Xue, D. Construction and Study of Vasopressor and Cardiac Injury Model in Zebrafish. Master's Thesis, Shanxi Medical University, Taiyuan, China, 2016.
20. Berman, N.; Lectura, M.; Thurman, J.; Reinecke, J.; Raff, A.C.; Melamed, M.L.; Reinecke, J.; Quan, Z.; Evans, T.; Meyer, T.W.; et al. A zebrafish model for uremic toxicity: Role of the complement pathway. *Blood Purif.* **2013**, *35*, 265–269. [CrossRef]
21. Brown, M.A.; Magee, L.A.; Kenny, L.C.; Karumanchi, S.A.; McCarthy, F.P.; Saito, S.; Hall, D.R.; Warren, C.E.; Adoyi, G.; Ishaku, S. Hypertensive Disorders of Pregnancy: ISSHP Classification, Diagnosis, and Management Recommendations for International Practice. *Hypertension* **2018**, *72*, 24–43. [CrossRef]
22. Yang, Y.; Cao, J.; Xu, X.; Xing, W.; Liu, Z.; Xu, J.; Shi, Y.; Wang, M.; Wang, G.; Yang, J. Distribution, excretion and toxicity of protocatechualdehyde in animals. *Jiangsu Med.* **1979**, *10*, 16–17+19. [CrossRef]
23. Zhou, S.Y.; Chen, J.P.; Liu, Z.D.; Zhou, J.R.; Liu, Y.; Liu, S.H.; Tian, C.W.; Chen, C.Q. Progress in the study of chemical composition and pharmacological effects of Yam bean root. *Chin. Herb. Med.* **2021**, *52*, 1510–1521.
24. Jang, S.M.; Bae, S.H.; Choi, W.K.; Park, J.B.; Kim, D.; Min, J.S.; Yoo, H.; Kang, M.; Ryu, K.H.; Bae, S.K. Pharmacokinetic properties of trifolirhizin, (-)-maackiain, (-)-isophorone and 2-(2,4-dihydroxy phenyl)-5,6-methylenedioxybenzofuran after intravenous and oral administration of Sophora tonkinensis extract in rats. *Xenobiotica* **2015**, *45*, 1092–1104. [CrossRef] [PubMed]
25. Duan, J.; Hu, H.; Li, Q.; Jiang, L.; Zou, Y.; Wang, Y.; Sun, Z. Combined toxicity of silica nanoparticles and methylmercury on the cardiovascular system in zebrafish (*Danio rerio*) embryos. *Environ. Toxicol. Pharmacol.* **2016**, *44*, 120–127. [CrossRef] [PubMed]

26. Duan, J.; Yu, Y.; Li, Y.; Li, Y.; Liu, H.; Jing, L.; Yang, M.; Wang, J.; Li, C.; Sun, Z. Low-dose exposure of silica nanoparticles induces cardiac dysfunction via neutrophil-mediated inflammation and cardiac contraction in zebrafish embryos. *Nanotoxicology* **2016**, *10*, 575–585. [CrossRef] [PubMed]
27. Han, Y.; Zhang, J.P.; Qian, J.Q.; Hu, C.Q. Cardiotoxicity evaluation of anthracyclines in zebrafish (*Danio rerio*). *J. Appl. Toxicol.* **2015**, *35*, 241–252. [CrossRef] [PubMed]
28. Han, Y.; Li, X.; Yan, M.; Yang, M.; Wang, S.; Pan, J.; Li, L.; Tan, J. Oxidative damage induces apoptosis and promotes calcification in disc cartilage endplate cell through ROS/MAPK/NF-κB pathway: Implications for disc degeneration. *Biochem. Biophys. Res. Commun.* **2019**, *516*, 1026–1032. [CrossRef]
29. Shen, R.; Yu, Y.; Lan, R.; Yu, R.; Yuan, Z.; Xia, Z. The cardiovascular toxicity induced by high doses of gatifloxacin and ciprofloxacin in zebrafish. *Environ. Pollut.* **2019**, *254*, 112861. [CrossRef]
30. Miao, W.; Zhu, X.; Xu, Y.; Jiang, Y.; Shao, L. Derivation of dose conversion factors for zebrafish and rodents based on experimental data. *Chin. Sci. Technol. J. Database (Full Text. Version) Nat. Sci.* **2022**, *3*, 61–69.
31. Rofaani, E.; Mardani, M.W.; Yutiana, P.N.; Amanda, O.; Darmawan, N. Differentiation of mesenchymal stem cells into vascular endothelial cells in 3D culture: A mini-review. *Mol. Biol. Rep.* **2024**, *51*, 781. [CrossRef]
32. Hu, Y.Y. PI3K/Akt/GSK-3β and Mitochondrial ATP-Sensitive Potassium Channels Mediate the Protective Effect of Procyanidins against Myocardial Ischemia-Reperfusion Injury. Ph.D. Thesis, Shandong University, Jinan, China, 2013.
33. Han, J.; Xuan, J.; Hu, H.; Chen, Z. Relationship between the effects of hypericin preconditioning to attenuate myocardial ischemia-reperfusion injury in rats and the PI3K/Akt signalling pathway. *Chin. J. Tradit. Chin. Med.* **2015**, *40*, 118–123.
34. Díaz, R.; Goyal, A.; Mehta, S.R.; Afzal, R.; Xavier, D.; Pais, P.; Chrolavicius, S.; Zhu, J.; Kazmi, K.; Liu, L.; et al. Glucose-insulin-potassium therapy in patients with ST-segment elevation myocardial infarction. *JAMA* **2007**, *298*, 2399–2405. [CrossRef]
35. Raghunath, A.; Perumal, E. Analysis of Lethality and Malformations During Zebrafish (*Danio rerio*) Development. *Methods Mol. Biol.* **2018**, *1797*, 337–363. [PubMed]
36. Sun, L.; Cui, K.; Xing, F.; Liu, X. Akt dependent adult hippocampal neurogenesis regulates the behavioral improvement of treadmill running to mice model of post-traumatic stress disorder. *Behav. Brain Res.* **2020**, *379*, 112375. [CrossRef]
37. Vicent, L.; Cinca, J.; Vazquez-García, R.; Gonzalez-Juanatey, J.R.; Rivera, M.; Segovia, J.; Pascual-Figal, D.; Bover, R.; Worner, F.; Delgado-Jiménez, J.; et al. Discharge treatment with angiotensin-converting enzyme inhibitor/angiotensin receptor blocker after a heart failure hospitalization is associated with a better prognosis irrespective of left ventricular ejection fraction. *Intern. Med. J.* **2019**, *49*, 1505–1513. [CrossRef] [PubMed]
38. McMurray, J.J.; Packer, M.; Desai, A.S.; Gong, J.; Lefkowitz, M.; Rizkala, A.R.; Rouleau, J.L.; Shi, V.C.; Solomon, S.D.; Swedberg, K.; et al. Baseline characteristics and treatment of patients in prospective comparison of ARNI with ACEI to determine the impact on global mortality and morbidity in heart failure trial (PARADIGM-HF). *Eur. J. Heart Fail.* **2014**, *16*, 817–825. [CrossRef] [PubMed]
39. He, Y. Study on Exosome-Derived Mir-320a Regulating PIK3CA against Myocardial Fibrosis in Chronic Heart Failure by Wenzhong Yiqi Fang. Master's Thesis, Guangxi Traditional Chinese Medical University, Nanning, China, 2019.
40. Wu, R.C.; Ayhan, A.; Maeda, D.; Kim, K.R.; Clarke, B.A.; Shaw, P.; Chui, M.H.; Rosen, B.; Shih Ie, M.; Wang, T.L. Frequent somatic mutations of the telomerase reverse transcriptase promoter in ovarian clear cell carcinoma but not in other major types of gynecological malignancy. *J. Pathol.* **2014**, *232*, 473–481. [CrossRef] [PubMed]
41. Embi, N.; Rylatt, D.B.; Cohen, P. Glycogen synthase kinase-3 from rabbit skeletal muscle. Separation from cyclic-AMP-dependent protein kinase and phosphorylase kinase. *Eur. J. Biochem.* **1980**, *107*, 519–527. [CrossRef]
42. Men, R.; Wang, Y.; Zhang, L.; Men, L.; Lan, W.; Meng, Q.; Yu, J. Mechanism of action of metoprolol combined with clopidogrel in mice with myocardial ischemia-reperfusion injury. *West. Med.* **2024**, *36*, 365–371.
43. Fang, X.; Yu, S.X.; Lu, Y.; Bast, R.C., Jr.; Woodgett, J.R.; Mills, G.B. Phosphorylation and inactivation of glycogen synthase kinase 3 by protein kinase A. *Proc. Natl. Acad. Sci. USA* **2000**, *97*, 11960–11965. [CrossRef]
44. Zhu, H.; Zhang, W.; Zhao, Y.; Shu, X.; Wang, W.; Wang, D.; Yang, Y.; He, Z.; Wang, X.; Ying, Y. GSK3β-mediated tau hyperphosphorylation triggers diabetic retinal neurodegeneration by disrupting synaptic and mitochondrial functions. *Mol. Neurodegener.* **2018**, *13*, 62. [CrossRef]
45. Takahashi-Yanaga, F. Roles of Glycogen Synthase Kinase-3 (GSK-3) in Cardiac Development and Heart Disease. *J. Uoeh* **2018**, *40*, 147–156. [CrossRef]
46. Zhou, B.P.; Deng, J.; Xia, W.; Xu, J.; Li, Y.M.; Gunduz, M.; Hung, M.C. Dual regulation of Snail by GSK-3beta-mediated phosphorylation in control of epithelial-mesenchymal transition. *Nat. Cell Biol.* **2004**, *6*, 931–940. [CrossRef] [PubMed]
47. Götschel, F.; Kern, C.; Lang, S.; Sparna, T.; Markmann, C.; Schwager, J.; McNelly, S.; von Weizsäcker, F.; Laufer, S.; Hecht, A.; et al. Inhibition of GSK3 differentially modulates NF-kappaB, CREB, AP-1, and beta-catenin signaling in hepatocytes, but fails to promote TNF-alpha-induced apoptosis. *Exp. Cell Res.* **2008**, *314*, 1351–1366. [CrossRef] [PubMed]
48. Li, H.; Zha, Y.; Du, F.; Liu, J.; Li, X.; Zhao, X. Contributions of PARP-1 rs1136410 C>T polymorphism to the development of cancer. *J. Cell Mol. Med.* **2020**, *24*, 14639–14644. [CrossRef]
49. Deng, S.; Dai, G.; Chen, S.; Nie, Z.; Zhou, J.; Fang, H.; Peng, H. Dexamethasone induces osteoblast apoptosis through ROS-PI3K/AKT/GSK3β signaling pathway. *Biomed. Pharmacother.* **2019**, *110*, 602–608. [CrossRef] [PubMed]
50. Wang, X.; Zou, W.; Li, J.; Cai, G.; Liu, K.; Jia, K.; Wang, T.; Peng, Y. Mechanistic study on the myocardial protective effect of cardiostatin on MIRI rats based on PI3K/Akt/GSK-3β signaling pathway. *J. Chin. Med.* **2020**, *48*, 6–11. [CrossRef]

51. Li, S. Study on the Protective Mechanism of Myocardial Ischemia-Reperfusion Injury via ALKBH5/GSK3β/mTOR Signaling Pathway by Quick-Acting Heart-Saving Pill. Master's Thesis, Shanghai University of Traditional Chinese Medicine, Shanghai, China, 2021.
52. Huang, J.; Lei, Y.; Hua, X.; Zhou, H.; Zhu, X. The intervention of miR-208a based on down-regulation of PI3K/AKT/GSK3β signaling pathway in acute myocardial infarction model rats. *Hebei Med.* **2022**, *44*, 3530–3533+3537.
53. Sinha, K.; Das, J.; Pal, P.B.; Sil, P.C. Oxidative stress: The mitochondria-dependent and mitochondria-independent pathways of apoptosis. *Arch. Toxicol.* **2013**, *87*, 1157–1180. [CrossRef]
54. Burgos-Aceves, M.A.; Cohen, A.; Smith, Y.; Faggio, C. MicroRNAs and their role on fish oxidative stress during xenobiotic environmental exposures. *Ecotoxicol. Environ. Saf.* **2018**, *148*, 995–1000. [CrossRef]
55. Burgos-Aceves, M.A.; Cohen, A.; Paolella, G.; Lepretti, M.; Smith, Y.; Faggio, C.; Lionetti, L. Modulation of mitochondrial functions by xenobiotic-induced microRNA: From environmental sentinel organisms to mammals. *Sci. Total Environ.* **2018**, *645*, 79–88. [CrossRef]

Disclaimer/Publisher's Note: The statements, opinions and data contained in all publications are solely those of the individual author(s) and contributor(s) and not of MDPI and/or the editor(s). MDPI and/or the editor(s) disclaim responsibility for any injury to people or property resulting from any ideas, methods, instructions or products referred to in the content.

toxics

MDPI

Article

Actin Dysregulation Mediates Nephrotoxicity of Cassiae Semen Aqueous Extracts

Jinlan Yang [1,†], Sheng Xiao [1,†], Ludi Li [1], An Zhu [1], Wusheng Xiao [1] and Qi Wang [1,2,3,*]

1 Department of Toxicology, School of Public Health, Peking University, Beijing 100191, China; yangjinlan@bjmu.edu.cn (J.Y.); sheng_xiao@pku.edu.cn (S.X.); liludi@bjmu.edu.cn (L.L.); zhuan@fjmu.edu.cn (A.Z.); wxiao@bjmu.edu.cn (W.X.)
2 Key Laboratory of State Administration of Traditional Chinese Medicine (TCM) for Compatibility Toxicology, Peking University, Beijing 100191, China
3 Beijing Key Laboratory of Toxicological Research and Risk Assessment for Food Safety, Peking University, Beijing 100191, China
* Correspondence: wangqi@bjmu.edu.cn
† These authors contributed equally to this work.

Abstract: *Cassiae* semen, commonly consumed as roasted tea, has been widely used for both medicinal purposes and dietary supplements. In this study, we investigated the nephrotoxic effects and underlying mechanisms of *Cassiae* semen aqueous extracts (CSAEs) using computational and animal models. Both male and female Sprague Dawley rats were treated with 4.73–47.30 g/kg (body weight) of CSAEs by oral gavage twice a day for 7–28 days. We found that serum and urinary biomarkers of kidney injury and kidney coefficients were increased in a dose-dependent manner, and were accompanied by morphological alterations in the kidneys of CSAEs-treated rats. Computational and molecular docking approaches predicted that the three most abundant components of CSAEs—obtusifolin, aurantio-obtusin, and obtusin—exhibited strong affinity for the binding of F-actin, ROCK1, and Rac1, and the RhoA–ROCK pathway was identified as the most likely regulatory mechanism mediating the nephrotoxicity of CSAEs. Consistently, immunofluorescence staining revealed F-actin and cytoskeleton were frequently disturbed in renal cells and brush borders at high doses of CSAEs. Results from gene expression analyses confirmed that CSAEs suppressed the key proteins in the RhoA–ROCK signaling pathway and consequently the expression of F-actin and its stabilization genes. In summary, our findings suggest that Cassiae semen can depolymerize and destabilize actin cytoskeleton by inhibition of the RhoA–ROCK pathway and/or direct binding to F-actin, leading to nephrotoxicity. The consumption of *Cassiae* semen as a supplement and medicine warrants attention.

Keywords: *Cassiae* semen; nephrotoxicity; RhoA–ROCK pathway; cytoskeleton

1. Introduction

Cassiae semen, a herb consumed as a roasted tea and a class of traditional Chinese medicine (TCM), is widely used in eastern Asia for weight control and treatment of hyperlipidemia, dizziness, constipation, and eye diseases [1–4]. Traditionally, *Cassiae* semen is defined as a low toxic agent [4]. However, the safety of *Cassiae* semen remains controversial. For example, hepatotoxicity has been reported in rats after a 90-day administration of extract mixed into the fodder [5]. Nephrotoxicity manifested by pigment deposition, atrophy, or regeneration of renal tubules has also been found in rats after administration of *Cassiae* semen (10 g/kg body weight (B.W.)) [6]. These lines of evidence support the necessity to reevaluate the safety of *Cassiae* semen.

To date, over 70 components have been isolated and identified from *Cassiae* semen, approximately 53 of which are biologically active and structurally distinct anthraquinones

(AQs) [1]. We previously revealed that after oral administration of *Cassiae* semen, obtusifolin, *Epi*-9-dehydroxyeurotinone-β-D-glucopyranoside (EDG), aurantio-obtusin, obtusin, 2-O-methyl-9-dehydroxyeurotinone (OMD), rhein, questin, emodin, and cassiaside were the nine most abundant components in plasma of rats [7]. Aurantio-obtusin, one major AQ ingredient of *Cassiae* semen, was shown to induce hepatotoxicity through enhanced reactive oxygen species (ROS) production, apoptosis, and ferroptosis [8]. Qin et al. found that after administration of aurantio-obtusin, a major anthraquinone compound of *Cassiae* semen at a dose of 200 mg/kg B.W., metabolites of aurantio-obtusin were detected and identified in the heart, liver, spleen, lungs and kidneys [9]. In a tissue distribution study of obtusifolin, after intragastric administration of 1.3 mg/kg B.W., obtusifolin was rapidly distributed into tissues, with the highest distribution in the liver, followed by lung, heart, kidney, spleen, and brain [10]. Yang et al. also observed the presence of chrysophanol, emodin, aloe-emodin, rhein, physcion, obtusifolin, and aurantio-obtusin in plasma after oral administration 1.25 g/kg B.W. of *Cassiae* semen extract, and the time to reach the maximum plasma concentration varied from 0.167 to 0.5 h [11]. Nephrotoxicity can be another problem of *Cassiae* semen, and the toxic molecules are worth exploring. Some components of TCMs, such as aristolochic acids, alkaloids, anthraquinones, and flavonoids, have been reported to cause kidney injury [12,13]. An adverse outcome pathway (AOP) identified loss of tubular cells and tubular vacuolization as key events in kidney toxicity [14]. Other mechanisms were also involved, such as the direct perturbations of cellular or subcellular organelle function, cell death (apoptosis and necrosis), calcium dysregulation and cytoskeleton malfunction [6]. Since the form of aqueous extracts mimics more closely its consumption as roasted tea and decoction, it is worthwhile to study the influences of *Cassiae* semen aqueous extracts (CSAEs) on kidney functions and the potential mechanisms.

Actin is one of the most abundant cytoskeleton proteins to support cellular structure and functions [15]. Actin cytoskeletal dynamics, which regulates intracellular calcium (Ca^{2+}) concentration, is controlled by nuclear factor of activated T cells (NFAT)-dependent transcriptional activity [16] and by Rho GTPases via the RhoA–ROCK signaling pathway [17,18]. More importantly, cytoskeletal dynamics is also involved in cell death pathways, such as apoptosis [19] and necrosis [20]. It has been reported that actin destabilization is one of the factors mediating nephrotoxicity [21]. However, the intrinsic interaction between the main ingredients of CSAEs and cytoskeleton and their role in the renal toxicity of *Cassiae* semen remains obscure.

In this study, we aimed to elucidate the dose- and time-dependent effects and their underlying mechanisms of CSAEs-induced nephrotoxicity in rat models and computational approaches.

2. Materials and Methods

2.1. Chemicals and Materials

Ultrapure water was prepared by a Milli-Q system (Millipore, Bedford, MA, USA). Creatinine (Cr) and blood urea nitrogen (BUN) assay kits were purchased from Sichuan Maccura Biotechnology Co., Ltd. (Chengdu, China). Anti-ROCK1 (phospho T455 + S456; Cat. # ab97592), anti-myosin light chain (phospho S20; Cat. # Ab2480), anti-cofilin (phospho S3; Cat. # ab 12866), and F-actin staining kit (green fluorescence; Cat. # ab112125) were purchased from Abcam (Cambridge, UK). Anti-RhoA (26C4) (Cat. # sc-418) and anti-GAPDH (Cat. # A19056) were purchased from Santa Cruz Biotechnology (Santa Cruz, CA, USA) and Abclonal (Wuhan, China), respectively.

2.2. Preparation of *Cassiae* Semen Aqueous Extracts (CSAEs)

Cassiae semen (Anguo Qi An Pharmaceutical Co., Ltd., Anguo, China) was prepared using the seeds of *Senna obtusifolia* (L.) H. S. Irwin & Barneby (*S. obtusifolia*). Specifically, the seeds of *S. obtusifolia* were immersed in eightfold volumes of distilled water for 30 minutes (min) and then boiled for 60 min. The residue was mixed with fourfold volumes of distilled water, decocted for 30 min, and the entire process was repeated twice. All the collected supernatants were filtered through eight layers of gauze and condensed to obtain different concentrations of CSAEs (0.158, 0.525, and 1.577 g/mL).

2.3. Animal Treatment

A total of 32 male and 32 female Sprague Dawley (SD) rats (180–200 g) aged 8–12 weeks were obtained from the Department of Laboratory Animal Science at Peking University Health Science Center (Beijing, China). These rats were randomly divided into four treatment groups, with eight rats/sex/group. Typically, the dose level for a toxicology study should be 10- to 30-folds that of the therapeutic dose to ensure the safety of human consumption. The doses we used are based on the following calculations. According to the guidelines in the *Chinese Pharmacopoeia* (2020), the intake of *Cassiae* semen is limited to 15 g per day: 15 g/60 kg = 0.25 g/kg for humans (the average body weight of an adult is assumed as 60 kg). For the adjustment of interspecies difference (human-to-animal) in body size, a parameter value of 6.3 was used (body weight approach). Therefore, the equivalent dose for rats is $0.25 \times 6.3 = 1.575$ g/kg. To mimic the long-term and low-dose exposure in humans using a short-term animal toxicity study, we chose the 3-, 10- and 30-fold equivalent doses, which were equivalent to 4.73 g/kg, 15.75 g/kg, and 47.30 g/kg. All animals were administered by gavage twice a day for 28 consecutive days. Control animals were treated with solvent (distilled water). Animals were housed under a controlled light intensity of 200 Lx with a 12 h/12 h light/dark cycle, temperature of 25 °C ± 1 °C, and 55–60% humidity. All experimental procedures were conducted according to an approved protocol by the Animal Experimental Ethical Committee of Peking University (LA2017227, Beijing, China) and under the guidelines of the Association for Assessment and Accreditation of Laboratory Animal Care International (AAALAC).

2.4. Serum Biochemical Parameters

Elevated levels of Cr and BUN are the most commonly used markers of kidney injury. Serum Cr and BUN levels were detected on days 0, 7, 14, and 28 of CSAEs treatment using a serum biochemistry analyzer (Hitachi, Tokyo, Japan). Blood was collected via the orbital venous plexus, kept at room temperature for 30 min for coagulation, and then centrifuged at 3000× *g* for 10 min (1630 RCF, MF300, Incheon, Republic of Korea).

2.5. Urinalysis

The urinary calbindin, kidney injury molecule 1 (KIM-1), osteopontin (OPN), neutrophil gelatinase-associated lipocalin (NGAL), cystatin C, and β-2-microglobulin (β2M) levels were early indications of kidney injury. Urinary samples were collected 12 h after the last treatment on the day, immediately centrifuged at 3000× *g* for 10 min (1630 RCF, MF300, Incheon, Republic of Korea), and then tested by a Milliplex Luminex 200TM and Milliplex® Map Kit following the manufacturer's instructions (Cat. # RKTX2MAG-37K and RKTX1MAG-37K, EMD Millipore, Billerica, MA, USA). Calbindin, KIM-1, and OPN levels were tested on days 7, 14, and 28, and β2M, cystatin C, and NGAL/lipocalin 2 levels were tested on day 28 of CSAEs treatment.

2.6. Histopathological Examinations

Rats were sacrificed on day 28 and the left kidney were collected. Kidneys were fixed in 4% paraformaldehyde, sequentially dehydrated with ethanol and xylene, embedded in paraffin, sectioned at 5 μm thickness, and stained with hematoxylin and eosin (H&E) for histology. The H&E-stained kidney sections were analyzed under an optical microscope (Olympus, Tokyo, Japan) to examine morphological changes.

2.7. Fluorescent Staining of Cellular Cytoskeleton

Kidneys embedded in paraffin were sliced into sections of 4 μm thickness, deparaffinized and hydrated, and then rinsed in distilled water and phosphate-buffered saline (PBS) 3 times. Tissue sections were incubated in 0.5% Triton X-100 for 30 min to allow permeabilization and then with green fluorescent phalloidin conjugate for 1 h followed by rinsing with 1× PBS. Images were recorded using a confocal laser-scanning microscope (Nikon, Tokyo, Japan) with an FITC emission filter (488/520 nm).

2.8. Molecular Docking

Cytoscape (version 3.7.2) software was used to construct a composition–target interaction network model with the nine most abundant components of CSAEs identified in rat blood and key proteins of four renal injury pathways. Nodes in the network represent compounds or proteins. If a protein is a potential target for a specific CSAEs compound, the nodes are linked by edges.

To explore the potential mechanism of kidney injury caused by CSAEs, the key proteins of different kidney injury pathways (apoptosis, necrosis, calcium regulation, and cytoskeleton regulation) were the central focus, and the 3D structures of these proteins were retrieved from the Protein Data Bank (PDB). The interactions between these proteins and the nine major components in CSAEs (Figure 1) were predicted using SYBYL-X 2.0 software (Tripos, St. Louis, MO, USA). Before docking, the proteins were prepared by removal of water molecules, metal ions, and solvent molecules, repair of side chains and side chain amides, and addition of hydrogen atoms. The nine major components, the ligands of proteins, were prepared by the addition of Gasteiger–Hückel charges in the Tripos force field to attain minimum energy status. Using SYBYL-X 2.0 software, a total score was used as a comprehensive evaluation of hydrophobic complementarity, polar complementarity, solvation terms, and entropic terms. When a total score is higher than 7, the interaction between the protein and molecule is considered as stable.

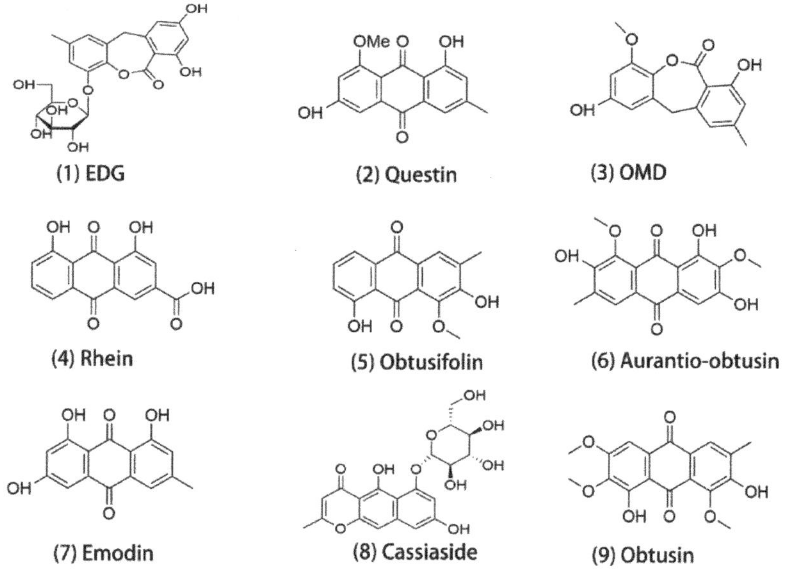

Figure 1. Structures of the 9 major components identified in rat plasma after 28 days of CSAEs administration. EDG, *Epi*-9-dehydroxyeurotinone-*β*-D-glucopyranoside; OMD, 2-*O*-methyl-9-dehydroxyeurotinone.

2.9. RNA Isolation and RT-qPCR

Quantitative reverse-transcription polymerase chain reaction (RT-qPCR) was performed to examine the expression of genes related to the RhoA–ROCK pathway. Total ribonucleic acid (RNA) was isolated from kidney tissues using TRIzol reagent (Invitrogen, Carlsbad, CA, USA). Subsequently, complementary deoxyribonucleic acid (cDNA) was synthesized from 10 μL of total RNA using a reverse-transcriptase reaction. To quantify the relative messenger RNA (mRNA) expression, the primers were synthesized, as shown in Table S1, with *Gapdh* used as the internal reference. Relative mRNA expression was calculated using the $2^{-\Delta\Delta Ct}$ method, and the fold change was normalized to the expression levels of control animals.

2.10. Western Blotting

Total protein was extracted from kidneys by RIPA buffer supplemented with proteinase inhibitors and phosphatase inhibitors and then centrifuged at 14,000× *g* for 5 min at 4 °C. The protein concentration in the supernatant was measured using the BCA method and denatured at 100 °C for 10 min. Equal amounts of protein (15 μg) were separated on a 4–15% precast gel and then electrophoretically transferred to polyvinylidene difluoride membranes at 220 mA for 120 min. The membranes were blocked with 5% bovine serum albumin in Tris-buffered saline with 0.1% Tween 20 (TBST) buffer for 120 min at room temperature and then rinsed three times in TBST for 10 min. The membranes were incubated with primary antibodies in TBST overnight at 4 °C, and then blots were probed by incubation with a secondary antibody for 120 min at room temperature. Finally, the proteins were visualized using ECL chemiluminescence solution and imaged by a Tanon 4500 System (Tanon, Shanghai, China).

2.11. Statistical Analysis

Data analyses were performed using SPSS 22.0 software (IBM, New York, NY, USA). All data are presented as means ± standard deviation (SD), and statistical significance was tested by one-way analysis of variance (ANOVA) followed by a least-significant difference test (LSD) for multiple comparisons as appropriate. A p value < 0.05 was considered statistically significant.

3. Results

3.1. Administration of CSAEs Induces Nephrotoxicity in Rats

To evaluate the effects of *Cassiae* semen on renal functions, rats were treated with different doses of CSAEs for 7–28 days. Renal injury was examined by the measurement of serum and urine biomarkers. Increases in Cr and BUN are critical manifestations of acute kidney injury. We did not observe obvious dose- or time-dependent effects in either male or female rats. However, when compared to the control group at days 7, 14, and 28, the levels of Cr and BUN in male rats treated with medium dose and the BUN levels in female rats treated with low dose were significantly elevated (Figure 2). According to the RIFLE criteria, a 1.5-fold increase in Cr level indicates an increased risk of renal injury and a 2-fold increase indicates renal injury [22]. We thus postulated that CSAEs may cause mild damage to kidneys, which led us to further investigate using urinalysis.

Then, we analyzed urinary levels of renal damage marker proteins KIM-1, OPN, calbindin, β2M, cystatin C, and NGAL (Figures 3 and 4, Table S2). Compared to control rats, urinary levels of KIM-1, OPN, and calbindin proteins were markedly increased in male rats treated with 15.75 or 47.30 g/kg of CSAEs for 7 to 28 days (Figure 3A,C,E). In female rats, a significant rise in KIM-1 protein level was noted at day 7 of CSAEs treatment, which became comparable with control animals at later time points (Figure 3B). By contrast, similar to male rats, the urinary levels of OPN and calbindin proteins remained significantly higher for all three treatment durations when compared to time-matched control rats (Figure 3D,F).

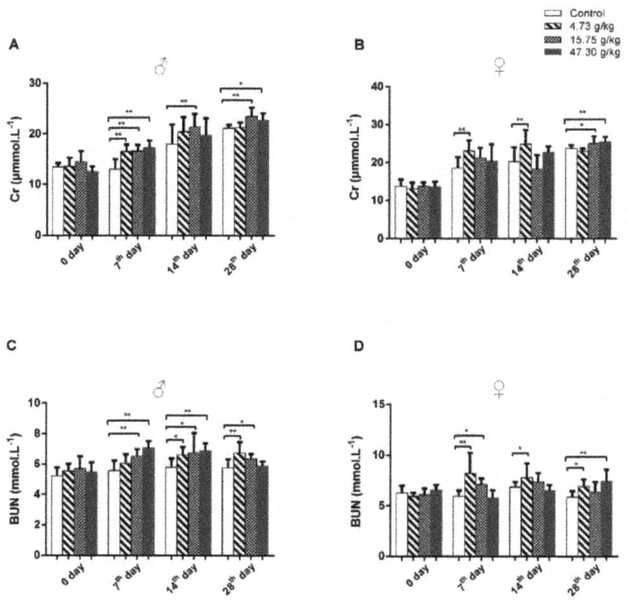

Figure 2. CSAEs increased serum Cr and BUN levels in rats. Male and female SD rats were treated with CSAEs (4.73, 15.75, and 47.3 g/kg/day) for 7—28 days. Serum was collected after the final treatment at each time point. (**A**,**B**) Serum Cr levels in male (**A**) and female (**B**) rats; (**C**,**D**) serum BUN levels in male (**C**) and female (**D**) rats. * and ** indicate $p < 0.05$ and $p < 0.01$, respectively, when compared with the vehicle control rats; $n = 8$ in each sex.

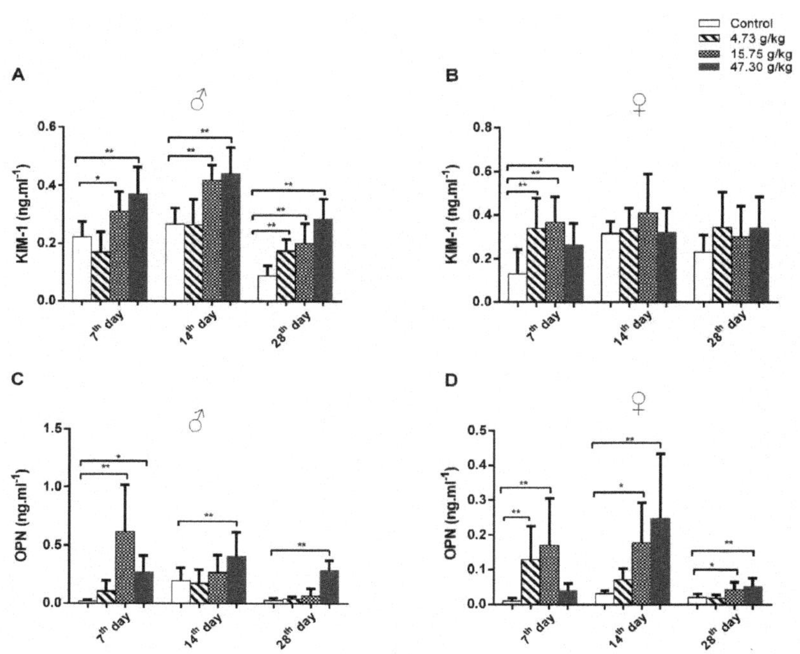

Figure 3. *Cont.*

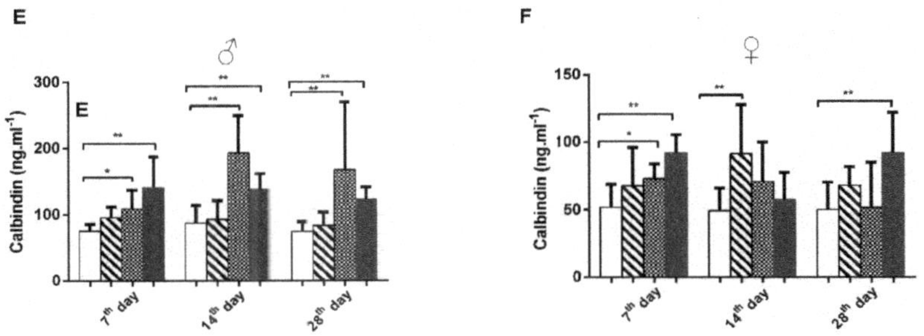

Figure 3. CSAEs increased urinary KIM−1, OPN, and calbindin protein levels in rats. Male and female SD rats were treated with CSAEs (4.73, 15.75, and 47.3 g/kg/day). Urine was collected after the final treatment on days 7, 14, and 28. (**A**,**C**,**E**) Levels of KIM−1, OPN, and calbindin in male rats; (**B**,**D**,**F**) results of the female rats. * and ** indicate $p < 0.05$ and $p < 0.01$, respectively, when compared with the vehicle control rats; $n = 8$ in each sex.

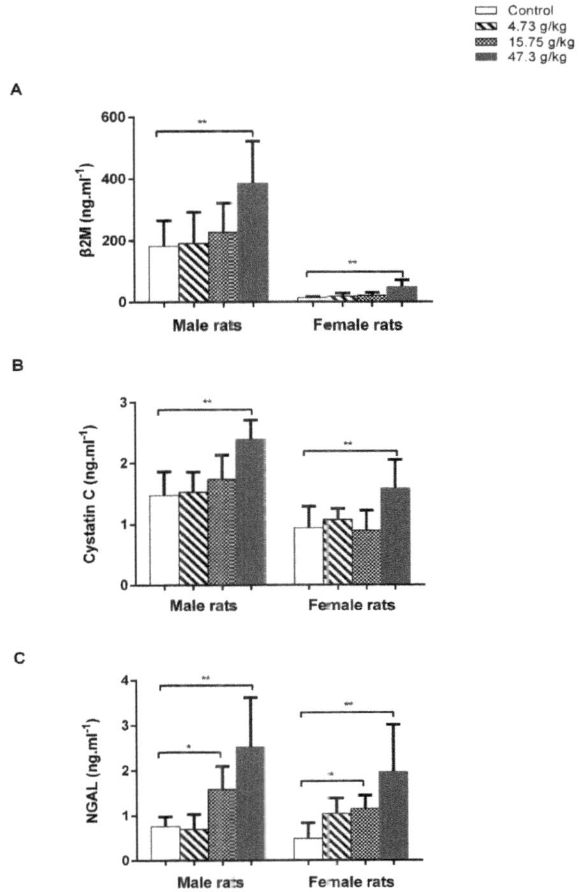

Figure 4. CSAEs−induced elevation in β2M, cystatin C, and NGAL levels in urine. Male and female SD rats were treated with AECS (4.73, 15.75, and 47.3 g/kg/day). Urine was collected after the final treatment on day 28. β2M (**A**), cystatin C (**B**), and NGAL (**C**) levels were measured by assay kits. * and ** indicate $p < 0.05$ and $p < 0.01$, respectively, when compared with the vehicle control rats; $n = 8$ in each sex.

We further determined the urinary levels of β2M, cystatin C, and NGAL on day 28 of CSAEs treatment. Results showed that treatment of CSAEs, particularly at the highest dose (47.30 g/kg), caused obvious increases in the levels of these three marker proteins in both male and female animals (Figure 4). Interestingly, we noted a significant difference in the urinary β2M levels between male and female rats at basal and CSAEs-treated conditions, while there was no such difference for cystatin C and NGAL proteins (Figure 4). Tsuji et al. compared the urinary biomarker excretion levels between male and female rats at 5, 7, 9, and 12 weeks of age, and revealed higher excretion levels of β2-microglobulin (β2-MG) in male rats than female rats [23], in line with our findings. Despite such sex differences in absolute amounts, both male and female rats showed the same pattern, but with changes by different extents in nephrotoxicity markers after the administration of CSAEs. Together, these data demonstrate that high doses of CSAEs treatment cause renal damage as early as day 7 in both male and female rats.

3.2. Changes in Organ Coefficients and Histopathology by CSAEs Administration

As presented in Figure 5, compared to the control group, the organ coefficients of the kidneys were significantly increased in all treatment groups of both male and female rats. These increased approximately 25% in male and female rats treated with the highest dose (47.30 g/kg) of CSAEs.

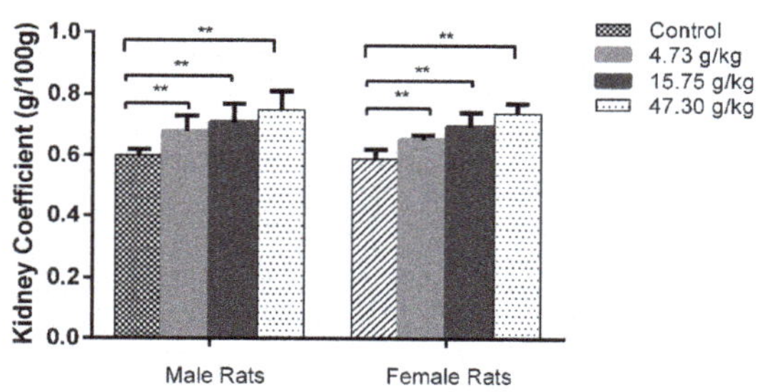

Figure 5. Kidney coefficients of male and female rats after a 28-day repeated oral dose toxicity study of AECS. ** $p < 0.01$ compared with the control ($n = 8$).

The histopathological changes in kidney tissues after CSAEs treatment were presented in Figure 6. Compared to the well-characterized normal kidney tissue structures in control rats, morphological changes in the kidney were evident in all treatment groups and both sexes, as evidenced by larger and swelling glomeruli, shrunken or even disappearance of glomerular capsules, tubular dilatation and congestion, and the presence of protein cast or granular cast in the renal tubular lumen. Thus, these results also support the presence of renal toxicity in CSAEs-treated rats. As there is no obvious difference between male and female rats in most biochemical and histopathological markers, only male rats were employed for the following mechanistic investigation.

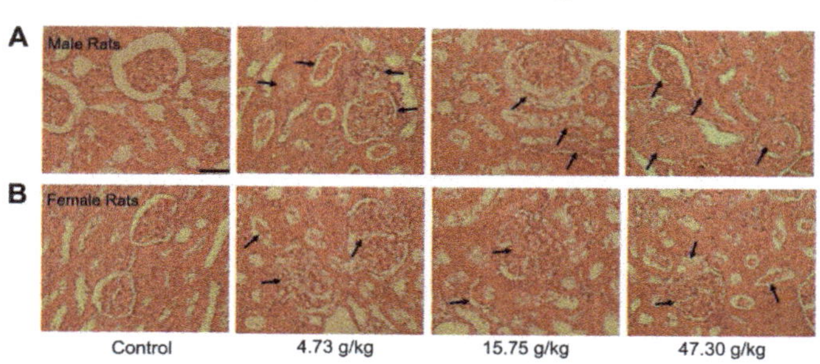

Figure 6. Representative histopathological images of male (**A**) and female (**B**) rats after administration of CSAEs for 28 days. Arrows indicate the damaged glomerulus tubes. Scale bar = 50 μm; $n = 8$.

3.3. Molecular Docking Predicts the Potential Mechanisms of CSAEs-Induced Kidney Injury

To examine the underlying mechanisms mediating CSAEs-induced nephrotoxicity, we applied an in silico approach to evaluate the molecular interactions between nine major components in CSAEs and the key regulatory proteins of four pathways known for their involvement in kidney injury. As shown in Figure 7 and Table S3, there were 14, 7, 13, and 12 proteins in the RhoA–ROCK pathway, apoptosis pathway, calcium regulation pathway, and necrosis pathway, respectively, which correspondingly generated 51, 9, 45, and 36 compound–protein complexes with a total score higher than 7 in these four pathways. Of note, the percentage of target proteins for the nine major components in the Rho and Rho-associated coiled-coil protein kinase (ROCK) pathway was greater than that in the other three pathways. The overall docking situation was shown in Table S4. These results indicate a direct interaction between the nine major components in CSAEs and the RhoA–ROCK pathway.

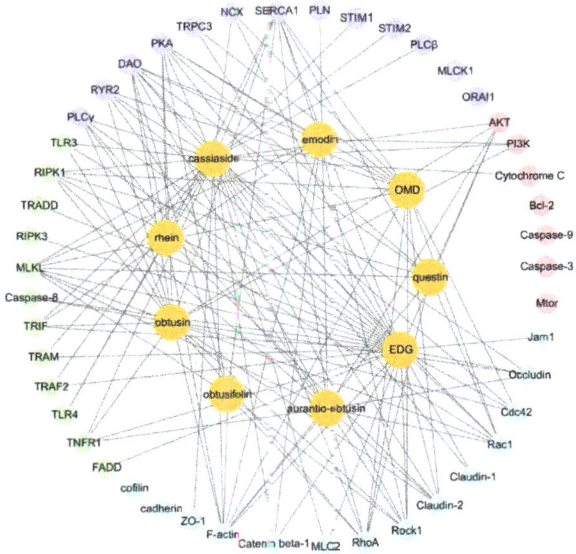

Figure 7. Cytoscape shows the interactions between 9 major components of CSAEs and 4 known kidney injury pathways. The RhoA–ROCK pathway, apoptosis pathway, calcium regulation pathway, and necrosis pathway are represented by blue, pink, purple, and green, respectively.

We next examined how the RhoA–ROCK pathway could possibly interact with the components of CSAEs. Since obtusifolin, aurantio-obtusin, and obtusin were the three most abundant components of CSAEs, we focused on these compounds for exemplary illustration. Intriguingly, all of obtusifolin, aurantio-obtusin, and obtusin were found to directly bind to F-actin, ROCK1, occludin, and Rac1 proteins through the formation of different degrees of hydrogen bonds and hydrophobic bonds (Figures 8–10 and Table S5). Specifically, obtusin and aurantio-obtusin bonded with Rac1 via hydrogen bonds formed by the interaction with Ala159 (A) and Lys116 (A). Obtusin and obtusifolin bound to ROCK1 via hydrogen bonds formed by the interaction with Phe87 (C) and Ala86 (C). Obtusin and obtusifolin bound to F-actin via hydrogen bonds formed by interactions with Asp153 (A), Gln136 (A), Gly14 (A), and Leu15 (A), while aurantio-obtusin interacted with Lys335 (A) and Glu213 (A). Thus, these computational predictions imply that the RhoA–ROCK signaling pathway and F-actin could be potential targets of CSAEs.

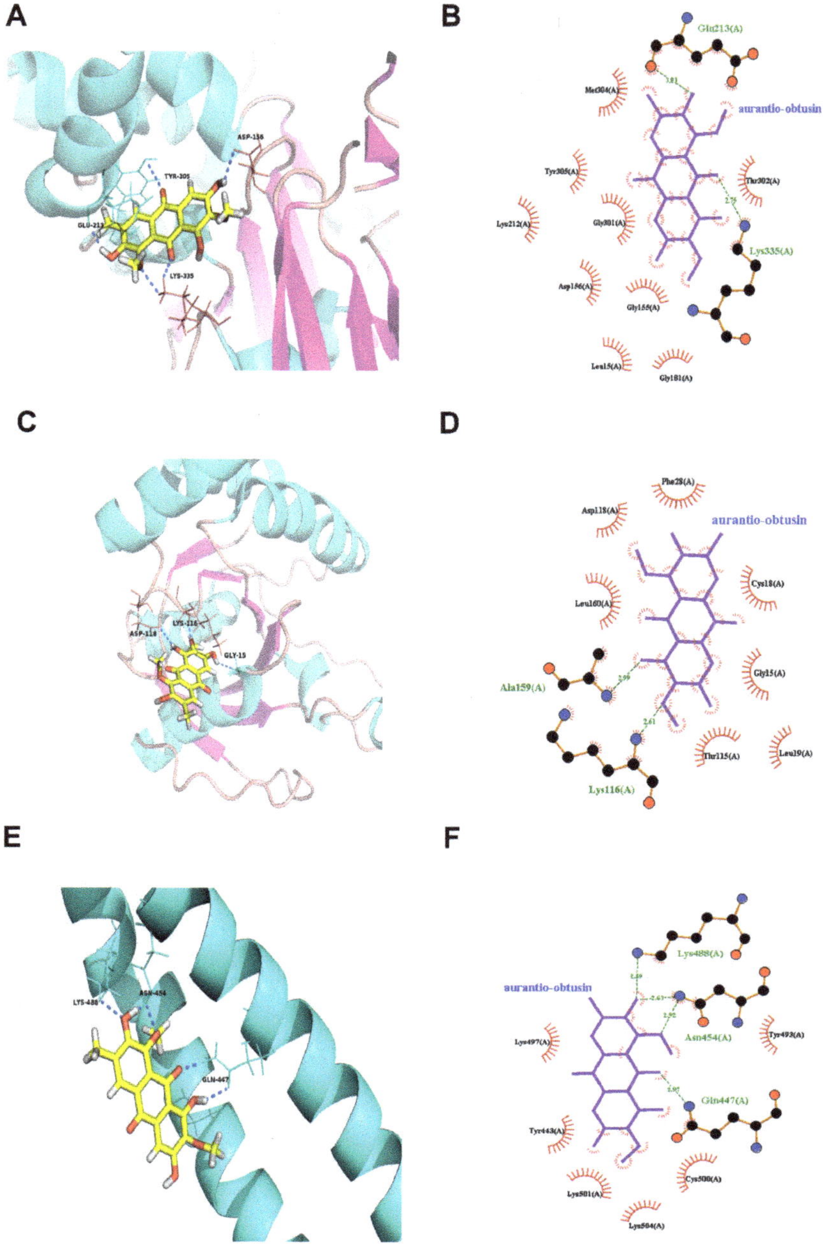

Figure 8. Molecular docking of aurantio-obtusin into the active sites of human F-actin (**A**,**B**), Rac1 (**C**,**D**), and occludin (**E**,**F**). The 3D structure is shown in panels (**A**,**C**,**E**), while the 2D structure is shown in panels (**B**,**D**,**F**).

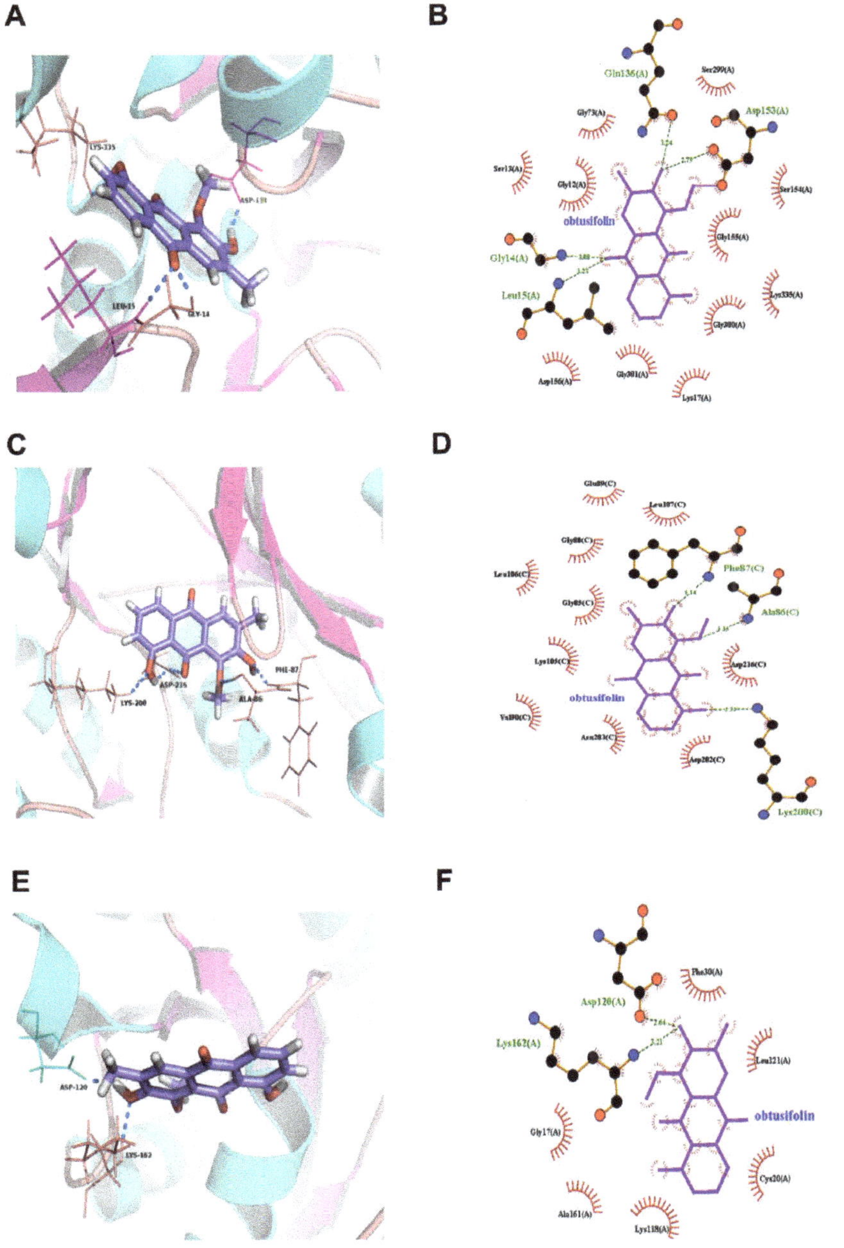

Figure 9. Molecular docking of obtusifolin into the active sites of human F-actin (**A**,**B**), Rock1 (**C**,**D**), and RhoA (**E**,**F**). The 3D structure is shown in panels (**A**,**C**,**E**), while the 2D structure is shown in panels (**B**,**D**,**F**).

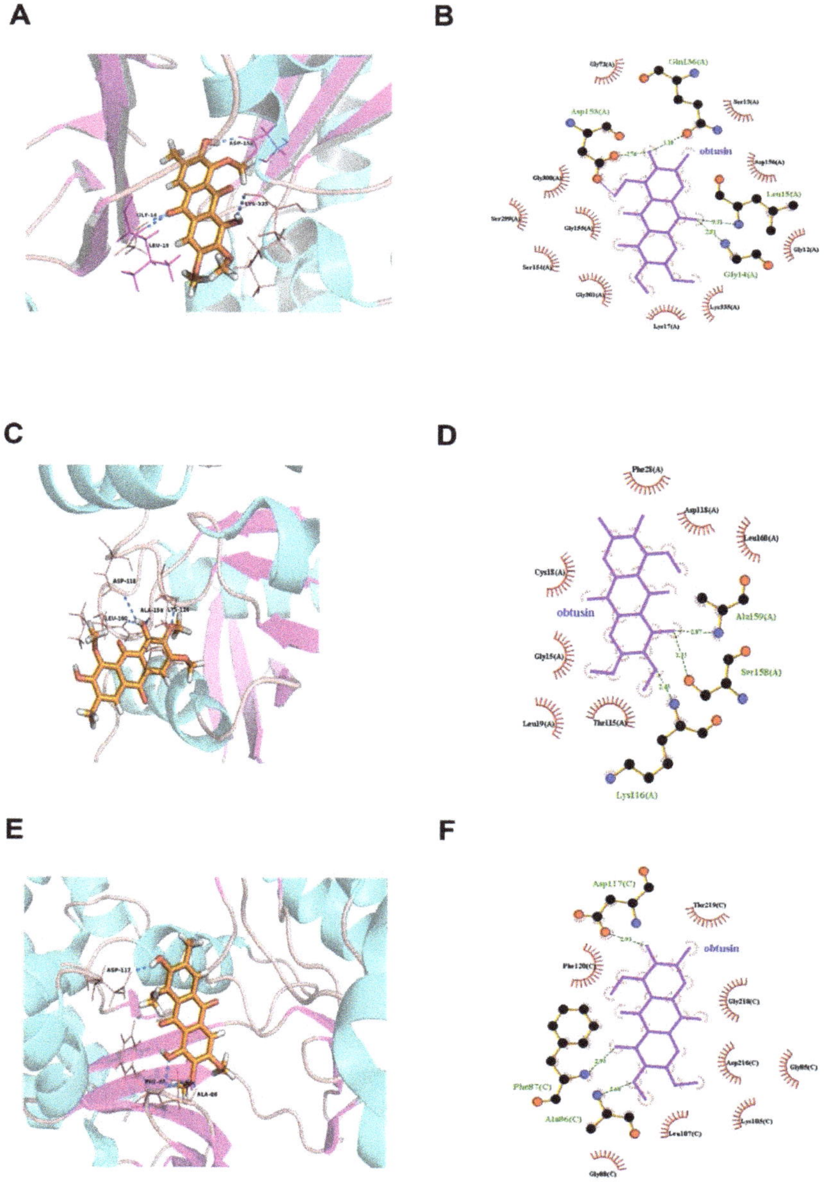

Figure 10. Molecular docking of obtusin into the active sites of human F-actin (**A**,**B**), Rac1 (**C**,**D**), and Rock1 (**E**,**F**). The 3D structure is shown in panels (**A**,**C**,**E**), while the 2D structure is presented in panels (**B**,**D**,**F**).

3.4. F-Actin Protein Expression Was Inhibited in the Kidneys of CSAEs-Treated Rats

To validate the in silico prediction findings, F-actin expression was determined in rat kidneys after 28 days of administration of CSAEs. Results from immunofluorescence staining showed that compared to intact cytoskeleton and membrane structure as well as clear brush borders in the proximal tubules of control rats, F-actin expression was significantly suppressed in the kidneys of CSAEs-treated rats, which was accompanied by disrupted membrane and brush borders in renal cells (Figure 11). Together with computational prediction, these results identify that F-actin is a toxic action target of CSAEs.

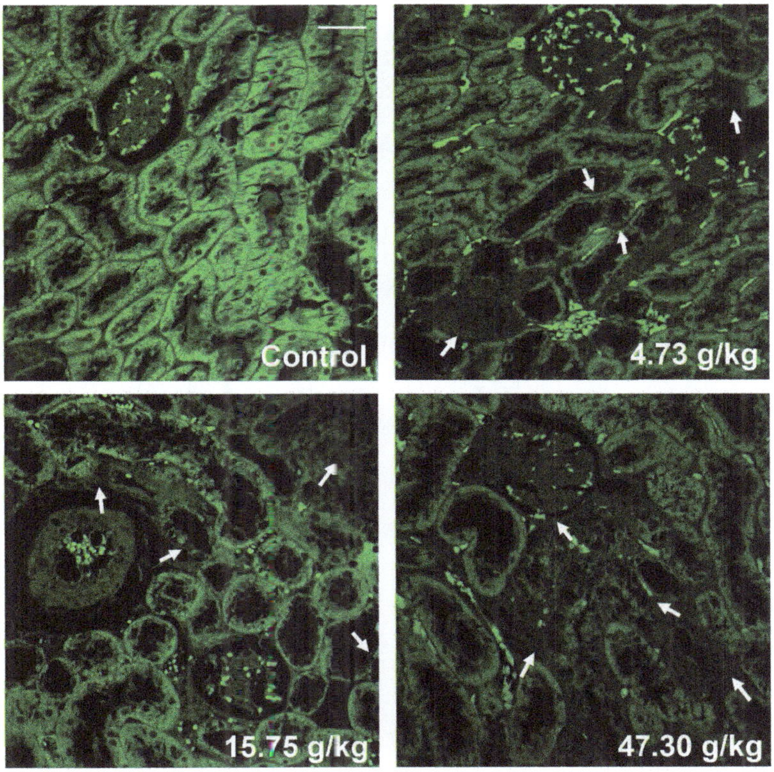

Figure 11. Immunofluorescence staining showing F-actin expression was inhibited in kidney tissues in CSAEs-treated rats. Alexa 488 phalloidin staining for F-actin (green) in the kidneys of male rats after administration of CSAEs for 28 days. The injury sites are indicated by white arrows. Scale bar = 50 μm; *n* = 8.

3.5. The RhoA–ROCK Pathway Is Inhibited by CSAEs

To elucidate the molecular mechanisms mediating F-actin disruption by CSAEs, we focused on the RhoA–ROCK pathway, since cytoskeleton formation is partially controlled by the activity of this pathway and our in silico analyses suggested possible interactions between CSAEs and regulatory proteins of this pathway. Actin filament assembly/disassembly can be regulated by cofilins that integrate transmembrane signals to coordinate the spatial and temporal organization of actin filaments [24]. These transmembrane signals mainly involve cell–cell junctions, such as ZO-1, occludin, claudin, and JAMs [25]. As expected, the mRNA expressions of *RhoA*, *Rac1*, *ROCK1*, *actin*, *cofilin*, *CDC42*, *ZO-1*, and *JAM1* were significantly and dose-dependently downregulated in renal tissues of rats treated with higher doses of CSAEs (15.75 and 47.30 g/kg) (Figure 12A–C). Similar effects were also observed in *JAM4* and *occludin* mRNA expression, despite their mRNA levels being significantly induced in rats treated with low-dose CSAEs (4.73 g/kg), and the expression of *claudin-1* mRNA was also stimulated by CSAEs (Figure 12A).

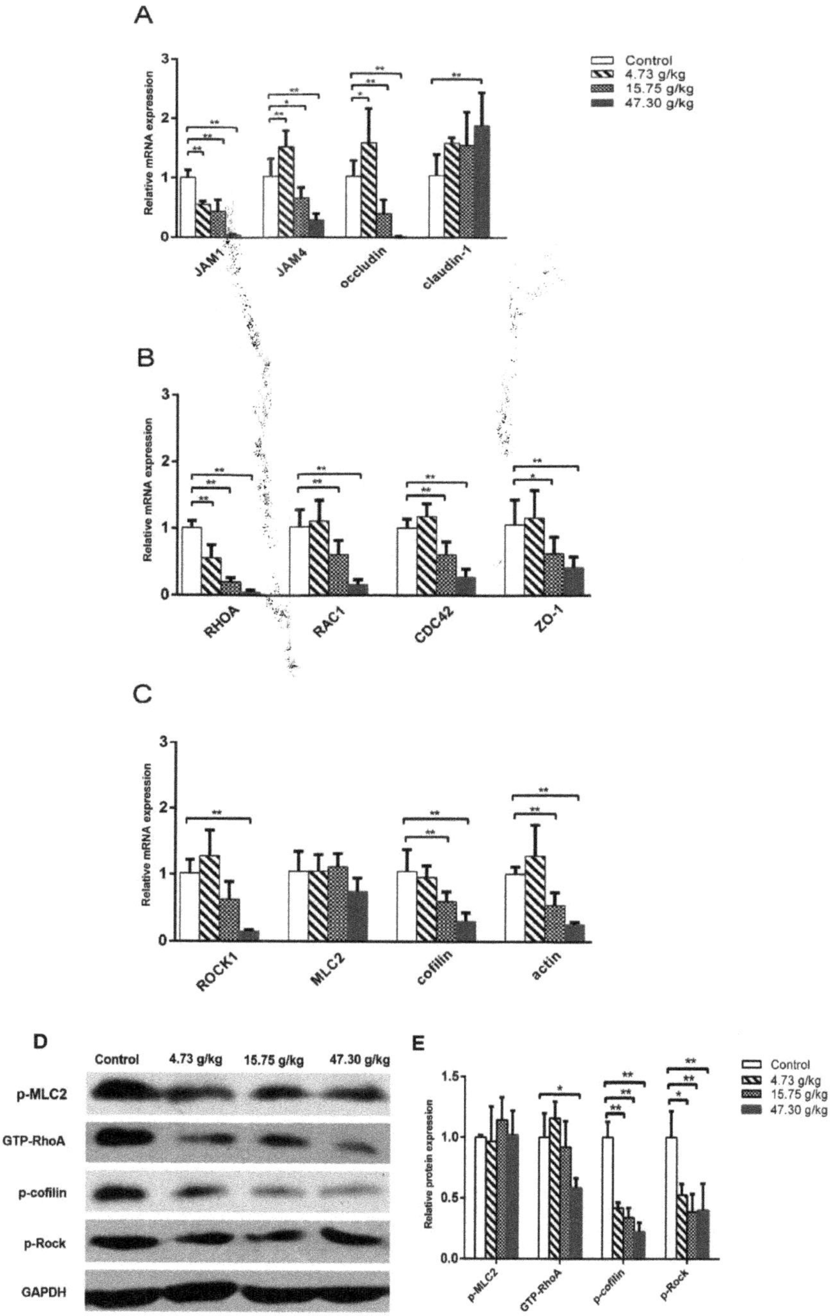

Figure 12. Effects of CSAEs on the expression of key regulatory genes of F-actin formation, assembly, and stabilization in the kidneys. Male SD rats were treated with CSAEs at the indicated doses for 28 days. The mRNA expression (**A–C**) was normalized to *Gapdh* mRNA, and protein expression (**D**) was normalized by GAPDH protein. Fold change (**E**) was calculated relative to untreated control rats. * and ** indicate $p < 0.05$ and $p < 0.01$, respectively, when compared with the vehicle control rats, n = 3.

In line with the mRNA expression profile, kidney tissue from CSAEs-treated rats expressed lower levels of GTP-RhoA protein and phosphorylated ROCK and cofilin proteins than that of control rats, while no changes were observed in phosphorylated levels of MLC2 protein (Figure 12D,E). The results suggest that CSAEs can inhibit the RhoA–ROCK–cofilin pathway, leading to disruption of actin depolymerization and F-actin stabilization and consequently renal toxicity.

4. Discussion

In earlier studies, Lee et al. [26] reported that *Cassia tora* Linn seed ethanol extract exhibited no treatment-related adverse effects, even at doses of over 2000 mg/kg/day in both sexes in rats, and no target organs were identified. Gao et al. [5] investigated the subchronic toxicity of ethanol extract of *Cassiae* semen. They detected increasing levels of BUN in 25, 35, and 45 g/kg B.W. dose groups and pigmentation in the kidney in 45 g/kg B.W. group, but they did not detect the main components of ethanol extract. Pei et al. [6] observed pigment deposition in the epithelial cells of the renal proximal convoluted tubules and atrophy or regeneration of renal tubules in SD rats after treatment with 10 g/kg B.W./day of freeze-dried powdered *Cassiae* semen, whose main compounds are anthraquinones, for 26 weeks. They also found that the male rats were more sensitive to freeze-dried powdered *Cassiae* semen than the female rats. Our findings were distinct from the observations of that study. In the present study, we obtained new findings in both renal effects and action mechanisms in rats treated with 4.73–47.30 g/kg B.W. of CSAEs for 28 days, and concluded that obtusifolin, aurantio-obtusin, and obtusin may disrupt the cytoskeleton by interacting with F-actin, Rac1, and ROCK1 after 28 days of administration of CSAEs.

The increase in Cr and BUN in serum indicated the risk of renal injury, while the increase in KIM-1, cystatin C, and β2M in urine and the changes in kidney histopathology indicated that CSAEs caused dysfunction of glomerular filtration and tubular damage. Brush borders, which are developed by kidney tubule epithelial cells, increase the cell surface and are required for the digestion and absorption of lumen components, which are vital to tubular reabsorption. Brush borders are mainly constituted by microvilli, and are single apical poles rich in cylindrical membrane protrusions. Each microvillus has an actin bundle backbone that is composed of 19 actin filaments [27]. F-actin staining demonstrated the disappearance of the brush border, which indicated that dysregulation of the actin cytoskeleton could be the main cause of kidney injury after 28 days of CSAEs administration.

Few experimental studies have shed new light on molecular and cellular mechanisms of *Cassiae* semen-induced nephrotoxicity. Huang et al. found that the mitochondrial pathway is involved in the nephrotoxicity induced by rhein, emodin, and aurantio-obtusin [28]. However, our previous study indicated that obtusifolin, aurantio-obtusin, and obtusin have high plasma concentrations and can accumulate in rat plasma after 28 days of administration of CSAEs [7]. In addition, apoptosis and necrosis are often related to mitochondrial dysfunction in the kidney [29], suggesting that the apoptosis pathway and necrosis pathway may not be core pathways. Therefore, obtusifolin, aurantio-obtusin, and obtusin were regarded as major nephrotoxicity components in CSAEs and may be involved in another pathway. In this study, according to the results of the composition–target interaction network model, most key regulatory proteins are related to the Rho–ROCK pathway, and actin is closely related to the RhoA–ROCK pathway.

We first explored the effects of *Cassiae* semen on regulating the actin cytoskeleton using molecular docking. The results indicated that the components in *Cassiae* semen are more likely to directly regulate the actin cytoskeleton through interaction between the key proteins in the RhoA–ROCK pathways, especially the proteins F-actin, Rac1, ROCK1, and occludin. The RhoA–ROCK signaling has been extensively investigated since it is critically involved in cell growth, differentiation, migration, cell contraction, adhesion, inflammation, and survival from apoptosis [30,31]. Rho GTPases act as molecular switches in the cell by cycling between the inactive GDP-bound state and the active GTP-bound state. The activation of RhoA stimulates ROCK, the downstream effector that phosphorylates LIM kinase (LIMK), myosin light chain (MLC), and cofilin, subsequently impacting some cellular processes [32], such as actin cytoskeleton remodeling, cell adhesion and migration, reactive oxygen species (ROS) formation, and cell apoptosis [33]. A study showed that inactivation of the Rho–ROCK1 pathway was associated with significant improvement in proteinuria and tubulointerstitial fibrosis, and could affect kidney function in small congenic regions (e.g., RBF and GFR) [34]. Another study revealed that in canine kidney cells, apoptosis could be induced through mitochondrial malfunction and cytoskeleton disassembly [21].

Therefore, we turned to the molecular level to see whether the RhoA–ROCK pathway played the most important role in our model. Results of RT-PCR and Western blot showed that GTP-RhoA, and p-cofilin, but not p-MLC-2, were downregulated at the protein level, while mRNAs related to upstream proteins (ZO-1, RAC1, JAM1, JAM4, occludin, claudin, and CDC42) were downregulated as well. This indicated that *Cassiae* semen preferred to impact the activity of cofilin rather than MLC2. It has reported that ROCK can promote the increase of intracellular Ca^{2+} concentration through the activation of Ca^{2+}/calmodulin-dependent MLCK, resulting in the phosphorylation of MLC2 [35]. Thus, we speculate that the calcium regulation pathway can also be a secondary pathway. Whether cofilin promotes actin assembly or disassembly depends on the concentration of cofilin relative to actin and the relative concentrations of other actin-binding proteins. When the ratio of cofilin/actin subunits in the filament is low (less than 1%), persistent filament severing occurs. Cofilin severs rapidly but transiently at higher cofilin/actin molar ratios because it binds to F-actin cooperatively and stabilizes F-actin in a twisted form as it saturates the severed pieces [36]. As an actin depolymerizing factor, cofilin can be blocked by activating the RhoA–LIMK–cofilin pathway [37], and dephosphorylation of cofilin enhances the activation to induce apoptosis [38]. In the present study, we demonstrated that *Cassiae* semen can interact with transmembrane signals, impact the RhoA–ROCK pathway, and lead to a change in cofilin and actin cytoskeleton, and that the main components of CSAEs can influence actin by the RhoA–ROCK pathway or bind directly to F-actin. It has been shown that the Rho family small G protein Rac–GTP signaling pathway phosphorylates LIMK1 at Thr508 and LIMK2 at Thr505 by p21-activated kinases 1 and 4, which further led to phosphorylation of cofilin at Ser3 [39]. Activated cofilin converts the polymer F-actin into monomer G-actin, which in turn affects the formation of the cytoskeleton. The loss of p-cofilin decreased the stability of F-actin. However, the exact molecular initiation event is still worthy of further investigation because CSAEs are a mixture. Our findings indicate the disruption of actin as a key event of CSAEs-mediated nephrotoxicity in rats.

In conclusion, we demonstrated that *Cassiae* semen can cause nephrotoxicity after 28 days of repeated administration in rats and that the potential action mechanisms were the abnormal structure of glomeruli and tubules, especially tubules, which manifested as the disappearance of F-actin (Figure 13). Taking together the results of molecular docking and the nephrotoxicity mechanism, *Cassiae* semen impacts actin cytoskeleton depolymerization and filament stabilization by interacting with the RhoA–ROCK pathway and/or directly binding to F-actin.

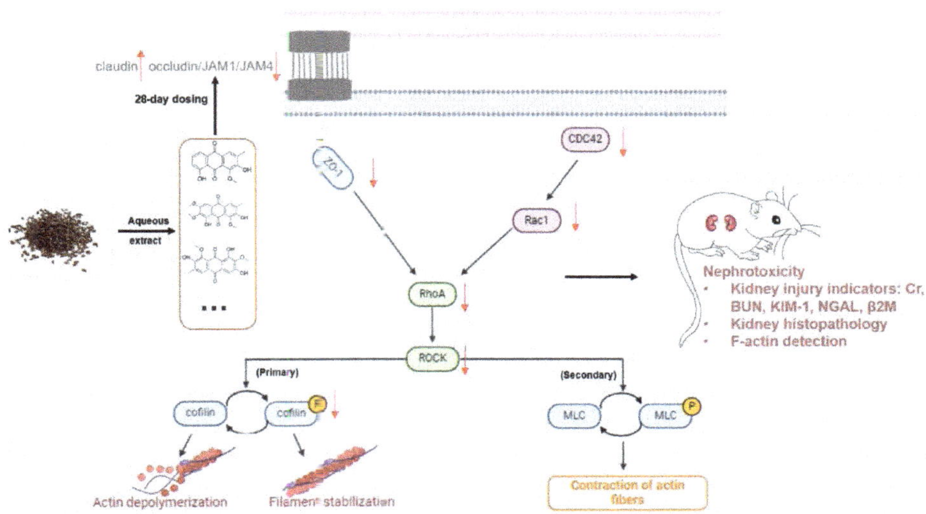

Figure 13. Schematic illustration showing dysregulation of actin dynamics by CSAEs via the RhoA–ROCK signaling pathway.

Supplementary Materials: The following supporting information can be downloaded at https://www.mdpi.com/article/10.3390/toxics12080556/s1. Table S1: Primer sequences; Table S2: The meaning of kidney injury indicators; Table S3: The target proteins in different renal injury pathways; Table S4: The interactions between 9 major components and 4 kidney injury pathways by molecular docking; Table S5: Molecular interactions between 3 anthraquinones extracted from Cassiae Semen and proteins of RhoA–ROCK.

Author Contributions: J.Y.: conceptualization, formal analysis, investigation, visualization, writing—original draft. S.X.: formal analysis, visualization, writing—original draft, writing—review and editing. L.L.: formal analysis, writing—original draft, writing—review and editing. A.Z.: investigation, writing—review and editing. W.X.: writing—review and editing. Q.W.: conceptualization, funding acquisition, project administration, supervision, writing—review and editing. All data were generated in-house, and no paper mill was used. All authors agree to be accountable for all aspects of work, ensuring integrity and accuracy. All authors have read and agreed to the published version of the manuscript.

Funding: This research was funded by the China Special Research Project of Traditional Chinese Medicine, grant number [201507004-1].

Institutional Review Board Statement: The animal study protocol was approved by the Animal Experimental Ethical Committee of Peking University (LA2017227, Beijing, China).

Informed Consent Statement: Not applicable.

Data Availability Statement: All data are available upon reasonable request to the corresponding author.

Conflicts of Interest: The authors declare no conflicts of interest.

References

1. Dong, X.; Fu, J.; Yin, X.; Yang, C.; Zhang, X.; Wang, W.; Du, X.; Wang, Q.; Ni, J. Cassiae semen: A review of its phytochemistry and pharmacology (Review). *Mol. Med. Rep.* **2017**, *16*, 2331–2346. [CrossRef]
2. Yuen, H.; Hong Yang, A.W.; Hung, A.; Lenon, G.B. How does traditional knowledge of Cassiae semen shed light on weight management?—A classical and modern literature review. *J. Ethnopharmacol.* **2021**, *268*, 113572. [CrossRef]
3. Xie, W.; Zhao, Y.; Du, L. Emerging approaches of traditional Chinese medicine formulas for the treatment of hyperlipidemia. *J. Ethnopharmacol.* **2012**, *140*, 345–367. [CrossRef]

4. Chen, Y.; Chen, X.; Yang, X.; Gao, P.; Yue, C.; Wang, L.; Wu, T.; Jiang, T.; Wu, H.; Tang, L.; et al. Cassiae Semen: A comprehensive review of botany, traditional use, phytochemistry, pharmacology, toxicity, and quality control. *J. Ethnopharmacol.* **2023**, *306*, 116199. [CrossRef]
5. Gao, P.; Sui, H.; Liu, H.B.; Zhi, Y.; Wang, H.L.; Yang, H.; Yu, Z.; Liu, C.X. A 90-day subchronic toxicity study on Semen Cassiae ethanol extract. *Chin. J. Food Hyg.* **2004**, *16*, 410–415.
6. Pei, Y.; Wei, R.; Sun, J.; Gao, H. Safety assessment of freeze-dried powdered Cassiae Semen: Evaluation of chronic toxicity (26-week) in Sprague-Dawley rats. *Toxicol. Rep.* **2017**, *4*, 143–150. [CrossRef]
7. Yang, J.; Zhu, A.; Xiao, S.; Zhang, T.; Wang, L.; Wang, Q.; Han, L. Anthraquinones in the aqueous extract of Cassiae semen cause liver injury in rats through lipid metabolism disorder. *Phytomedicine* **2019**, *64*, 153059. [CrossRef]
8. Hu, M.; Zhong, Y.; Liu, J.; Zheng, S.; Lin, L.; Lin, X.; Liang, B.; Huang, Y.; Xian, H.; Li, Z.; et al. An adverse outcome pathway-based approach to assess aurantio-obtusin-induced hepatotoxicity. *Toxicology* **2022**, *478*, 153293. [CrossRef]
9. Qin, S.-H.; Xu, Y.; Li, K.-L.; Gong, K.-Y.; Peng, J.; Shi, S.-L.; Yan, F.; Cai, W. Identification of Metabolites of Aurantio-Obtusin in Rats Using Ultra-High-Performance Liquid Chromatography-Q-Exactive Orbitrap Mass Spectrometry with Parallel Reaction Monitoring. *J. Anal. Methods Chem.* **2021**, *2021*, 6630604. [CrossRef]
10. Huang, Z.; Sun, Q.; Hao, W.; Zhao, J. Pharmacokinetics and tissue distribution study of obtusifolin in rats by liquid chromatography-tandem mass spectrometry. *Biomed. Chromatogr.* **2021**, *35*, e5009. [CrossRef]
11. Yang, C.; Wang, S.; Guo, X.; Sun, J.; Liu, L.; Wu, L. Simultaneous determination of seven anthraquinones in rat plasma by Ultra High Performance Liquid Chromatography-tandem Mass Spectrometry and pharmacokinetic study after oral administration of Semen Cassiae extract. *J. Ethnopharmacol.* **2015**, *169*, 305–313. [CrossRef]
12. Luyckx, V.A. Nephrotoxicity of alternative medicine practice. *Adv. Chronic Kidney Dis.* **2012**, *19*, 129–141. [CrossRef]
13. Yang, B.; Xie, Y.; Guo, M.; Rosner, M.H.; Yang, H.; Ronco, C. Nephrotoxicity and Chinese Herbal Medicine. *Clin. J. Am. Soc. Nephrol.* **2018**, *13*, 1605–1611. [CrossRef]
14. Mally, A.; Jarzina, S. Mapping Adverse Outcome Pathways for Kidney Injury as a Basis for the Development of Mechanism-Based Animal-Sparing Approaches to Assessment of Nephrotoxicity. *Front. Toxicol.* **2022**, *4*, 863643. [CrossRef]
15. Dominguez, R.; Holmes, K.C. Actin structure and function. *Annu. Rev. Biophys.* **2011**, *40*, 169–186. [CrossRef]
16. Descazeaud, V.; Mestre, E.; Marquet, P.; Essig, M. Calcineurin regulation of cytoskeleton organization: A new paradigm to analyse the effects of calcineurin inhibitors on the kidney. *J. Cell. Mol. Med.* **2012**, *16*, 218–227. [CrossRef]
17. Burridge, K.; Wennerberg, K. Rho and Rac take center stage. *Cell* **2004**, *116*, 167–179. [CrossRef]
18. Cai, R.; Wang, Y.; Huang, Z.; Zou, Q.; Pu, Y.; Yu, C.; Cai, Z. Role of RhoA/ROCK signaling in Alzheimer's disease. *Behav. Brain Res.* **2021**, *414*, 113481. [CrossRef]
19. Shi, J.; Wei, L. Rho kinase in the regulation of cell death and survival. *Arch. Immunol. Ther. Exp.* **2007**, *55*, 61–75. [CrossRef]
20. Tomasella, A.; Blangy, A.; Brancolini, C. A receptor-interacting protein 1 (RIP1)-independent necrotic death under the control of protein phosphatase PP2A that involves the reorganization of actin cytoskeleton and the action of cofilin-1. *J. Biol. Chem.* **2014**, *289*, 25699–25710. [CrossRef]
21. Lee, J.Y.; Lee, J.; Lee, S.H.; Hwang, J.H.; Suh, H.N. Pelargonium sidoides extract mediates nephrotoxicity through mitochondrial malfunction and cytoskeleton destabilization. *Toxicol. Res.* **2023**, *39*, 601–609. [CrossRef]
22. Bellomo, R.; Ronco, C.; Kellum, J.A.; Mehta, R.L.; Palevsky, P. Acute renal failure—Definition, outcome measures, animal models, fluid therapy and information technology needs: The Second International Consensus Conference of the Acute Dialysis Quality Initiative (ADQI) Group. *Crit. Care* **2004**, *8*, R204–R212. [CrossRef]
23. Tsuji, S.; Sugiura, M.; Tsutsumi, S.; Yamada, H. Sex differences in the excretion levels of traditional and novel urinary biomarkers of nephrotoxicity in rats. *J. Toxicol. Sci.* **2017**, *42*, 615–627. [CrossRef]
24. Bamburg, J.R.; Bernstein, B.W. Roles of ADF/cofilin in actin polymerization and beyond. *F1000 Biol. Rep.* **2010**, *2*, 62. [CrossRef]
25. Hartsock, A.; Nelson, W.J. Adherens and tight junctions: Structure, function and connections to the actin cytoskeleton. *Biochim. Biophys. Acta* **2008**, *1778*, 660–669. [CrossRef]
26. Lee, M.-J.; Nho, J.-H.; Yang, B.-D.; Park, H.; Lee, H.-J.; Lee, K.-H.; Jang, J.-H.; Jung, H.-K.; Kim, S.-R.; Cho, H.-W.; et al. Subchronic toxicity evaluation of ethanol extract of *Cassia tora* L. seeds in rats. *Regul. Toxicol. Pharmacol.* **2019**, *109*, 104487. [CrossRef]
27. Brown, J.W.; McKnight, C.J. Molecular model of the microvillar cytoskeleton and organization of the brush border. *PLoS ONE* **2010**, *5*, e9406. [CrossRef]
28. Huang, Q.; Fan, M.; Ji, F.; Wang, Y.; Ding, H.; Xu, J.; Wang, X.; Liu, B.; Wang, B.; Yu, X.; et al. The safety evaluation of Shenze Shugan capsule and mechanism of apoptosis induced by five potentially nephrotoxic components. *J. Ethnopharmacol.* **2024**, *324*, 117777. [CrossRef]
29. Silva, J.P.; Araújo, A.M.; de Pinho, P.G.; Carmo, H.; Carvalho, F. Synthetic Cannabinoids JWH-122 and THJ-2201 Disrupt Endocannabinoid-Regulated Mitochondrial Function and Activate Apoptotic Pathways as a Primary Mechanism of In Vitro Nephrotoxicity at In Vivo Relevant Concentrations. *Toxicol. Sci.* **2019**, *169*, 422–435. [CrossRef]
30. Chen, K.; Zhang, W.; Chen, J.; Li, S.; Guo, G. Rho-associated protein kinase modulates neurite extension by regulating microtubule remodeling and vinculin distribution. *Neural Regen. Res.* **2013**, *8*, 3027–3035. [CrossRef]
31. Strassheim, D.; Gerasimovskaya, E.; Irwin, D.; Dempsey, E.C.; Stenmark, K.; Karoor, V. RhoGTPase in Vascular Disease. *Cells* **2019**, *8*, 551. [CrossRef]

32. Budzyn, K.; Marley, P.D.; Sobey, C.G. Targeting Rho and Rho-kinase in the treatment of cardiovascular disease. *Trends Pharmacol. Sci.* **2006**, *27*, 97–104. [CrossRef]
33. Riento, K.; Ridley, A.J. Rocks: Multifunctional kinases in cell behaviour. *Nat. Rev. Mol. Cell Biol.* **2003**, *4*, 446–456. [CrossRef]
34. Williams, J.M.; Johnson, A.C.; Stelloh, C.; Dreisbach, A.W.; Franceschini, N.; Regner, K.R.; Townsend, R.R.; Roman, R.J.; Garrett, M.R. Genetic variants in Arhgef11 are associated with kidney injury in the Dahl salt-sensitive rat. *Hypertension* **2012**, *60*, 1157–1168. [CrossRef]
35. Moreno, C.A.; Sobreira, N.; Pugh, E.; Zhang, P.; Steel, G.; Torres, F.R.; Cavalcanti, D.P. Homozygous deletion in MYL9 expands the molecular basis of megacystis-microcolon-intestinal hypoperistalsis syndrome. *Eur. J. Hum. Genet.* **2018**, *26*, 669–675. [CrossRef]
36. Andrianantoandro, E.; Pollard, T.D. Mechanism of actin filament turnover by severing and nucleation at different concentrations of ADF/cofilin. *Mol. Cell* **2006**, *24*, 13–23. [CrossRef]
37. Qiao, Y.; Chen, J.; Lim, Y.B.; Finch-Edmondson, M.L.; Seshachalam, V.P.; Qin, L.; Jiang, T.; Low, B.C.; Singh, H.; Lim, C.T.; et al. YAP Regulates Actin Dynamics through ARHGAP29 and Promotes Metastasis. *Cell Rep.* **2017**, *19*, 1495–1502. [CrossRef]
38. Chen, B.; Lin, W.; Qi, W.; Li, S.; Hong, Z.; Zhao, H. Cofilin Inhibition by Limk1 Reduces Rod Formation and Cell Apoptosis after Ischemic Stroke. *Neuroscience* **2020**, *444*, 64–75. [CrossRef]
39. Bernard, O. Lim kinases, regulators of actin dynamics. *Int. J. Biochem. Cell Biol.* **2007**, *39*, 1071–1076. [CrossRef]

Disclaimer/Publisher's Note: The statements, opinions and data contained in all publications are solely those of the individual author(s) and contributor(s) and not of MDPI and/or the editor(s). MDPI and/or the editor(s) disclaim responsibility for any injury to people or property resulting from any ideas, methods, instructions or products referred to in the content.

toxics

MDPI

Article

Risk Factors of Optic Neuropathy in Ethambutol Users: Interaction with Isoniazid and Other Associated Conditions of Toxic Optic Neuropathy

Jiyeong Kim [1] and Seong Joon Ahn [2,*]

[1] Department of Pre-Medicine, College of Medicine, and Biostatistics Lab, Medical Research Collaborating Center (MRCC), Hanyang University, Seoul 04763, Republic of Korea; kimzi@hanyang.ac.kr
[2] Department of Ophthalmology, Hanyang University Hospital, Hanyang University College of Medicine, Seoul 04763, Republic of Korea
* Correspondence: ahnsj81@gmail.com; Tel.: +82-2-2290-8574; Fax: +82-2-2291-8517

Abstract: (1) Background: To investigate the risk factors associated with optic neuropathy (ON) and validate the hypothesis that concomitant isoniazid use and other causes of toxic ON affect the development of ON in ethambutol users. (2) Methods: This cohort study identified ethambutol users who initiated ethambutol therapy between January 2015 and December 2021 and had no ON prior to ethambutol therapy. ON incidence up to 31 December 2022 was evaluated. The users were grouped on the basis of the presence of ON. Demographic and clinical characteristics were investigated for risk factor analyses of ON. Odds ratios (ORs) were calculated using multivariate logistic regression analyses. (3) Results: Among 204,598 ethambutol users, 5277 (2.6%) patients developed ON over the study period. Patients with ON included a higher percentage of women and had a higher mean age than patients without ON. In the multivariate analyses, the risk factors for ON and visual impairment included sex, age, cumulative dose, extrapulmonary indications for ethambutol use, and systemic conditions such as diabetes, hypertension, hyperlipidemia, diabetes, kidney disease, and liver disease. Malnutrition or nutritional disorders significantly increased the risk of ON (OR = 1.27, 95% confidence interval [CI] = 1.19–1.34), whereas concomitant isoniazid use decreased the risk (OR = 0.78, 95% CI = 0.72–0.86). (4) Conclusion: An increased risk of ON in patients with systemic diseases and nutritional deficiency was identified, whereas concomitant isoniazid use was associated with a decreased risk of ON. Patients with these risk factors should be carefully monitored to minimize the vision-threatening ON.

Keywords: ethambutol; optic neuropathy; risk factors

1. Introduction

Ethambutol, a key anti-tuberculosis medication, can induce optic neuropathy (ON), potentially leading to significant vision loss [1,2]. This adverse effect, known as ethambutol-induced ON (EON), often manifests as painless, progressive vision loss and can result in irreversible blindness if not promptly detected and managed [1,2]. Studies report that ON incidence ranges from 0.5% to 6% among ethambutol users, with older age, renal impairment, and daily dose >15 mg/kg implicated as potential risk factors [1–5]. The concomitant use of other anti-tuberculosis drugs, such as isoniazid, has been suggested as a contributing factor [6].

Isoniazid, another cornerstone of tuberculosis therapy, is known for its neurotoxic potential, which primarily manifests as peripheral neuropathy [7]. This side effect is attributed to the drug's interference with pyridoxine (vitamin B6) metabolism, leading to a functional deficiency in the nerves [8]. Pyridoxine is essential for neurotransmitter synthesis, and its depletion can result in various neurological diseases such as peripheral neuropathy [8,9]. Although isoniazid is more commonly associated with peripheral neuropathy, there is growing concern that its neurotoxic effects might also affect the optic nerve, thus potentially compounding the risk of EON when isoniazid is used in combination with ethambutol [10].

However, ON can stem from various sources, including exposure to toxic substances and nutritional deficiencies [11]. For instance, alcohol consumption is linked to toxic ON and may exacerbate the risk of EON because of its metabolic effects [12]. Heavy smoking and nutritional deficiencies, such as vitamin deficiencies, are also associated with ON [11,13]. The prolonged use of ethambutol has been linked to deficiencies in vitamins E and B1, potentially exacerbating optic neuropathy by interacting with the nutritional cause of optic nerve damage [11]. Additionally, the combination of ethambutol with isoniazid and other nutritional or systemic factors that lead to toxic ON may further complicate ON development [1,6], making considering these interactions crucial to clinical management. Several studies suggest that the concurrent use of ethambutol and isoniazid and the presence of other risk factors, such as metabolic or nutritional deficiencies, could increase the susceptibility to ON [6,10,14], although the evidence is inconclusive, highlighting the need for careful monitoring and early intervention.

Given these associations, we hypothesized that concomitant isoniazid use and metabolic/nutritional deficiencies could serve as risk factors for EON, although this association has not been validated. Our study aims to validate this hypothesis by exploring systemic diseases/comorbidity data in a nationwide cohort of ethambutol users in South Korea by using a national health claims database. We specifically focused on understanding the interplay between ethambutol, isoniazid, and other potential conditions associated with ON.

2. Materials and Methods

2.1. Study Design and Population

This nationwide cohort study utilized the Health Insurance Review and Assessment Service (HIRA) database, which is a health claims database in South Korea covering approximately 50 million individuals (97% of the overall population). The database comprises comprehensive data on medication records, demographic details, and medical diagnoses utilizing the Korean Standard Classification of Diseases (either the seventh or eighth revision), which is slightly modified from the International Statistical Classification of Diseases and Related Health Problems, Tenth Revision (ICD-10) [15].

Ethambutol users who initiated therapy between 1 January 2013 and 31 December 2021 were identified for inclusion in the study cohort. To focus on users who began the drug between 1 January 2015 and 31 December 2021, we excluded those receiving an ethambutol prescription between 1 January 2013 and 31 December 2014. This exclusion criterion was based on the assumption that the absence of ethambutol prescriptions for two years prior to 2015 indicates no history of ethambutol use before 2015, given its continuous prescription for treatment in typical tuberculosis patients, as employed in previous studies on drug toxicity [15,16]. Ethambutol initiation was defined as the first prescription fill date within the study period. Among the included patients, those with pre-existing ON or a diagnosis of multiple sclerosis were excluded to ensure that the analyzed cohort was devoid of pre-existing ON or other frequently encountered causes of optic neuritis/neuropathy. The cohort for final inclusion consisted of 204,598 ethambutol users and was followed from the date of ethambutol initiation until 31 December 2022 to evaluate the occurrence of ON. Figure 1 shows the inclusion/exclusion criteria and the number of subjects after applying the criteria. This research acquired approval from the Institutional Review Board of Hanyang University Hospital (file no. 2023-11-008) and adhered to the Declaration of Helsinki. The need for informed consent was waived because of the retrospective nature of our study and the utilization of anonymized data.

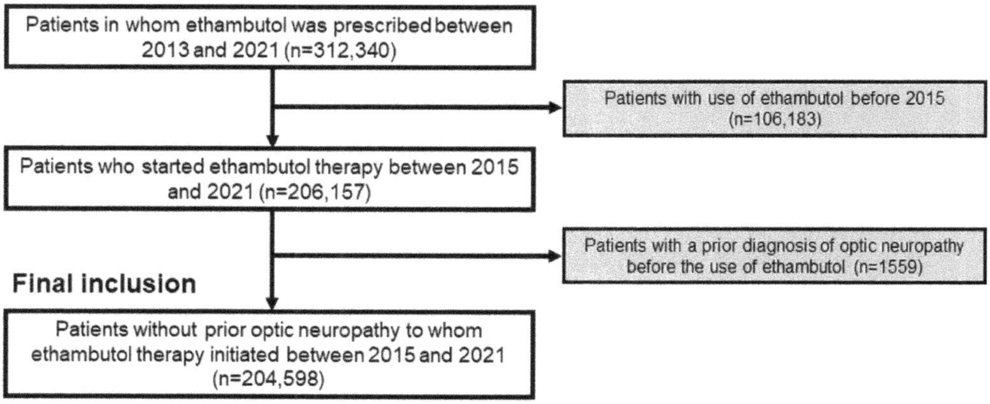

Figure 1. A flowchart of the study population and inclusion/exclusion criteria in this study.

2.2. Exposure and Outcome Assessments

Information on age, sex, systemic diseases (such as diabetes, hypertension, hyperlipidemia, kidney disease, and liver disease), and medication history (particularly ethambutol and isoniazid use) were extracted from the HIRA database. Additionally, the potential causes of toxic ON, such as alcohol, tobacco, and nutritional deficiencies, were assessed. Given that there were no specific data on the uptake of alcohol or tobacco from the database, information on alcohol- or tobacco-related disorders or alcohol or tobacco dependence was identified on the basis of ICD-10 codes. Supplementary Table S1 shows a summary of the diagnostic codes used for this study.

The occurrence of ON, which is the primary outcome of this study, was identified using the diagnostic codes of several categories of ON within the database, including codes for overall ON (ICD-10 codes H46, H47.7, and H47.2), optic neuritis/ON (ICD-10 code H46), and optic atrophy (ICD-10 code 47.2), and a concomitant prescription of ethambutol. Furthermore, visual impairment was assessed as a secondary outcome by using relevant diagnostic codes, including visual impairment or blindness (ICD-10 codes H54.0 and H54.4).

2.3. Statistical Analysis

Descriptive statistics were used to summarize the demographic and clinical characteristics of the study population. Categorical variables were presented as frequencies and percentages, whereas continuous variables were reported as means with standard deviations or medians with interquartile ranges as appropriate. Multivariate logistic regression analyses were conducted to determine the adjusted odds ratios (ORs) for the risk of ON associated with each characteristic while controlling for potential confounding variables. Covariates for multivariate logistic regression analyses included age, sex, cumulative dose of ethambutol, diabetes, hypertension, hyperlipidemia, kidney disease, liver disease, malnutrition/nutritional deficiency, alcohol-related diseases, and tobacco-related diseases as covariates. These factors were selected on the basis of study results indicating their association to ON or their significance to the pharmacokinetics of ethambutol therapy (i.e., liver disease and kidney disease). The same analyses were performed to identify risk factors with visual impairment/blindness. Baseline (at the time of ethambutol initiation) predictive factors, which were associated with late ON development during the observation period, were also assessed, and hazard ratios (HRs) were calculated for each factor by adjusting for other confounding variables. The HRs of clinical variables such as age; sex; daily dose of ethambutol; indication of ethambutol use; and systemic diseases such as diabetes, hypertension, hyperlipidemia, kidney disease, liver disease, malnutrition/nutritional deficiency, alcohol-related diseases, and tobacco-related diseases at baseline were calculated using the

Cox proportional hazards model. All analyses were performed using SAS version 9.4 (SAS Institute Inc., Cary, NC, USA), and a two-sided *p*-value of less than 0.05 was considered statistically significant.

3. Results

3.1. Demographic and Clinical Characteristics

Table 1 summarizes the demographic and clinical characteristics of the 204,598 ethambutol users included in this study. The cohort consisted of 118,427 males (57.9%) and 86,171 females (42.1%). The mean age was 60.1 years, and the majority of users were aged between 50 and 80 years, with 22.1%, 17.5%, and 17.2% of users in the 70–80, 50–59, and 60–69 age groups, respectively. A significant portion of the cohort had systemic diseases: 34.9% had diabetes mellitus, 45.4% had hypertension, 48.4% had hyperlipidemia, 18.8% had kidney disease, and 47.1% had liver disease.

Table 1. Demographic and clinical information of ethambutol users included in this study.

Characteristics	Overall Users (n = 204,598)
Sex	
Male/female	118,427 (57.9%):86,171 (42.1%)
Mean age (±SD), years	60.1 ± 19.0
<30	17,560 (8.6%)
30–39	16,453 (8.0%)
40–49	23,454 (11.5%)
50–59	35,707 (17.5%)
60–69	35,168 (17.2%)
70–80	45,152 (22.1%)
≥80	31,104 (15.2%)
Systemic diseases	
Diabetes mellitus	71,392 (34.9%)
Hypertension	92,843 (45.4%)
Hyperlipidemia	99,016 (48.4%)
Kidney disease	38,405 (18.8%)
Liver disease	96,261 (47.1%)
Malnutrition or other nutritional deficiency	51,150 (25.0%)
Alcohol-related disorders	121 (0.1%)
Tobacco-related disorders	194 (0.1%)
Indication for ethambutol use	
Pulmonary tuberculosis	156,962 (76.7%)
Extrapulmonary tuberculosis	22,722 (11.1%)
Others	24,914 (12.2%)
Combined use of isoniazid (%)	180,874 (88.4%)
Mean duration of ethambutol use (±SD), months	12.1 ± 11.7
Less than 3 months	42,636 (20.8%)
3–6 months	27,315 (13.4%)
6 months–1 year	44,022 (21.5%)
1–1.5 years	46,603 (22.8%)
1.5–2 years	22,212 (10.9%)
2 years or longer	21,810 (10.7%)
Mean daily dose of ethambutol (±SD), mg/day	902.9 ± 193.5
Less than 750 mg	11,266 (5.5%)
750–1000 mg	137,517 (67.2%)
1000–1250 mg	51,877 (25.4%)
1250 mg or greater	3938 (1.9%)
Mean cumulative dose of ethambutol (±SD), g	315.7 ± 301.1
Less than 200 g	83,270 (40.7%)
200–400 g	60,021 (29.3%)
400–600 g	36,239 (17.7%)
600 g or greater	25,068 (12.3%)

SD, standard deviation.

Regarding the indication for ethambutol use, the majority (76.7%) were treated for pulmonary tuberculosis. A significant proportion of users (88.4%) were on combined isoniazid therapy. The mean duration of ethambutol use was 12.1 months, and the mean daily dose of ethambutol was 902.9 mg.

3.2. Comparison of Clinical Characteristics between Patients with and without ON

Among the 204,598 ethambutol users, 5277 (2.6%) developed overall ON. Table 2 presents a comparison of the demographic and clinical characteristics between ethambutol users with ON and those without ON. Female patients were significantly more likely to develop ON ($p < 0.001$). The mean age of patients with ON was slightly higher at 60.8 years than that of patients without ON at 60.1 years ($p = 0.010$). Systemic diseases were more prevalent among patients with ON; these included diabetes mellitus, hypertension, hyperlipidemia, liver diseases, kidney diseases, and malnutrition or other nutritional deficiencies (all $p < 0.001$). Alcohol- and tobacco-related disorders were rare but showed a statistically significant difference between the two groups ($p < 0.001$ for both). In terms of ethambutol use, patients with ON had a higher cumulative dose than those without ON ($p < 0.001$).

Table 2. Demographic and clinical characteristics of patients with and without overall optic neuropathy.

Characteristics	Without Optic Neuropathy (n = 199,321)	With Optic Neuropathy (n = 5277)	p-Value
Sex			
Female (%)	83,455 (41.9%)	2716 (51.5%)	<0.001
Mean age (±SD), years	60.1 ± 19.1	60.8 ± 17.5	0.010
Systemic diseases			
Diabetes mellitus (%)	69,102 (34.7%)	2290 (43.4%)	<0.001
Hypertension (%)	90,034 (45.2%)	2809 (53.2%)	<0.001
Hyperlipidemia (%)	95,686 (48.0%)	3330 (63.1%)	<0.001
Liver diseases (%)	37,104 (18.6%)	1301 (24.7%)	<0.001
Kidney diseases (%)	93,291 (46.8%)	2970 (56.3%)	<0.001
Malnutrition or other nutritional deficiency	49,381 (24.8%)	1769 (33.5%)	<0.001
Alcohol-related disorders (F10, Z72.1, T51)	118 (0.1%)	3 (0.1%)	<0.001
Tobacco-related disorders (F17, Z72.0, T65.2	188 (0.1%)	6 0.1(%)	<0.001
Indication for ethambutol use			
Pulmonary tuberculosis (%)	153,228 (76.9%)	3734 (70.8%)	<0.001
Cumulative dose of ethambutol (± SD), g	312.9 ± 297.8	418.2 ± 392.4	<0.001
Mean (median) duration of ethambutol use, months	12.0 (10.8)	15.9 (12.3)	<0.001
Mean daily dose of ethambutol (± SD), mg/day	902.5 ± 193.5	919.3 ± 191.7	<0.001

3.3. Risk Factors of Several ON Conditions and Visual Impairment

Table 3 presents the risk factors for various ON conditions in ethambutol users obtained by univariate and multivariate logistic regression analyses. For overall ON, female sex was a significant risk factor (OR = 1.51, 95% confidence interval [CI] = 1.43–1.60). Age also showed a slight but significant association (OR = 1.002, 95% CI = 1.000–1.003). Systemic diseases such as diabetes, hypertension, hyperlipidemia, kidney disease, liver disease, and malnutrition/nutritional disorders were all significantly associated with increased risk of overall ON. Interestingly, the concomitant use of isoniazid was associated with a decreased risk (OR = 0.78, 95% CI = 0.72–0.86).

Table 3. Risk factors for several optic neuropathy conditions on logistic regression analyses in ethambutol users.

Factors	Overall Optic Neuropathy				Optic Neuropathy/Optic Neuritis				Optic Atrophy			
	Univariate		Multivariate		Univariate		Multivariate		Univariate		Multivariate	
	OR (95% CI)	p	OR (95% CI)	p	OR (95% CI)	p	OR (95% CI)	p	OR (95% CI)	p	OR (95% CI)	p
Sex *	1.47 (1.39–1.56)	<0.001	1.51 (1.43–1.60)	<0.001	1.58 (1.49–1.69)	<0.001	1.50 (1.42–1.59)	<0.001	1.33 (1.18–1.50)	<0.001	1.50 (1.42–1.58)	<0.001
Age	1.002 (1.000–1.003)	0.017	0.998 (0.996–1.000)	0.018	0.999 (0.997–1.001)	0.206			1.02 (1.01–1.02)	<0.001	0.997 (0.995–0.999)	0.002
Monitoring period, months	1.02 (1.02–1.02)	<0.001	1.00 (1.00–1.01)	0.335	1.02 (1.02–1.02)	<0.001	1.00 (1.00–1.00)	0.391	1.01 (1.01–1.01)	<0.001	0.99 (0.98–0.99)	<0.001
Indications for ethambutol use †		<0.001		0.002		<0.001		0.001		0.240		
Extrapulmonary Tb	1.30 (1.19–1.41)		1.14 (1.05–1.24)		1.44 (1.31–1.58)		1.15 (1.06–1.25)		0.90 (0.73–1.10)			
Others	1.44 (1.34–1.56)		1.11 (1.02–1.22)		1.62 (1.48–1.76)		1.11 (1.01–1.21)		1.11 (0.93–1.33)			
Cumulative dose	1.001 (1.001–1.001)	<0.001	1.001 (1.000 1.001)	0.003	1.001 (1.001 1.001)	<0.001	1.001 (1.000–1.001)	0.002	1.000 (1.000–1.001)	<0.001	1.001 (1.001–1.002)	<0.001
Concomitant use of isoniazid	0.65 (0.61–0.70)	<0.001	0.78 (0.72–0.86)	<0.001	0.57 (0.52–0.62)	<0.001	0.79 (0.72–0.86)	<0.001	0.98 (0.81–1.18)	<0.001	0.75 (0.70–0.81)	<0.001
Diabetes	1.45 (1.37–1.53)	<0.001	1.14 (1.07–1.22)	<0.001	1.30 (1.22–1.38)	<0.001	1.13 (1.06–1.21)	<0.001	2.28 (2.02–2.57)	<0.001	1.14 (1.07–1.22)	<0.001
Hypertension	1.38 (1.31–1.46)	<0.001	1.12 (1.05–1.20)	0.001	1.25 (1.17–1.33)	<0.001	1.08 (1.02–1.15)	0.011	2.26 (1.99–2.56)	<0.001	1.12 (1.05–1.20)	0.001
Hyperlipidemia	1.85 (1.75–1.96)	<0.001	1.47 (1.38–1.58)	<0.001	1.74 (1.63–1.86)	<0.001	1.47 (1.38–1.57)	<0.001	2.47 (2.16–2.81)	<0.001	1.48 (1.39–1.58)	<0.001
Kidney disease	1.43 (1.34–1.53)	<0.001	1.19 (1.12–1.28)	<0.001	1.36 (1.26–1.46)	<0.001	1.19 (1.11–1.27)	<0.001	1.90 (1.66–2.16)	<0.001	1.20 (1.12–1.29)	<0.001
Liver disease	1.46 (1.39–1.55)	<0.001	1.47 (1.38–1.58)	<0.001	1.38 (1.29–1.47)	<0.001	1.15 (1.09–1.22)	<0.001	1.84 (1.62–2.08)	<0.001	1.14 (1.08–1.21)	<0.001
Malnutrition/nutritional disorders	1.53 (1.45–1.62)	<0.001	1.27 (1.19–1.34)	<0.001	1.56 (1.45–1.66)	<0.001	1.26 (1.19–1.34)	<0.001	1.58 (1.40–1.80)	<0.001	1.27 (1.20–1.35)	<0.001
Alcohol-related disorders	0.96 (0.31–3.02)	0.946			0.87 (0.22–3.51)	0.847			1.60 (0.23–11.39)	0.638		
Tobacco-related disorders	1.21 (0.54–2.72)	0.652			1.64 (0.73–3.70)	0.233			N/A	N/A		

N/A = not applicable. * Male as reference. † Pulmonary tuberculosis as reference.

For specific conditions such as optic neuritis/ON and optic atrophy, similar patterns were observed. Females had higher risk, and systemic conditions such as diabetes, hypertension, hyperlipidemia, kidney disease, liver disease, and malnutrition/nutritional disorders also posed significant risks. For optic atrophy, older age showed a strong association, and systemic diseases such as diabetes, hypertension, hyperlipidemia, kidney disease, liver disease, and malnutrition/nutritional disorders were significant risk factors. Remarkably, the protective effect of isoniazid was consistent across all conditions.

Table 4 presents the results of logistic regression analyses identifying risk factors for visual impairment among ethambutol users. In the multivariate analyses, age was significantly associated with an increased risk of visual impairment. Extrapulmonary tuberculosis and other indications for ethambutol use also showed significant associations. Among systemic diseases, diabetes, hypertension, hyperlipidemia, kidney disease, liver disease, and malnutrition or nutritional disorders were identified as significant risk factors. Whereas the concomitant use of isoniazid was significantly associated with a decreased risk of visual impairment (OR = 0.83, 95% CI = 0.71–0.97), it did not show a significant protective effect in the multivariate model.

Table 4. Risk factors for visual impairment on logistic regression analyses in ethambutol users.

Factors	Univariate		Multivariate	
	OR (95% CI)	*p*	OR (95% CI)	*p*
Sex *	1.05 (0.94–1.17)	0.417		
Age	1.02 (1.01–1.02)	<0.001	1.01 (1.01–1.02)	<0.001
Monitoring period, months	1.01 (1.01–1.01)	<0.001	1.00 (0.98–1.02)	0.858
Indications for ethambutol use †		<0.001		<0.001
Extrapulmonary Tb	1.26 (1.07–1.48)		1.32 (1.12–1.56)	
Others	1.42 (1.22–1.65)		1.34 (1.13–1.58)	
Cumulative dose	1.000 (1.000–1.001)	<0.001	1.000 (1.000–1.001)	0.214
Concomitant use of isoniazid	0.83 (0.71–0.97)	0.018	0.97 (0.81–1.16)	0.698
Diabetes	2.19 (1.97–2.44)	<0.001	1.33 (1.17–1.50)	<0.001
Hypertension	2.39 (2.13–2.67)	<0.001	1.40 (1.22–1.60)	<0.001
Hyperlipidemia	2.47 (2.20–2.77)	<0.001	1.53 (1.34–1.75)	<0.001
Kidney disease	2.03 (1.81–2.28)	<0.001	1.37 (1.21–1.55)	<0.001
Liver disease	1.68 (1.51–1.88)	<0.001	1.18 (1.05–1.33)	0.006
Malnutrition or nutritional disorders	1.71 (1.53–1.92)	<0.001	1.30 (1.16–1.46)	<0.001
Alcohol-related disorders	3.86 (1.23–12.17)	0.021	3.02 (0.95–9.55)	0.061
Tobacco-related disorders	0.79 (0.11–5.61)	0.810		

* Male as reference. † Pulmonary tuberculosis as reference.

3.4. Baseline Predictive Factors of ON and Visual Impairment in Ethambutol Initiators

Table 5 shows the baseline predictive factors associated with ON and visual impairment among patients initiating ethambutol therapy, together with the HR from the univariate and multivariate analyses. For ON, female sex showed HRs of 1.467 and 1.478 in the univariate and multivariate analyses, respectively. The daily ethambutol dose was significantly associated with an increased risk of ON in the multivariate analysis. Factors such as diabetes and hyperlipidemia also showed significant associations with ON. For visual impairment, older age and systemic conditions such as diabetes and hypertension were identified as significant risk factors in the multivariate analyses.

Table 5. Baseline (at the time of ethambutol initiation) predictive factors of optic neuropathy and visual impairment and their hazard ratios (HRs).

Factors	Optic Neuropathy				Visual Impairment			
	Univariate		Multivariate		Univariate		Multivariate	
	HR (95% CI)	*p*	HR (95% CI)	*p*	HR (95% CI)	*p*	HR (95% CI)	*p*
Sex *	1.457 (1.390–1.543)	<0.001	1.478 (1.399–1.563)	<0.001	0.692 (0.548–0.873)	0.002	0.630 (0.498–0.797)	<0.001
Age	1.002 (1.001–1.004)	0.002	1.000 (0.998–1.002)	0.950	1.031 (1.024–1.038)	<0.001	1.022 (1.014–1.030)	<0.001
Daily dose	1.000 (1.000–1.001)	<0.001	1.001 (1.000–1.001)	<0.001	1.000 (0.999–1.000)	0.150		
Indications for ethambutol use †		<0.001		<0.001		0.143		
Extrapulmonary Tb	1.296 (1.195–1.405)		1.204 (1.109–1.307)		0.996 (0.695–1.427)			
Others	1.458 (1.354–1.571)		1.151 (1.059–1.251)		1.358 (0.998–1.846)			
Concomitant use of isoniazid	0.630 (0.586–0.675)	<0.001	0.669 (0.620–0.723)	<0.001	1.018 (0.726–1.430)	0.916		
Diabetes	1.177 (1.115–1.243)	<0.001	1.147 (1.075–1.223)	<0.001	2.088 (1.669–2.613)	<0.001	1.311 (1.016–1.692)	0.037
Hypertension	1.081 (1.024–1.140)	0.005	0.952 (0.888–1.020)	0.160	2.948 (2.312–3.759)	<0.001	1.841 (1.372–2.471)	<0.001
Hyperlipidemia	1.302 (1.231–1.377)	<0.001	1.245 (1.163–1.333)	<0.001	1.591 (1.263–2.006)	<0.001	0.847 (0.645–1.113)	0.233
Kidney disease	1.108 (1.042–1.177)	0.001	1.003 (0.940–1.071)	0.918	1.533 (1.213–1.938)	<0.001	1.047 (0.816–1.342)	0.720
Liver disease	1.074 (1.017–1.134)	0.011	0.950 (0.893–1.010)	0.103	1.488 (1.183–1.873)	0.001	1.056 (0.819–1.361)	0.674
Malnutrition or nutritional disorders	1.072 (1.006–1.142)	0.032	0.985 (0.922–1.051)	0.641	1.540 (1.213–1.956)	<0.001	1.200 (0.938–1.534)	0.147

* Male as reference. † Pulmonary tuberculosis as reference.

4. Discussion

This nationwide study offers significant insights into the risk of ON and visual impairment during tuberculosis treatment and identified various risk factors, including demographic characteristics, systemic diseases, and other potential contributors to toxic ON. Specifically, female sex, older age, systemic diseases such as diabetes, hypertension, hyperlipidemia, kidney and liver diseases, and malnutrition or nutritional disorders significantly increased ON risk. Among them, older age and systemic diseases, including diabetes, hypertension, hyperlipidemia, kidney and liver diseases, and malnutrition, also increased the risk of visual impairment. Longer duration and higher cumulative doses of ethambutol were also linked to a higher incidence of ON, whereas concomitant isoniazid use reduced the risk. These findings suggest the complex mechanism of ON induced by ethambutol or the vulnerability of the optic nerve to diverse factors. This also emphasizes the clinical need for a thorough evaluation of risk factors for those receiving ethambutol therapy. Effective monitoring strategies are essential for mitigating the risk of vision-threatening adverse reactions in ethambutol users with risk factors.

Our findings reveal that ethambutol users were predominantly elderly, with a mean age exceeding 60 years. The prevalence of systemic diseases such as diabetes mellitus, hypertension, and hyperlipidemia underscores their common coexistence, which should be carefully evaluated in populations initiating ethambutol therapy for tuberculosis. The widespread use of combined isoniazid therapy in our cohort (88.4%) reflects the standard clinical practice of using combination therapy in tuberculosis management [17–19]. The diverse durations and doses of ethambutol highlight the heterogeneity of drug exposure and their potential effects on toxicity outcomes. These demographic and clinical characteristics provide crucial context for interpreting our cumulative incidence of ON (2.6%) and identified risk factors. These data also emphasize the need for tailored monitoring strategies and interventions to mitigate the risk of vision-threatening ON in high-risk populations.

There were significant differences between the clinical characteristics of ethambutol users who developed ON and those who did not. Female patients exhibited a higher susceptibility to ON, thus highlighting a gender disparity in risk, which was also found in other ocular toxicities due to systemic medications such as hydroxychloroquine retinopathy [20]. Moreover, patients who developed ON tended to be slightly older and have a greater prevalence of systemic diseases such as diabetes mellitus, hypertension, hyperlipidemia, liver disease, kidney disease, and malnutrition/nutritional deficiencies than their counterparts without ON. Notably, alcohol- and tobacco-related disorders also showed a notable difference between the groups. The findings also reveal that patients who developed ON had a higher cumulative dose and longer duration of ethambutol use, thus suggesting a potential dose-dependent relationship with ON development. Furthermore, a smaller proportion of patients with pulmonary tuberculosis were noted among those with ON, potentially suggesting differences in cumulative dose according to indications, as extrapulmonary tuberculosis is usually treated for a longer duration than pulmonary tuberculosis [18]. However, the significant differences observed from all explored characteristics in Table 2 can also be attributed to the large sample size and the heterogeneity of the two compared groups, as with a large number of subjects, it is easier to detect statistically significant differences. However, this also indicates that various confounding factors may have influenced the results. To address this, we performed multivariate analyses to account for these potential confounders (Tables 3–5).

Our risk factor analyses (Table 3), by adjusting several confounders, identified several risk factors. Most importantly, the association between higher cumulative doses of ethambutol further underscored the dose-dependent nature of ethambutol toxicity on optic nerve function. Furthermore, demographic features such as female and old age were associated with an increased risk of ON. This highlights the heightened need for monitoring and preventive strategies in female and old patients undergoing ethambutol therapy. Furthermore, advancing age was a significant risk factor for optic atrophy and visual impairment, thus highlighting the age-related vulnerability to more severe structural and visual outcomes among elderly patients, which was also confirmed in ethambutol users in a previous study [2]. Systemic diseases such as diabetes, hypertension, hyperlipidemia, liver disease, and kidney diseases were consistently identified as significant risk factors for ON and visual impairment. These findings emphasize the importance of considering comorbid conditions in risk assessment and management strategies of ON for ethambutol users. Interestingly, the protective effect of concomitant isoniazid use was consistently observed across different ON conditions but did not extend to reducing the risk of visual impairment.

In addition, malnutrition or nutritional disorders significantly increased the risk of ON in ethambutol users. Malnutrition or nutritional disorders significantly increase ON risk due to deficiencies in essential nutrients, namely, vitamins B1, B6, and B12, which are crucial for maintaining nerve health [21,22]. These neurotrophic vitamins play vital roles in neuronal function, and their deficiencies impair electron transport and reduce ATP production in nerve cells [22], exacerbating neurotoxic effects and increasing the susceptibility of the optic nerve to damage from toxic medications such as ethambutol.

Ethambutol has also been associated with inducing deficiencies in these neurotrophic vitamins, further increasing the risk of ON in malnourished individuals. Accordingly, some experts recommend a combination of vitamins, specifically Vitamin B12, along with B1 and B6, for the primary prevention of optic neuropathy in ethambutol users [23]. However, isoniazid, primarily linked to peripheral neuropathy rather than ON, is routinely administered with pyridoxine (vitamin B6) to prevent neurotoxic side effects, as some guidelines suggest [6,23]. This supplemental pyridoxine may also help mitigate the risk of EON by maintaining adequate vitamin B6 levels, thereby offering some protection to the optic nerve. Therefore, the confounding effect of vitamin supplements should be carefully considered and adjusted; however, assessing patient uptake of vitamin B6 from our health claims database is challenging, as it may come from over-the-counter supplements. Additionally, the presence of numerous codes for pyridoxine in our health claims databases (>1000), along with limitations on data retrieval from the HIRA database, complicated our comprehensive analysis of the effect of vitamin B6 on determining the true relationship between isoniazid and ethambutol-induced optic nerve toxicity. This should be carefully addressed in future studies in terms of mechanisms of optic nerve damage caused by ethambutol and its interaction with isoniazid and nutritional deficiency.

Although ethambutol is well documented for its potential to cause ON, the effect of isoniazid is often underrecognized. Isoniazid-induced ON, although less common than ethambutol-induced cases, can present similar symptoms such as decreased visual acuity, color vision deficits, and central scotomas [6,24]. The concomitant use of isoniazid and ethambutol has been believed to have an additive toxic effect, thus exacerbating the risk of ON [6]. However, our findings indicate that there was no synergistic effect between the two, suggesting that ethambutol and isoniazid may involve different mechanisms in causing ON. Mechanistically, EON is attributed to its metal chelation effects, particularly on copper and zinc, which disrupt mitochondrial function and cause cellular energy depletion. Zinc chelation also inhibits lysosomal activation, thus affecting cellular waste processing [1,25]. Animal studies indicate that ethambutol-induced zinc deficiency may lead to myelin destruction and glial cell proliferation in optic nerves [26,27]. By contrast, the mechanism of isoniazid-associated ON is likely different from that of ethambutol because isoniazid is not known for its metal chelating properties.

Notably, by comparing the daily dose and duration of ethambutol use between those treated with ethambutol without isoniazid and those with ethambutol and isoniazid, we found that the combined isoniazid therapy significantly reduced ethambutol use duration. There were significant differences in the mean duration of ethambutol therapy (18.0 $\pm$ 18.6 months in those without isoniazid and 11.3 $\pm$ 10.2 months in those with isoniazid; $p < 0.001$). Although there were slight differences in the mean daily dose between the two groups (868.3 $\pm$ 202.7 mg in those without isoniazid vs. 907.5 $\pm$ 191.7 mg in those with combined isoniazid), the shorter duration of ethambutol in those treated with combined isoniazid and ethambutol therapy might explain the reduced risk of EON. However, to adjust for the effect of combined isoniazid on ethambutol dose reduction, we included the cumulative dose of ethambutol as a covariate in the multivariate analyses. Consequently, the protective effect of combined isoniazid on visual impairment was insignificant in the multivariate analyses (Table 4) but still significant for ON (Table 3). Accordingly, the protective effect of isoniazid should be validated in future studies, with careful consideration and adjustment of its effects on ethambutol dose reduction.

The findings on several key baseline factors associated with the development of ON and visual impairment have additional practical implications in treatment and monitoring decisions for patients initiating ethambutol therapy for tuberculosis (Table 5). Female sex and older age are consistent predictors of an increased risk of ON, as evidenced by significant HRs in both the univariate and multivariate analyses. The association with daily ethambutol dose further highlights the importance of monitoring toxicity in a dose-dependent manner through pharmacovigilance. Systemic conditions such as diabetes and hyperlipidemia also emerged as significant predictive factors, indicating the importance of considering these comorbidities when planning baseline monitoring.

However, our study has a few limitations. First, the retrospective design and reliance on health claims databases of this study inherently introduce typical biases such as selection bias and misclassification errors. For example, the use of diagnostic codes for identifying ON cases could lead to misclassification or underreporting, thus potentially affecting the accuracy of our incidence estimates, particularly given the lack of specificity in certain ON categories that require further validation. The daily dose divided by body weight should be considered to define the risk of retinopathy as a measure of drug exposure, as in previous studies [1,4]; however, information on body weight was not available in the HIRA database. Furthermore, due to the absence of pharmacogenetic data from the HIRA database, our study could not account for genetic factors contributing to ON development. As genetic predispositions, such as mitochondrial mutations associated with LHON or hereditary optic neuropathy, may affect the risk of EON [28–30], this is another limitation of our study. Future research incorporating pharmacogenetic analyses may provide more comprehensive risk factor analyses, thereby enhancing the precision of risk assessments and personalized interventions. Additionally, considering that the study population consisted exclusively of Koreans, our findings may not be fully generalizable to other populations with different healthcare systems and tuberculosis epidemiological profiles. The inclusion of several ON categories might lack specificity, for which further validation is required to confirm our findings. Furthermore, the absence of quantitative data on alcohol or tobacco use from our database limits our ability to definitively assess their association with ethambutol toxicity. Finally, we acknowledge that various conditions affecting the pharmacokinetics or distribution of ethambutol in the CNS and neurological diseases such as meningitis could be potential risk factors for EON, which we did not evaluate. These limitations underscore the need for a cautious interpretation of our findings and suggest avenues for improving future research in this area.

5. Conclusions

In conclusion, this nationwide study significantly enhances our understanding of the risk factors associated with ON and visual impairment in ethambutol users. Our findings show the significant association of demographic characteristics, systemic diseases, and drug exposure with ON and visual impairment in ethambutol users. This study also highlights the potential protective effects of isoniazid, although further investigation is needed to elucidate the underlying mechanisms and interactions between these drugs. This information needs to be utilized to refine risk assessment and monitoring schemes for ON and to enhance the ocular safety of ethambutol treatment in patients with tuberculosis.

Supplementary Materials: The following supporting information can be downloaded at: https://www.mdpi.com/article/10.3390/toxics12080549/s1, Table S1: Definitions and corresponding ICD-10 and Korean Classification of Disease (KCD)-7 or -8 codes used in this study.

Author Contributions: Conceptualization, S.J.A. and J.K.; methodology, S.J.A. and J.K.; validation, S.J.A. and J.K.; formal analysis, J.K.; investigation, S.J.A. and J.K.; resources, S.J.A. and J.K.; data curation, S.J.A. and J.K.; writing—original draft preparation, S.J.A. and J.K.; writing—review and editing, S.J.A.; visualization, S.J.A. and J.K.; supervision, S.J.A.; project administration, S.J.A.; funding acquisition, S.J.A. All authors have read and agreed to the published version of the manuscript.

Funding: This research received no external funding.

Institutional Review Board Statement: This study was approved by the Institutional Review Board (IRB) of Hanyang University Hospital (IRB file number: 2023-11-008).

Informed Consent Statement: The need/requirement for informed consent was waived by the IRB of Hanyang University Hospital because the retrospective study data were analyzed anonymously.

Data Availability Statement: Data and materials can be requested by e-mail and will be provided after consultation with the IRB.

Conflicts of Interest: The authors declare no conflicts of interest.

References

1. Chamberlain, P.D.; Sadaka, A.; Berry, S.; Lee, A.G. Ethambutol optic neuropathy. *Curr. Opin. Ophthalmol.* **2017**, *28*, 545–551. [CrossRef]
2. Chen, H.Y.; Lai, S.W.; Muo, C.H.; Chen, P.C.; Wang, I.J. Ethambutol-induced optic neuropathy: A nationwide population-based study from Taiwan. *Br. J. Ophthalmol.* **2012**, *96*, 1368–1371. [CrossRef] [PubMed]
3. Talbert Estlin, K.A.; Sadun, A.A. Risk factors for ethambutol optic toxicity. *Int. Ophthalmol.* **2010**, *30*, 63–72. [CrossRef] [PubMed]
4. Lee, E.J.; Kim, S.J.; Choung, H.K.; Kim, J.H.; Yu, Y.S. Incidence and clinical features of ethambutol-induced optic neuropathy in Korea. *J. Neuroophthalmol.* **2008**, *28*, 269–277. [CrossRef] [PubMed]
5. Yang, H.K.; Park, M.J.; Lee, J.H.; Lee, C.T.; Park, J.S.; Hwang, J.M. Incidence of toxic optic neuropathy with low-dose ethambutol. *Int. J. Tuberc. Lung Dis.* **2016**, *20*, 261–264. [CrossRef] [PubMed]
6. Sharma, P.; Sharma, R. Toxic optic neuropathy. *Indian J. Ophthalmol.* **2011**, *59*, 137–141. [CrossRef] [PubMed]
7. Badrinath, M.; Chen, P.; John, S. Isoniazid Toxicity. In *StatPearls*; StatPearls Publishing: Treasure Island, FL, USA, 2024.
8. Hadtstein, F.; Vrolijk, M. Vitamin B-6-Induced Neuropathy: Exploring the Mechanisms of Pyridoxine Toxicity. *Adv. Nutr.* **2021**, *12*, 1911–1929. [CrossRef] [PubMed]

9. Parra, M.; Stahl, S.; Hellmann, H. Vitamin B(6) and Its Role in Cell Metabolism and Physiology. *Cells* **2018**, *7*, 84. [CrossRef] [PubMed]
10. Jimenez-Lucho, V.E.; del Busto, R.; Odel, J. Isoniazid and ethambutol as a cause of optic neuropathy. *Eur. J. Respir. Dis.* **1987**, *71*, 42–45.
11. Baj, J.; Forma, A.; Kobak, J.; Tyczynska, M.; Dudek, I.; Maani, A.; Teresinski, G.; Buszewicz, G.; Januszewski, J.; Flieger, J. Toxic and Nutritional Optic Neuropathies-An Updated Mini-Review. *Int. J. Environ. Res. Public Health* **2022**, *19*, 3092. [CrossRef]
12. Donnadieu-Rigole, H.; Daien, V.; Blanc, D.; Michau, S.; Villain, M.; Nalpas, B.; Perney, P. The prevalence of optic neuropathy in alcoholic patients—A pilot study. *Alcohol. Clin. Exp. Res.* **2014**, *38*, 2034–2038. [CrossRef]
13. Margolin, E.; Blair, K.; Shemesh, A. Toxic and Nutritional Optic Neuropathy. In *StatPearls*; StatPearls Publishing: Treasure Island, FL, USA, 2024.
14. Rasool, M.; Malik, A.; Manan, A.; Aziz, K.; Mahmood, A.; Zaheer, S.; Shuja, N.; Qazi, M.H.; Kamal, M.A.; Karim, S. Determination of potential role of antioxidative status and circulating biochemical markers in the pathogenesis of ethambutol induced toxic optic neuropathy among diabetic and non-diabetic patients. *Saudi J. Biol. Sci.* **2015**, *22*, 739–743. [CrossRef]
15. Kim, J.; Kim, K.E.; Kim, J.H.; Ahn, S.J. Practice Patterns of Screening for Hydroxychloroquine Retinopathy in South Korea. *JAMA Netw. Open* **2023**, *6*, e2314816. [CrossRef]
16. Kim, J.; Kwon, H.Y.; Kim, J.H.; Ahn, S.J. Nationwide Usage of Pentosan Polysulfate and Practice Patterns of Pentosan Polysulfate Maculopathy Screening in South Korea. *Ophthalmol. Retin.* **2024**, *8*, 246–253. [CrossRef] [PubMed]
17. Nolan, C.M.; Goldberg, S.V. Treatment of isoniazid-resistant tuberculosis with isoniazid, rifampin, ethambutol, and pyrazinamide for 6 months. *Int. J. Tuberc. Lung Dis.* **2002**, *6*, 952–958. [PubMed]
18. World Health Organization. *WHO Consolidated Guidelines on Tuberculosis: Module 4: Treatment—Tuberculosis Care and Support*; WHO Guidelines Approved by the Guidelines Review Committee; World Health Organization: Geneva, Switzerland, 2022.
19. World Health Organization. *WHO Consolidated Guidelines on Tuberculosis: Module 4: Treatment—Drug-Resistant Tuberculosis Treatment*; WHO Guidelines Approved by the Guidelines Review Committee; World Health Organization: Geneva, Switzerland, 2020.
20. Jorge, A.M.; Melles, R.B.; Marmor, M.F.; Zhou, B.; Zhang, Y.; Choi, H.K. Risk Factors for Hydroxychloroquine Retinopathy and Its Subtypes. *JAMA Netw. Open* **2024**, *7*, e2410677. [CrossRef]
21. Lahoda Brodska, H.; Klempir, J.; Zavora, J.; Kohout, P. The Role of Micronutrients in Neurological Disorders. *Nutrients* **2023**, *15*, 4129. [CrossRef]
22. Baltrusch, S. The Role of Neurotropic B Vitamins in Nerve Regeneration. *BioMed Res. Int.* **2021**, *2021*, 9968228. [CrossRef]
23. Saxena, R.; Singh, D.; Phuljhele, S.; Kalaiselvan, V.; Karna, S.; Gandhi, R.; Prakash, A.; Lodha, R.; Mohan, A.; Menon, V.; et al. Ethambutol toxicity: Expert panel consensus for the primary prevention, diagnosis and management of ethambutol-induced optic neuropathy. *Indian J. Ophthalmol.* **2021**, *69*, 3734–3739. [CrossRef] [PubMed]
24. Kass, I.; Mandel, W.; Cohen, H.; Dressler, S.H. Isoniazid as a cause of optic neuritis and atrophy. *J. Am. Med. Assoc.* **1957**, *164*, 1740–1743. [CrossRef]
25. Heng, J.E.; Vorwerk, C.K.; Lessell, E.; Zurakowski, D.; Levin, L.A.; Dreyer, E.B. Ethambutol is toxic to retinal ganglion cells via an excitotoxic pathway. *Investig. Ophthalmol. Vis. Sci* **1999**, *40*, 190–196.
26. Yoon, Y.H.; Jung, K.H.; Sadun, A.A.; Shin, H.C.; Koh, J.Y. Ethambutol-induced vacuolar changes and neuronal loss in rat retinal cell culture: Mediation by endogenous zinc. *Toxicol. Appl. Pharmacol.* **2000**, *162*, 107–114. [CrossRef]
27. Chung, H.; Yoon, Y.H.; Hwang, J.J.; Cho, K.S.; Koh, J.Y.; Kim, J.G. Ethambutol-induced toxicity is mediated by zinc and lysosomal membrane permeabilization in cultured retinal cells. *Toxicol. Appl. Pharmacol.* **2009**, *235*, 163–170. [CrossRef]
28. Ikeda, A.; Ikeda, T.; Ikeda, N.; Kawakami, Y.; Mimura, O. Leber's hereditary optic neuropathy precipitated by ethambutol. *Jpn. J. Ophthalmol.* **2006**, *50*, 280–283. [CrossRef]
29. Guillet, V.; Chevrollier, A.; Cassereau, J.; Letournel, F.; Gueguen, N.; Richard, L.; Desquiret, V.; Verny, C.; Procaccio, V.; Amati-Bonneau, P.; et al. Ethambutol-induced optic neuropathy linked to OPA1 mutation and mitochondrial toxicity. *Mitochondrion* **2010**, *10*, 115–124. [CrossRef]
30. Seo, J.H.; Hwang, J.M.; Park, S.S. Antituberculosis medication as a possible epigenetic factor of Leber's hereditary optic neuropathy. *Clin. Exp. Ophthalmol.* **2010**, *38*, 363–366. [CrossRef]

Disclaimer/Publisher's Note: The statements, opinions and data contained in all publications are solely those of the individual author(s) and contributor(s) and not of MDPI and/or the editor(s). MDPI and/or the editor(s) disclaim responsibility for any injury to people or property resulting from any ideas, methods, instructions or products referred to in the content.

toxics

MDPI

Article

Rutaecarpine Aggravates Acetaminophen-Induced Acute Liver Injury by Inducing CYP1A2

Meiqi Wan [1], Hua Gao [1], Xiaoyan Liu [2,*] and Youbo Zhang [1,3,*]

[1] State Key Laboratory of Natural and Biomimetic Drugs, Key Laboratory of State Administration of Traditional Chinese Medicine for Compatibility Toxicology, Department of Natural Medicines, School of Pharmaceutical Sciences, Peking University, Beijing 100191, China; wanmeiqi2018@163.com (M.W.); gaohua_cpu@163.com (H.G.)

[2] Laboratory of Metabolism, Center for Cancer Research, National Cancer Institute, National Institutes of Health, Bethesda, MD 20892, USA

[3] Henan Engineering Research Center of Medicinal and Edible Chinese Medicine Technology, Henan University of Chinese Medicine, Zhengzhou 450046, China

* Correspondence: xiaoyan.liu2@nih.gov (X.L.); ybzhang@bjmu.edu.cn (Y.Z.)

Abstract: In this study, we investigated whether rutaecarpine could aggravate acetaminophen-induced acute liver damage in vivo and in vitro. CCK-8 and apoptosis assays were performed to verify the cytotoxicity of acetaminophen to L02 cells with or without rutaecarpine. The expression levels of the target proteins and genes were determined using Western blotting and qRT-PCR. The liver pathological changes were evaluated with hematoxylin and eosin staining, while the aspartate aminotransferase (AST) and alanine aminotransferase (AST) levels in plasma were measured to assess the liver damage. Our results revealed that pretreatment of the cell and mice with rutaecarpine significantly aggravated the acetaminophen-induced liver damage. Mechanistically, rutaecarpine induces the CYP1A2 protein, which accelerates the metabolism of acetaminophen to produce a toxic intermediate, N-acetyl-p-benzoquinone imine (NAPQI), leading to severe liver inflammation. Rutaecarpine exacerbated the liver damage by upregulating CYP1A2 and proinflammatory factors. These findings highlight the importance of carefully considering the dosage of rutaecarpine when combined with acetaminophen in drug design and preclinical trials.

Keywords: rutaecarpine; acetaminophen; hepatotoxicity; CYP1A2; inflammatory cytokines

1. Introduction

In recent years, the combination therapy of traditional Chinese medicine (TCM) and synthetic drugs has become increasingly common in clinical settings for the treatment of various diseases. Due to the diversity and complexity of the compounds in TCM, particular and ongoing attention should be paid to their side effects and safety when used in combination with synthetic drugs. The liver, which is rich in drug-metabolizing enzymes, is the primary organ responsible for many critical physiological functions, including drug metabolism and detoxification. However, some drugs can lead to hepatotoxicity, causing liver damage or acute and chronic liver failure, resulting in higher clinical drug toxicity-related incidence and mortality rates. As the prevalence of chemical drug use rises, there is growing concern over the escalating number of adverse reactions resulting from the concurrent use of Chinese and Western medications. Therefore, conducting research in this area is imperative.

An overdose of acetaminophen (APAP) is a major cause of acute liver failure (ALF) [1–3]. Some reports indicated that therapeutic doses of APAP can increase serum transaminases for a few days [4,5]. N-acetyl-p-benzoquinone imine (NAPQI) is a toxic intermediate and the main product of APAP via oxidation by cytochrome P450 enzymes (CYP2E1, CYP3A11 and CYP1A2). High production of NAPQI in the liver causes excessive depletion of glutathione (GSH) and production of NAPQI–protein adducts, ultimately leading to mitochondrial oxidative stress and acute liver inflammation [6–8].

Euodiae fructus (EF) is the dried unripe fruit of Euodia rutaecarpa (Juss.) Benth., Euodia rutaecarpa (Juss.) Benth. var. officinalis (Dode) Huang and Euodia rutaecarpa (Juss.) Benth. var. bodinieri (Dode) Huang. It has been used for centuries to treat gastrointestinal diseases, thermo-regulatory issues and headache in clinical settings [9,10]. However, the potentially hepatotoxic side effects of EF have been consistently reported [11–13]. Zhang et al. [14] found that the metabolic intermediate might contribute to the toxicity of the EF extract in L02 cells. The hepatotoxicity of the water extract was higher than that of the ethanol extract and volatile oil of EF, with all forms exhibiting dose-dependent toxicity in rats [15]. The clinical hepatotoxicity of EF is usually caused by consuming unprocessed materials or overdosing, with the potential mechanisms involving the activation or up-regulation of inflammatory factors, mitochondrial injury and peroxidation damage [16]. Phytochemical and pharmacological evaluations have shown that indolo-quinazoline alkaloids, such as rutaecarpine (Rut) and evodiamine (Evo), and quinolone alkaloids, such as 1-methyl-2-nonyl-4(1H)-quinolone (Mnq), 1-methyl-2-undecyl-4(1H)-quinolone (Muq), and evocarpine (Evc), are the main bioactive ingredients of EF [12,17–19].

Some studies have suggested that CYP3A4 plays a role in the metabolic activation and dehydrogenation of Evo and Rut, leading to potential liver toxicities in humans through the formation of electrophilic intermediates [20,21].

The impact of Rut on hepatotoxicity remains uncertain, while some evidence indicates that Rut may protect against acetaminophen-induced liver damage by enhancing Nrf2-mediated antioxidant enzyme activity [22]. However, other reports suggest that Rut could worsen drug-induced liver injury, such as acetaminophen-induced hepatotoxicity, by altering the acetaminophen pharmacokinetics [23], inhibiting CYP activity [24], and increasing the levels of AST and ALT in mouse serum through regulation of CYP3A4 [20,25]. This study aims to investigate whether Rut exacerbates acetaminophen-induced DILI by establishing in vivo and in vitro liver damage models. The findings seek to clarify the potential hepatotoxic effects of Rut in combination with acetaminophen and provide insights into the safety of using Chinese and Western medicines together.

2. Materials and Methods

2.1. Chemicals and Reagents

Rut was isolated in our lab with a purity > 98%, and the structure was identified by NMR and high-resolution mass spectrometry (Figure 1a). Acetaminophen (APAP) and α-Naphthoflavone were provided by Sigma Chemical Co. (St. Louis, MO, USA). TRIzol reagent was obtained from Thermo-Fisher Scientific (Halethorpe, MD). Moreover, 5×qRT Super Mix and Mon-Amp TM SYBR Green qPCR mix (Low ROX) were purchased from Monad (Suzhou, Jiangsu, China). RIPA Lysis Buffer was provided by Beyotime (Shanghai, China). RPMI-1640 cell culture medium and fetal bovine serum (FBS) were obtained from Gibco-BRL (Grand Island, NY, USA). Anti-cytochrome P450 1A2 (ab22717) and anti-β-actin (ab8227) were obtained from Abcam (Cambridge, Cambridgeshire, UK). The assay kit for apoptosis and the Cell Counting Kit-8 (CCK-8) were purchased from Meilunbio (Dalian, China).

2.2. Culture of Cell Lines

The human normal liver cell line L02 was provided by Beijing University of Chinese Medicine. The cells were cultivated in a humidified atmosphere in 5% CO_2 at 37 °C in RPMI-1640 (containing 10% FBS and 1% penicillin/streptomycin).

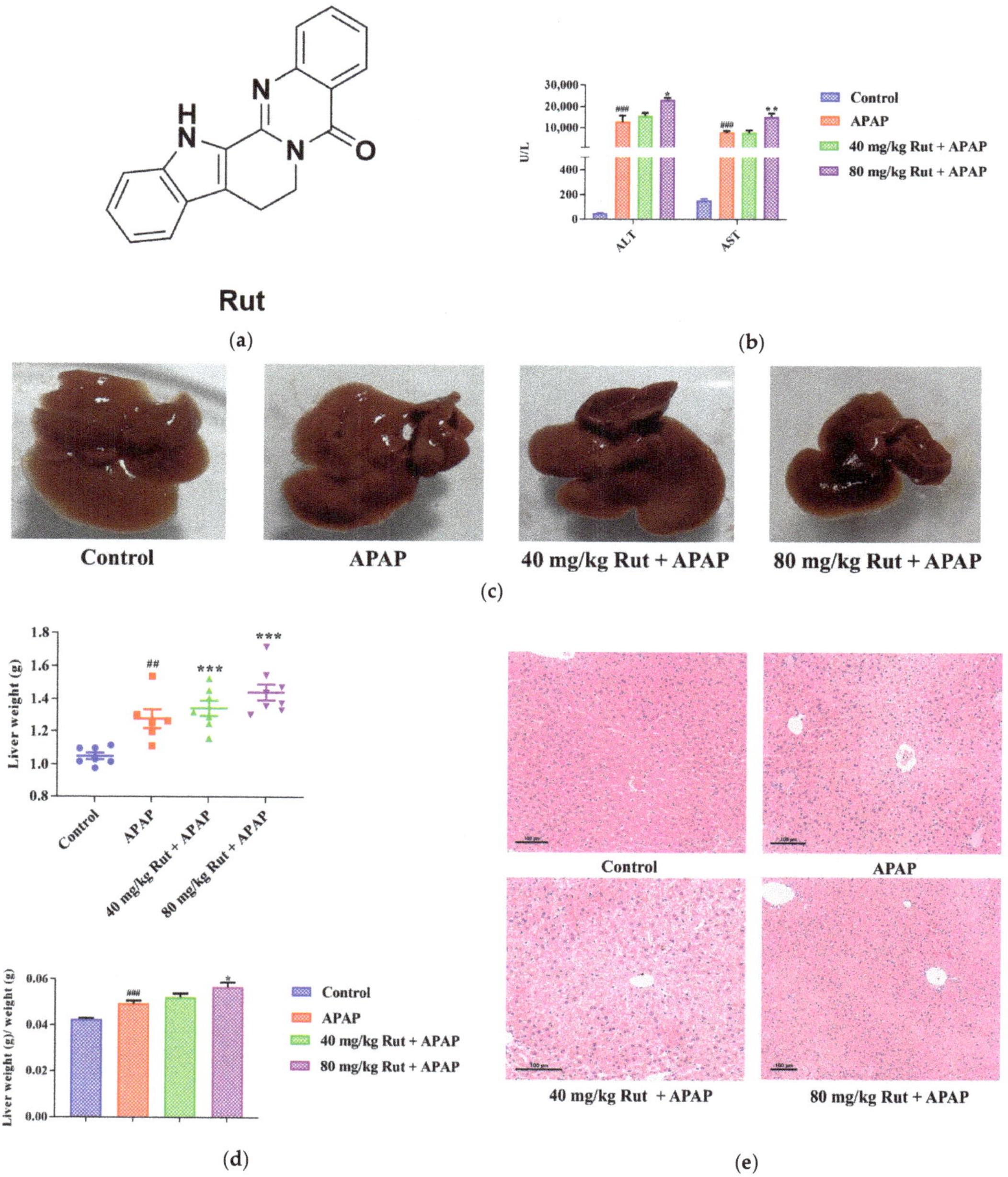

Figure 1. Effects of APAP and APAP + Rut on liver damage in mouse liver. (**a**) The chemical structure of Rut. (**b**) The activities of ALT and AST in mouse serum, data are presented as mean ± SEM (n = 5), statistical difference: compared with control, $^{###}$ $p < 0.001$; with APAP group, * $p < 0.05$ and ** $p < 0.01$. (**c**) Morphological changes in mouse liver. (**d**) The liver index of mouse, data are presented as mean ± SEM (n = 5), statistical difference: compared with control, $^{##}$ $p < 0.01$, $^{###}$ $p < 0.001$; with APAP group * $p < 0.05$, *** $p < 0.001$. (**e**) H&E staining of mouse liver, original scale: 10×. Rut pretreatment exacerbated liver injury.

2.3. Cell Viability Assay

The cytotoxicity of Rut and APAP was measured by the CCK-8 kit. Briefly, cells were seeded into 96-well plates (8×10^6 cells/mL) in a CO_2 incubator at 37 °C for 24 h, then treated with different concentrations of Rut (20, 10, 5, 2.5, 1.25 and 0.625 μM) for 18 h. A range of concentrations of APAP (50, 25, 12.5, 6.25, 3.125 and 1.5625 mM) were subsequently added to the medium and treated for 6 h at 37 °C. Afterwards, the CCK-8 solution was added to each well with 10% of the original concentration and co-incubated for 4 h. The optical density (OD) value was measured at 450 nm using a microplate reader (Thermo Fisher Scientific, Waltham, MA, USA).

2.4. Apoptosis Assay

Briefly, L02 cells were seeded into 12-well plates with a density of 2.5×10^5 cells/mL and cultured for 24 h. The control group, model group (30 mM APAP), and two concentrations of Rut groups (2.5 μM and 10 μM) were set, respectively, with three replicate wells for each group. The cell suspensions were treated with the protocol for the apoptosis detection kit and detected by flow cytometry (Beckman Coulter, Fullerton, CA, USA).

2.5. Animal Studies

Male C57BL/6J (8 weeks old) mice were purchased from the Laboratory Animal Center of Peking University Health Science Center (Beijing, China). All the animal experiments were approved by the Biomedical Ethical Committee of Peking. The mice were housed in a specific pathogen-free environment controlled for temperature, light, and humidity (25 °C, 12-h light/dark cycle, 45–65%) for 1 week before the experiments.

Experiment 1: thirty-two mice were randomly divided into four groups (blank, APAP, 40 mg/kg Rut + APAP and 80 mg/kg Rut + APAP groups, $n = 8$). Rut was dissolved in corn oil and APAP was freshly dissolved in warm saline. The mice were administered 40 mg/kg Rut, 80 mg/kg Rut and corn oil by gavage once a day for 4 days (blank and APAP group were treated with corn oil), and treated with APAP (300 mg/kg) by intraperitoneal administration 1 h after the last drug treatment to induce hepatotoxicity (the blank group was administrated with saline). Finally, the mice were sacrificed by cervical dislocation and dissected after 24 h and a proportion of the liver tissues were fixed in 10% formalin solution, and the serum and residual liver tissues were stored at −80 °C for further use, respectively.

Experiment 2: twenty-five male mice were randomly divided into five groups ($n = 5$). The blank, APAP and 80 mg/kg Rut + APAP groups were processed in the same way as in experiment 1. Mice in the 80 mg/kg Rut + inhibitor (α-Naphthoflavone) + APAP group and inhibitor group were separately pretreated with 80 mg/kg Rut or corn oil by gavage for 4 consecutive days. At the last day after administration, the mice were given 120 mg/kg α-Naphthoflavone by gavage one hour later, and then injected intraperitoneally with APAP or saline, respectively. The collection of serum and liver samples was consistent with experiment 1.

2.6. Quantitative Real-Time Polymerase Chain Reaction (qRT-PCR)

The total RNA was reverse transcribed with reverse transcriptase based on the protocol provided with the kit. The primer sequences are shown in Supplementary Tables S1 and S2. Mon-Amp TM SYBR Green qPCR mix (Low ROX) was used for the qRT-PCR. The Ct values were compared with β-actin/GAPDH to calculate the relative gene expression levels.

2.7. Western Blot

The lysis of the liver tissues took place with RIPA lysis buffer (phosphatase and protease inhibitors added) to obtain the total proteins. A BCA Protein Assay Kit was applied for the protein quantification. After electrophoresis on the 10% SDS–PAGE gels, the proteins were transferred to a polyvinylidene difluoride (PVDF) membrane and blocked with 5% non-fat milk. The PVDF membrane were incubated with primary antibodies overnight at 4 °C on an orbital shaker with gentle shaking. After rinsing with TBST, the PVDF membrane was incubated with fluorescent secondary antibody (in 5% skim milk) for 1 h and rinsed with TBS three times. Finally, the Odyssey® CLx Infrared Imaging System (Gene Company Limited, LI-COR, Lincoln, NE, USA) was adopted to capture and quantify the protein bands.

2.8. Serum Aminotransferase Analysis and Histological Examination

The ALT and AST contents of the serum were tested by an automatic biochemical analyzer. H&E staining was executed for the formalin-fixed liver tissues (embedded in paraffin and 5 μm thick sections).

2.9. Statistical Analysis

In this research, the GraphPad Prism 7.0 software (GraphPad Software, San Diego, CA, USA) and SPSS 26 software (IBM SPSS Inc., Chicago, IL, USA) were the main tools used for data analysis. The data in the experiments are presented as the mean ± SEM. A two-tailed Student's *t*-test analyzed the differences between two groups, and a one-way ANOVA was used among multiple comparisons. A p value < 0.05 was considered to be statistically significant.

3. Results

3.1. Rut Aggravated the APAP-Induced Acute Liver Injury in Mice

3.1.1. Serum Transaminases, Hepatic Index and Histological Analysis

In this study, the serum transaminases, hepatic index and histological analysis were used to evaluate the level of liver damage in mice. The ALT and AST concentration changes in the serum showed that a single dose of APAP (300 mg/kg) exposure significantly increased the levels of both transaminases compared with to the blank group ($p < 0.001$), indicating the severe hepatotoxicity of APAP. Additionally, 80 mg/kg Rut (80 mg/kg Rut + APAP) remarkably increased the concentration levels of ALT and AST when administered to mice in combination with APAP ($p < 0.05$ and 0.01, respectively) (Figure 1b), while there was no significant difference between the 40 mg/kg Rut + APAP and APAP groups ($p > 0.05$). The liver tissue of the mice in the APAP group appeared turgid with a dark color, and the liver was further aggravated in the Rut-pretreated mice (Figure 1c). The liver weight and hepatic index were more elevated in the APAP group compared to the blank group ($p < 0.01$ and 0.001, respectively) and Rut (80 mg/kg Rut + APAP) could increase these changes significantly ($p < 0.001$ and 0.05, respectively) (Figure 1d), but the hepatic index of the mice had no significant changes in the 40 mg/kg + APAP group compared to that in APAP group. The H&E staining results revealed that livers from the APAP-treated mice exhibited extensive focal necrosis and cell membrane damage, and Rut pretreatment exacerbated these symptoms (Figure 1e). These results demonstrated that Rut could aggravate APAP-induced acute liver injury in a dose-dependent manner.

3.1.2. The Involvement of Cyp1a2 in Rut-Aggravated APAP-Induced Hepatotoxicity

NAPQI is a highly reactive metabolite of APAP, catalyzed by cytochrome P450. The overproduction of NAPQI depletes glutathione (GSH), leading to the formation of NAPQI-GSH adducts, which triggers mitochondrial oxidative stress and ultimately initiates liver injury. The 3-alkylindole moiety in Rut is dehydrogenated to an electrophile, 3-methyleneindolenine, which is catalyzed by cytochrome P450, and this compound subsequently binds with hepatic GSH to form 3-methyleneindolenine-GSH, causing hepatotoxicity.

To evaluate the effect of Rut on APAP-mediated hepatic damage, we examined the expression of Cyp2e1, Cyp1a2, and pro-inflammatory cytokines. The qRT-PCR results showed that APAP significantly induced hepatic mRNA expression of Il6 and Il-1β, indicating the presence of a inflammatory reaction in the mice liver. Rut pretreatment aggravated the APAP-mediated liver toxicity in a dose-dependent manner (Figure 2a). Additionally, the mRNA and protein expression levels of Cyp1a2 in the Rut-pretreated groups were significantly upregulated compared to the APAP groups, respectively (Figure 2a,b), while there was no significant change in the Cyp2e1 mRNA expression (Figure 2a). These results demonstrated that Rut increased the inflammatory response in mice administered APAP. The potential mechanism may involve the modulation of CYP1A2 expression.

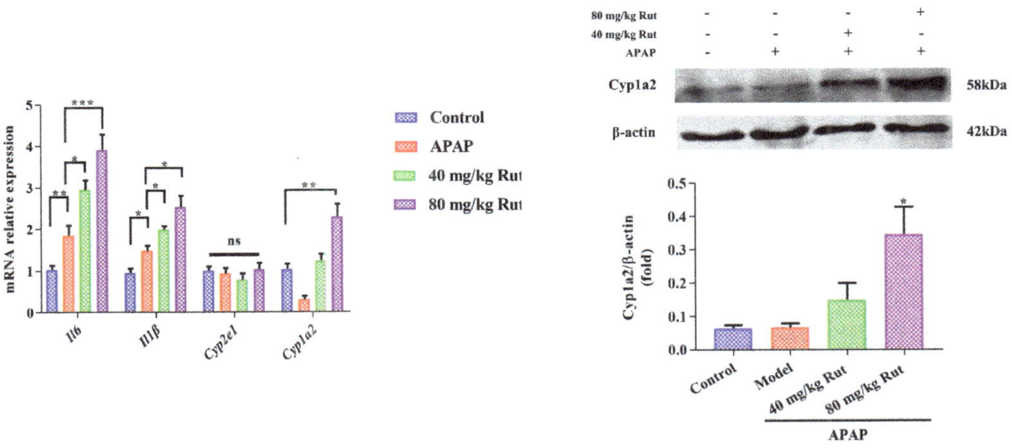

(a) (b)

Figure 2. Effects of APAP and APAP + Rut on mRNA and protein levels in mouse liver. (**a**) The mRNA expression of Cyp2e1, Cyp1a2, mIl6 and mIl-1β, data are presented as mean ± SEM ($n = 5$), statistical difference: ns (no significant difference), * $p < 0.05$, ** $p < 0.01$ and *** $p < 0.001$. (**b**) Protein level of Cyp1a2, results are indicated as means ± SEM ($n = 3$), significantly different compared with control, * $p < 0.05$.

3.2. CYP1A2 Inhibitor Reversed Rut Aggravation of APAP-Induced Hepatotoxicity

3.2.1. The Serum ALT and AST Levels and H&E Staining

The Cyp1a2 inhibitor (α-Naphthoflavone) was used to verify the effect of Cyp1a2 in relation to Rut aggravating APAP-mediated hepatotoxicity. The levels of ALT and AST, as well as the H&E staining, showed no significant pathological changes in mice liver when comparing the α-Naphthoflavone group with the control group, indicating that the inhibitor itself did not influence the results (Figure 3a,c). Compared to the control group, APAP significantly increased the concentrations of ALT and AST. When 80 mg/kg Rut was administered to mice in combination with APAP, these levels increased further. However, α-Naphthoflavone reversed these abnormal increases very significantly.

The histologic observations revealed that Rut exacerbated the hepatic damage in the APAP-administered mice, showing extensive focal necrosis, cell membrane damage, nuclear shrinkage, and significant inflammatory cell infiltration. In contrast, α-Naphthoflavone significantly alleviated these symptoms (Figure 3c). The results showed that the inhibition of CYP1A2 activity by α-Naphthoflavone ameliorated the liver injury caused by Rut and APAP, implying that CYP1A2 plays a critical role in Rut-aggravated APAP-mediated hepatotoxicity.

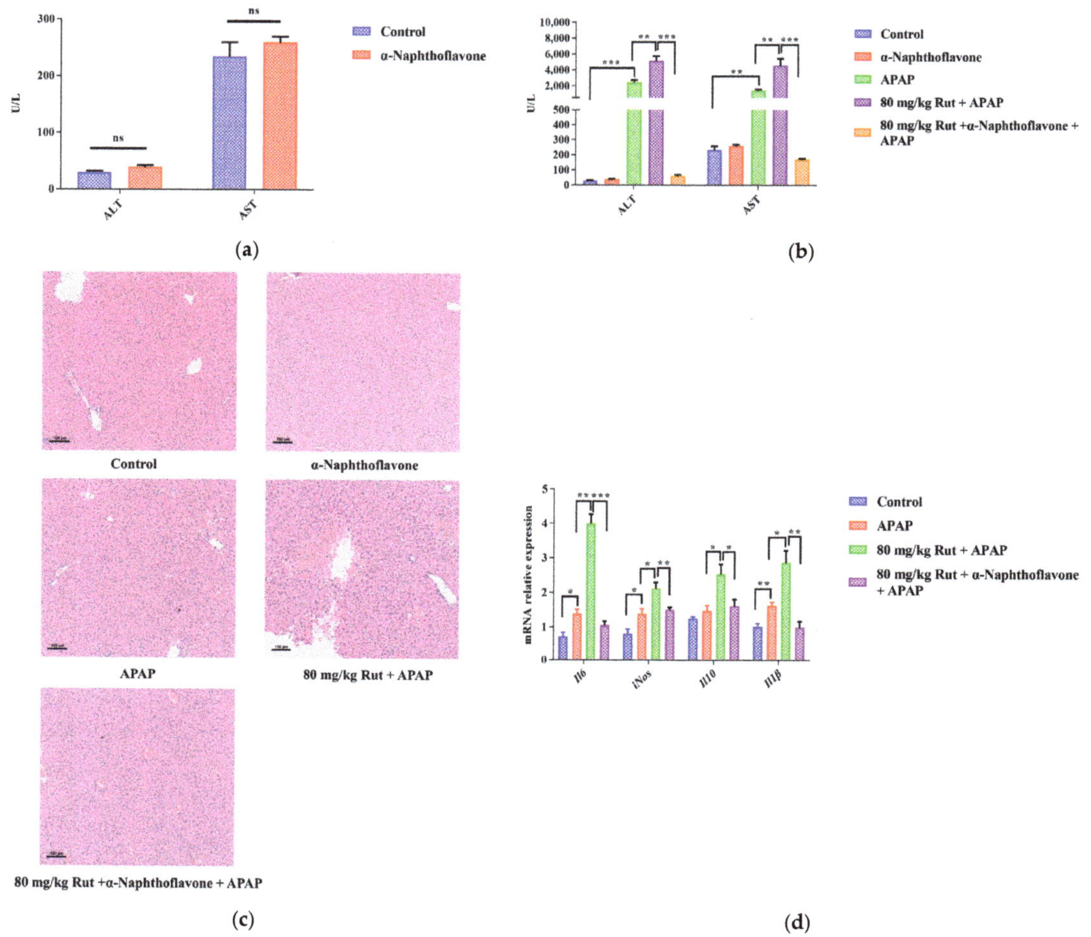

Figure 3. α-Naphthoflavone reversed the effects of Rut-aggravated APAP-induced acute liver injury. (**a**) The ALT and AST levels in mouse serum after treatment with α-Naphthoflavone. ns (no significant difference). (**b**) The ALT and AST levels in APAP/Rut-induced mouse serum with or without α-Naphthoflavone, data are presented as mean ± SEM (n = 5), statistical difference: ** $p < 0.01$ and *** $p < 0.001$. (**c**) H&E staining of mouse liver after treated α-Naphthoflavone, original scale: 10×. (**d**) The mRNA expression of mIl6, miNOS, mIl10 and mIl-1β, results are indicated as means ± SEM (n = 5), statistical difference: * $p < 0.05$, ** $p < 0.01$ and *** $p < 0.001$.

3.2.2. The Expression of Pro-Inflammatory Cytokines

The pro-inflammatory cytokines, including Il6, Il-1β and iNOS, as well as the anti-inflammatory cytokine, Il10, could directly reflect the extent of the liver damage. In this study, the mRNA expression levels of Il6, Il-1β, iNOS and Il-10 in mice liver increased in the APAP group, and Rut further upregulated the levels of these factors. However, treatment with α-Naphthoflavone significantly decreased the mRNA levels of these cytokines (Figure 3d). These findings indicated that Rut could aggravate APAP-induced liver inflammation via upregulating the mRNA expression of pro-inflammatory cytokines, and it is also related to the Cyp1a2 expression [26].

3.3. Rut Aggravated the APAP-Induced Acute Liver Injury In Vitro

3.3.1. Hepatocyte Injury Model In Vitro and Drug Concentration

The CCK-8 assay was conducted to determine the appropriate concentrations and dosages of APAP and Rut for modeling. According to the IC50 value, 30 mM of APAP increased the cell inhibition ratio to around 50% after being incubated with L02 cells for 6 h (Figure 4a). Rut showed significant cytotoxicity at a concentration of 20 μM, while the cell viability remained above 98% at 10 μM after 24 h of incubation. Based on these results, a simulated injury model was constructed with L02 cells co-cultured with 30 mM APAP for 6 h. Cells cocultured with 2.5 μM and 10 μM Rut for 24 h were used as the drug concentrations in the following experiments.

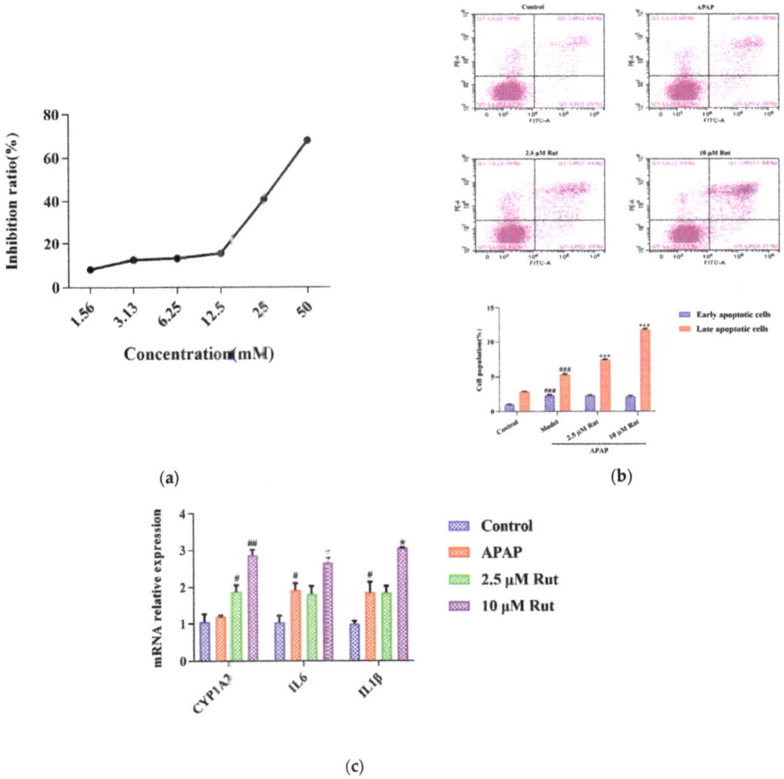

Figure 4. Rut aggravated the APAP-induced acute liver injury in vitro. (**a**) The relationship between the APAP concentration and L02 cell inhibition rate, 30 mM APAP is a suitable concentration for the model. (**b**) Apoptosis was detected by flow cytometry and date analysis, values are expressed as mean ± SEM (n = 3), statistical difference: compared with control, ### $p < 0.001$; with APAP group *** $p < 0.001$. (**c**) The mRNA expression of CYP1A2, IL6 and IL-1β, values are expressed as mean ± SEM (n = 3), statistical difference: compared with control, # $p < 0.05$ and ## $p < 0.01$; with APAP group * $p < 0.05$.

3.3.2. Rut Upregulates the Apoptosis Level of APAP-Induced Cells Injury

As shown in Figure 4b, flow cytometry analysis was used to evaluate whether Rut could exacerbate the apoptotic effect of APAP in L02 cells in vitro. The Annexin V/PI apoptosis assay revealed that the rates of the late stages of apoptosis in 40 mg/kg Rut + APAP group and 80 mg/kg Rut + APAP group were 7.46 ($p < 0.01$) and 11.98 ($p < 0.01$), respectively, which were significantly higher than in the APAP group. The results indicated that Rut increased the level of apoptosis in APAP-mediated cell injury.

3.3.3. Rut Upregulates the mRNA Expression of CYP1A2 and Pro-Inflammatory Factors In Vitro

To further evaluate whether CYP1A2 was involved in Rut exacerbating the APAP-induced cell injury, we measured the mRNA expression of CYP1A2, along with several pro-inflammatory factors. The result revealed that the mRNA expression of CYP1A2 in the APAP group did not significantly change compared to the blank group, indicating that APAP did not affect the expression level of CYP1A2. However, CYP1A2 was significantly upregulated in both the 2.5 and 10 μM Rut groups. The RT-PCR results of the pro-inflammatory factors showed that 10 μM Rut could remarkably upregulate the mRNA expression of Il6 and Il1β, while there was no significant difference between the 2.5 μM Rut group and the APAP group (Figure 4c). According to these results, CYP1A2 was involved in the process of Rut aggravating the APAP-mediated cells injury, which is consistent with the in vivo findings.

4. Discussion

The combination of traditional Chinese medicine (TCM) with synthetic drugs is a common clinical practice, which is increasingly popular due to the enhanced therapeutic effects achieved through multi-drug regimens. However, the complexity of TCM compositions can lead to adverse reactions when used in conjunction with synthetic drugs. Therefore, it is essential to conduct a comprehensive investigation into the toxic components of TCM, the potential toxic interactions with synthetic drugs, the metabolic enzyme systems involved in these reactions, and the underlying metabolic mechanisms. This study focuses on how Rut, a component of TCM, exacerbates APAP-induced acute liver damage by inducing the drug-metabolizing enzyme CYP1A2. The findings underscore the importance of understanding these drug interactions and their metabolic mechanisms to ensure the safe and effective use of combined TCM and synthetic drug therapies.

Hepatotoxicity can result from various factors, including excessive alcohol consumption, drugs, and viral infections. Among these, drug-induced toxicity is a major concern, with APAP overdose being the most common cause of acute liver injury.

APAP is commonly used as an antipyretic and analgesic, and it generally has few side effects at therapeutic doses. However, an overdose of APAP can lead to liver injury beginning as early as 3 h post-administration and progressing to severe hepatocyte death within 24 h in mouse models [27–30]. CYP2E1 and CYP1A2 are the primary cytochrome P450 enzymes responsible for metabolizing APAP into its metabolite, NAPQI. Elevated levels of NAPQI deplete GSH, leading to the formation of NAPQI-GSH adducts. This process triggers mitochondrial oxidative stress and ultimately causes acute liver inflammation [31].

APAP overdose can cause serious hepatic injury, as characterized by high serum level of ALT/AST, which are indicators of significant hepatotoxicity [32,33]. Previous reports have suggested that Rut pretreatment can ameliorate hepatocyte damage by inhibiting the expression of CYP2E1, reducing ALT/AST release and decreasing GSH consumption [34–36]. In contrast to these findings, our study demonstrated that Rut pretreatment of mice and L02 cells could exacerbate the APAP-mediated acute liver injury. This exacerbation occurs through the upregulation of both the mRNA and protein expressions of CYP1A2, which enhances the formation of the toxic metabolite NAPQI from APAP. Our results indicate that while Rut has previously been reported to mitigate liver damage under certain conditions, it can also aggravate APAP-induced acute liver injury by modulating CYP1A2 expression and promoting the toxicity of APAP.

Liver damage is always associated with the overexpression of pro-inflammatory factors, while a reduction in these factors is often related to the protection or restoration of hepatic function. Therefore, the inflammatory response is a crucial aspect of the mechanism underlying hepatotoxicity caused by APAP [27,37]. The APAP metabolite NAPQI can activate pro-inflammatory cytokines, such as IL-1β, IL-6, TNF-α, COX-2, and iNOS, leading to a significant inflammatory response [37]. In our study, we found that Rut exacerbates APAP-induced liver inflammation by further increasing the expression of Il-1β, Il-6, and iNOS, both in vivo and in vitro. These results suggest that Rut upregulates pro-inflammatory factors and aggravates APAP-induced liver inflammation. This process is linked to the upregulation of CYP1A2, which enhances the production of NAPQI and thereby intensifies the inflammatory response. A piece of more obvious evidence is that the exacerbation of APAP-induced hepatotoxicity by RUT can be mitigated by the CYP1A2-specific inhibitor α-Naphthoflavone. Unfortunately, the interaction of α-Naphthoflavone with APAP in hepatotoxicity was not involved in this study. However, the specific mechanisms through which Rut modulates CYP1A2 expression and influences inflammatory responses require further investigation to fully understand its role in APAP-induced liver injury and to explore the relationship between metabolic enzymes and inflammatory processes.

5. Conclusions

In summary, Rut exacerbates APAP-mediated liver damage by upregulating CYP1A2 and increasing the levels of pro-inflammatory factors. These results underscore the importance of carefully considering the dosage of Rut when used in combination with APAP. This study offers valuable insights for exploring the mechanisms of drug interactions in clinical practice, particularly in the context of combining TCM with synthetic pharmaceuticals.

Supplementary Materials: The following supporting information can be downloaded at https://www.mdpi.com/article/10.3390/toxics12070515/s1. Table S1: The primer for the mouse; Table S2: The primer for the human.

Author Contributions: The authors contributed to this work as follows: Y.Z. acquired funding for the research; Y.Z. designed the experiments; M.W., H.G. and X.L. performed the experiments and analyzed the data; M.W. wrote the primary manuscript; and Y.Z. and X.L. revised the manuscript. All authors have read and agreed to the published version of the manuscript.

Funding: This project was supported by the National Key R&D Program of China (2018YFC1704500, 2018YFC1704506).

Institutional Review Board Statement: This study was conducted in accordance with the guidelines of the Biomedical Ethical Committee of Peking, LA2021276.

Informed Consent Statement: Not applicable.

Data Availability Statement: The data underlying this article will be shared on reasonable request to the corresponding author.

Acknowledgments: We thank Daxeshkumar Patel for helping to revise the manuscript.

Conflicts of Interest: The authors declare that they have no conflicts of interests.

References

1. EASL Clinical Practice Guidelines: Drug-induced liver injury. *J. Hepatol.* **2019**, *70*, 1222–1261. [CrossRef] [PubMed]
2. Lee, W.M. Drug-induced acute liver failure. *Clin. Liver Dis.* **2013**, *17*, 575–586, viii. [CrossRef] [PubMed]
3. Shehu, A.I.; Ma, X.; Venkataramanan, R. Mechanisms of Drug-Induced Hepatotoxicity. *Clin. Liver Dis.* **2017**, *21*, 35–54. [CrossRef] [PubMed]
4. Larson, A.M.; Polson, J.; Fontana, R.J.; Davern, T.J.; Lalani, E.; Hynan, L.S.; Reisch, J.S.; Schiødt, F.V.; Ostapowicz, G.; Shakil, A.O.; et al. Acetaminophen-induced acute liver failure: Results of a United States multicenter, prospective study. *Hepatology (Baltimore Md.)* **2005**, *42*, 1364–1372. [CrossRef]
5. Watkins, P.B.; Kaplowitz, N.; Slattery, J.T.; Colonese, C.R.; Colucci, S.V.; Stewart, P.W.; Harris, S.C. Aminotransferase elevations in healthy adults receiving 4 grams of acetaminophen daily: A randomized controlled trial. *JAMA* **2006**, *296*, 87–93. [CrossRef]
6. Lee, S.S.; Buters, J.T.; Pineau, T.; Fernandez-Salguero, P.; Gonzalez, F.J. Role of CYP2E1 in the hepatotoxicity of acetaminophen. *J. Biol. Chem.* **1996**, *271*, 12063–12067. [CrossRef] [PubMed]
7. Manyike, P.T.; Kharasch, E.D.; Kalhorn, T.F.; Slattery, J.T. Contribution of CYP2E1 and CYP3A to acetaminophen reactive metabolite formation. *Clin. Pharmacol. Ther.* **2000**, *67*, 275–282. [CrossRef]
8. Cheung, C.; Yu, A.M.; Ward, J.M.; Krausz, K.W.; Akiyama, T.E.; Feigenbaum, L.; Gonzalez, F.J. The cyp2e1-humanized transgenic mouse: Role of cyp2e1 in acetaminophen hepatotoxicity. *Drug Metab. Dispos. Biol. Fate Chem.* **2005**, *33*, 449–457. [CrossRef] [PubMed]
9. Yu, H.; Jin, H.; Gong, W.; Wang, Z.; Liang, H. Pharmacological actions of multi-target-directed evodiamine. *Molecules* **2013**, *18*, 1826–1843. [CrossRef]

10. Tsai, T.H.; Lee, T.F.; Chen, C.F.; Wang, L.C. Thermoregulatory effects of alkaloids isolated from Wu-chu-yu in afebrile and febrile rats. *Pharmacol. Biochem. Behav.* **1995**, *50*, 293–298. [CrossRef]
11. Liao, W.Q.; Li, B.; Li, L.; Zhao, J.N. Study on molecular mechanism of Euodiae Fructus on liver toxicity in MICE. *Zhongguo Zhong Yao Za Zhi = Zhongguo Zhongyao Zazhi = China J. Chin. Mater. Medica* **2014**, *39*, 4865–4868.
12. Li, W.; Sun, X.; Liu, B.; Zhang, L.; Fan, Z.; Ji, Y. Screening and identification of hepatotoxic component in Evodia rutaecarpa based on spectrum-effect relationship and UPLC-Q-TOFMS. *Biomed. Chromatogr. BMC* **2016**, *30*, 1975–1983. [CrossRef] [PubMed]
13. Cai, Q.; Wei, J.; Zhao, W.; Shi, S.; Zhang, Y.; Wei, R.; Zhang, Y.; Li, W.; Wang, Q. Toxicity of Evodiae fructus on rat liver mitochondria: The role of oxidative stress and mitochondrial permeability transition. *Molecules* **2014**, *19*, 21168–21182. [CrossRef] [PubMed]
14. Zhang, W.; Wang, M.; Song, H.; Gao, C.; Wang, D.; Hua, H.; Pan, Y.; Liu, X. CYP3A4 inducer aggravates big flower Evodiae Fructus-induced hepatotoxicity whereas limonin attenuates its hepatotoxicity. *J. Ethnopharmacol.* **2021**, *264*, 113277. [CrossRef]
15. Zhang, M.; Gao, M.; Wu, S.; Zhou, L.; Cao, L.; Qiao, R.; Zhong, M.; Yang, L.; Yuan, J. Hepatotoxicity Comparison of Crude and Licorice-Processed Euodiae Fructus in Rats with Stomach Excess-Cold Syndrome. *Front. Pharmacol.* **2021**, *12*, 756276. [CrossRef] [PubMed]
16. Cohen, S.M.; Heywood, E.; Pillai, A.; Ahn, J. Hepatotoxicity Associated with the Use of white Flood, a Nutritional Supplement. *J. Pract. Gastroenterol.* **2012**, *10*, 45–47.
17. Qian, P.; Jin, H.W.; Yang, X.W. New limonoids from Coptidis Rhizoma-Euodiae Fructus couple. *J. Asian Nat. Prod. Res.* **2014**, *16*, 333–344. [CrossRef] [PubMed]
18. Yang, X.W.; Zhang, H.; Li, M.; Du, L.J.; Yang, Z.; Xiao, S.Y. Studies on the alkaloid constituents of Evodia rutaecarpa (Juss) Benth var. bodinaieri (Dode) Huang and their acute toxicity in mice. *J. Asian Nat. Prod. Res.* **2006**, *8*, 697–703. [CrossRef] [PubMed]
19. Zhang, Y.; Yan, T.; Sun, D.; Xie, C.; Zheng, Y.; Zhang, L.; Yagai, T.; Krausz, K.W.; Bisson, W.H.; Yang, X.; et al. Structure-Activity Relationships of the Main Bioactive Constituents of Euodia rutaecarpa on Aryl Hydrocarbon Receptor Activation and Associated Bile Acid Homeostasis. *Drug Metab. Dispos. Biol. Fate Chem.* **2018**, *46*, 1030–1040. [CrossRef]
20. Wen, B.; Roongta, V.; Liu, L.; Moore, D.J. Metabolic activation of the indoloquinazoline alkaloids evodiamine and rutaecarpine by human liver microsomes: Dehydrogenation and inactivation of cytochrome P450 3A4. *Drug Metab. Dispos. Biol. Fate Chem.* **2014**, *42*, 1044–1054. [CrossRef] [PubMed]
21. Zhang, W.; Guo, J.; Wang, D.; Ren, S.; Hua, H.; Morikawa, T.; Pan, Y.; Liu, X. Effect of CYP3A inducer/inhibitor on pharmacokinetics of five alkaloids in Evodiae Fructus. *Chem. Biol. Interact.* **2020**, *327*, 109146. [CrossRef] [PubMed]
22. Choi, J.H.; Jin, S.W.; Lee, G.H.; Han, E.H.; Hwang, Y.P.; Jeong, H.G. Rutaecarpine Protects against Acetaminophen-Induced Acute Liver Injury in Mice by Activating Antioxidant Enzymes. *Antioxidants* **2021**, *10*, 86. [CrossRef]
23. Lee, S.K.; Bista, S.R.; Jeong, H.; Kim, D.H.; Kang, M.J.; Jahng, Y.; Jeong, T.C. The effects of rutaecarpine on the pharmacokinetics of acetaminophen in rats. *Arch. Pharmacal Res.* **2007**, *30*, 1629–1634. [CrossRef] [PubMed]
24. Zhang, F.L.; He, X.; Zhai, Y.R.; He, L.N.; Zhang, S.C.; Wang, L.L.; Yang, A.H.; An, L.J. Mechanism-based inhibition of CYPs and RMs-induced hepatoxicity by rutaecarpine. *Xenobiotica Fate Foreign Compd. Biol. Syst.* **2015**, *45*, 978–989. [CrossRef] [PubMed]
25. Liu, Y.; Liu, C.; Liu, Y.; Ge, Q.; Sun, C. Cytochrome P450 Mediated Bioactivation of Rutaevin, a Bioactive and Potentially Hepatotoxic Component of Evodia Rutaecarpa. *Chem. Res. Toxicol.* **2020**, *33*, 3054–3064. [CrossRef] [PubMed]
26. Dunvald, A.D.; Järvinen, E.; Mortensen, C.; Stage, T.B. Clinical and Molecular Perspectives on Inflammation-Mediated Regulation of Drug Metabolism and Transport. *Clin. Pharmacol. Ther.* **2022**, *112*, 277–290. [CrossRef] [PubMed]
27. Zhang, J.; Song, Q.; Han, X.; Zhang, Y.; Zhang, Y.; Zhang, X.; Chu, X.; Zhang, F.; Chu, L. Multi-targeted protection of acetaminophen-induced hepatotoxicity in mice by tannic acid. *Int. Immunopharmacol.* **2017**, *47*, 95–105. [CrossRef] [PubMed]
28. Wang, X.; Liu, J.; Zhang, X.; Zhao, S.; Zou, K.; Xie, J.; Wang, X.; Liu, C.; Wang, J.; Wang, Y. Seabuckthorn berry polysaccharide extracts protect against acetaminophen induced hepatotoxicity in mice via activating the Nrf-2/HO-1-SOD-2 signaling pathway. *Phytomedicine Int. J. Phytother. Phytopharm.* **2018**, *38*, 90–97. [CrossRef]
29. Yan, M.; Ye, L.; Yin, S.; Lu, X.; Liu, X.; Lu, S.; Cui, J.; Fan, L.; Kaplowitz, N.; Hu, H. Glycycoumarin protects mice against acetaminophen-induced liver injury predominantly via activating sustained autophagy. *Br. J. Pharmacol.* **2018**, *175*, 3747–3757. [CrossRef]
30. Wang, Z.; Hu, J.N.; Yan, M.H.; Xing, J.J.; Liu, W.C.; Li, W. Caspase-Mediated Anti-Apoptotic Effect of Ginsenoside Rg5, a Main Rare Ginsenoside, on Acetaminophen-Induced Hepatotoxicity in Mice. *J. Agric. Food Chem.* **2017**, *65*, 9226–9236. [CrossRef] [PubMed]
31. Jaeschke, H.; McGill, M.R.; Ramachandran, A. Oxidant stress, mitochondria, and cell death mechanisms in drug-induced liver injury: Lessons learned from acetaminophen hepatotoxicity. *Drug Metab. Rev.* **2012**, *44*, 88–106. [CrossRef] [PubMed]
32. Xie, W.; Jiang, Z.; Wang, J.; Zhang, X.; Melzig, M.F. Protective effect of hyperoside against acetaminophen (APAP) induced liver injury through enhancement of APAP clearance. *Chem. Biol. Interact.* **2016**, *246*, 11–19. [CrossRef] [PubMed]
33. Wang, W.; Guan, C.; Sun, X.; Zhao, Z.; Li, J.; Fu, X.; Qiu, Y.; Huang, M.; Jin, J.; Huang, Z. Tanshinone IIA protects against acetaminophen-induced hepatotoxicity via activating the Nrf2 pathway. *Phytomedicine Int. J. Phytother. Phytopharm.* **2016**, *23*, 589–596. [CrossRef] [PubMed]
34. Zhang, J.; Zhang, S.; Bi, J.; Gu, J.; Deng, Y.; Liu, C. Astaxanthin pretreatment attenuates acetaminophen-induced liver injury in mice. *Int. Immunopharmacol.* **2017**, *45*, 26–33. [CrossRef]

35. Lv, H.; Xiao, Q.; Zhou, J.; Feng, H.; Liu, G.; Ci, X. Licochalcone A Upregulates Nrf2 Antioxidant Pathway and Thereby Alleviates Acetaminophen-Induced Hepatotoxicity. *Front. Pharmacol.* **2018**, *9*, 147. [CrossRef] [PubMed]
36. Xu, X.Y.; Hu, J.N.; Liu, Z.; Zhang, R.; He, Y.F.; Hou, W.; Wang, Z.Q.; Yang, G.; Li, W. Saponins (Ginsenosides) from the Leaves of Panax quinquefolius Ameliorated Acetaminophen-Induced Hepatotoxicity in Mice. *J. Agric. Food Chem.* **2017**, *65*, 3684–3692. [CrossRef] [PubMed]
37. Yang, C.; Yi, J.; Gong, X.; Ge, P.; Dai, J.; Lin, L.; Xing, Y.; Zhang, L. Anti-oxidative and anti-inflammatory benefits of the ribonucleoside analogue 5-azacitidine in mice with acetaminophen-induced toxic hepatitis. *Int. Immunopharmacol.* **2017**, *48*, 91–95. [CrossRef]

Disclaimer/Publisher's Note: The statements, opinions and data contained in all publications are solely those of the individual author(s) and contributor(s) and not of MDPI and/or the editor(s). MDPI and/or the editor(s) disclaim responsibility for any injury to people or property resulting from any ideas, methods, instructions or products referred to in the content.

toxics

MDPI

Article

Ribosomal Dysregulation in Metastatic Laryngeal Squamous Cell Carcinoma: Proteomic Insights and CX-5461's Therapeutic Promise

Miao Gao †, Ting Liu †, Kairui Hu, Songling Chen, Shixin Wang, Di Gan, Zhihan Li and Xiaohuang Lin *

Key Laboratory of Ministry of Education for Gastrointestinal Cancer, School of Basic Medical Sciences, Fujian Medical University, Fuzhou 350108, China; miaomiao055@163.com (M.G.); liuting8026@fjmu.edu.cn (T.L.); hkr59625@fjmu.edu.cn (K.H.); chensongling@fjmu.edu.cn (S.C.); wangshixin@stu.fjmu.edu.cn (S.W.); gandi@stu.fjmu.edu.cn (D.G.); lizhihan@stu.fjmu.edu.cn (Z.L.)

* Correspondence: linxiaohuang@fjmu.edu.cn

† These authors contributed equally to this work.

Abstract: One of the main barriers to the successful treatment of laryngeal squamous cell carcinoma (LSCC) is postoperative progression, primarily due to tumor cell metastasis. To systematically investigate the molecular characteristics and potential mechanisms underlying the metastasis in laryngeal cancer, we carried out a TMT-based proteomic analysis of both cancerous and adjacent non-cancerous tissues from 10 LSCC patients with lymph node metastasis (LNM) and 10 without. A total of 5545 proteins were quantified across all samples. We identified 57 proteins that were downregulated in LSCC with LNM, which were enriched in cell adhesion pathways, and 69 upregulated proteins predominantly enriched in protein production pathways. Importantly, our data revealed a strong correlation between increased ribosomal activity and the presence of LNM, as 18 ribosomal subunit proteins were found to be upregulated, with RPS10 and RPL24 being the most significantly overexpressed. The potential of ribosomal proteins, including RPS10 and RPL24, as biomarkers for LSCC with LNM was confirmed in external validation samples (six with LNM and six without LNM) using Western blotting and immunohistochemistry. Furthermore, we have confirmed that the RNA polymerase I inhibitor CX-5461, which impedes ribosome biogenesis in LSCC, also decreases the expression of RPS10, RPL24, and RPS26. In vitro experiments have revealed that CX-5461 moderately reduces cell viability, while it significantly inhibits the invasion and migration of LSCC cells. It can enhance the expression of the epithelial marker CDH1 and suppress the expression of the mesenchymal markers CDH2, VIM, and FN at a dose that does not affect cell viability. Our study broadens the scope of the proteomic data on laryngeal cancer and suggests that ribosome targeting could be a supplementary therapeutic strategy for metastatic LSCC.

Keywords: LSCC; Lymph node metastasis; Proteomics; Ribosome; CX-5461

1. Introduction

Head and neck cancers (HNCs) are ranked as the sixth most common type of cancer worldwide, they encompass a diverse range of tumors classified by their site of origin [1,2]. Laryngeal carcinoma (LC) represents a substantial fraction of HNCs, accounting for one third of all such cases [3]. Laryngeal squamous cell carcinoma (LSCC) is estimated to constitute approximately 85% to 95% of all cases of LC [4,5]. Despite advancements in its treatment, the five-year overall survival rate for laryngeal cancer hovers around 50%, primarily due to the occurrence of distant metastases and the development of therapy-resistant local and regional recurrences [6,7]. It is widely acknowledged that the presence of metastasis at the time of diagnosis is a critical prognostic factor for patients with LSCC [7,8].

The initial spread of head and neck squamous cell carcinoma (HNSCC) typically targets the neck lymph nodes [9,10]. Most patients with LSCC present with advanced stages of the disease, and over 60 percent are predisposed to lymph node metastasis (LNM), which is a crucial factor in their prognosis [11]. The presence, number, distribution, and extranodal extension of lymph node metastases are all critical in assessing the risk of distant disease and patient survival. An ipsilateral single-node metastasis can reduce survival rates by half, and contralateral or bilateral involvement can decrease survival by an additional 50% [12,13]. Consequently, preventing and inhibiting lymph node metastasis should be integral to strategies aimed at controlling tumor progression.

Lymph node metastasis is a multi-step process that encompasses invasion, lymphangiogenesis, the spread of cancer cells through lymphatic channels, their transit into the lymph nodes, and their subsequent settlement and proliferation [14]. Over the last few decades, a range of biomarkers implicated in the metastatic cascade of HNSCC have been identified [15]. Key among these are matrix metalloproteinases (MMPs), which are critical enzymes that degrade and remodel the extracellular matrix (ECM), thus facilitating tumor invasion and metastasis [16,17]. CD44, functioning as a cell surface receptor, not only binds to but also potentiates the activity of MMPs [18]. Furthermore, proangiogenic factors, including VEGF and IL-8, along with chemokine receptor-7 (CCR7), have been implicated in the promotion of metastatic disease [19]. Recent findings also suggest a correlation between elevated levels of miR-23a [20] and EPCAM in laryngeal cancer [13], which is associated with an increased risk of lymph node metastasis and poorer prognostic outcomes. There is still a noticeable gap in in-depth omics-level analyses that could elucidate the molecular mechanisms and identify reliable biomarkers of lymph node metastasis in LSCC.

The metastasis of tumor cells is a complex process involving numerous genes, with increasing evidence suggesting that ribosomal proteins (RPs) play a pivotal role [21]. The proliferation in cancer cells demands accelerated protein production, requiring enhanced ribosome biogenesis. This enhancement can be driven by altered signaling, metabolic shifts, and changes in non-coding RNA, leading to increased RNA Pol I (RNA polymerase I) activity [22]. Studies have revealed that RPs such as RPL15 are key in advancing metastasis, particularly in circulating tumor cells (CTCs), through the amplification of protein translation [23]. Moreover, reducing RPL27A or RPL15 in vitro can hinder the movement of breast cancer cells [24]. La-related protein 6 (LARP6) has also been recognized for its role in epithelial–mesenchymal transition (EMT) through affecting the localization of ribosomal proteins (RPs), thereby aiding cell migration [25]. In addition to cytoplasmic ribosomal proteins, the abnormal expression of mitochondrial ribosomal proteins may also promote the invasion and metastasis of tumors [26]. For example, MRPS16 promotes the migration and invasion of glioma cells by activating the PI3K/Akt/Snail axis [27]. The protein levels of MRPL15, MRPL13, and MRPL54 are associated with the recurrence, distant metastasis, and prognosis of breast cancer [28]. Additionally, MRPL38 is more abundant in most metastatic cancer cell lines [29]. Such studies underscore the critical role of ribosomal protein variations in modulating the transition of cancer cells to a state of enhanced migration and invasion.

In this study, we conducted a tandem mass tag (TMT)-based whole-cell proteomic analysis of LSCC to obtain a comprehensive view of the proteins that are dysregulated and their association with lymph node metastasis. A proteome-based bioinformatics analysis highlighted the importance of ribosomal proteins in LSCC's metastasis to the lymph nodes. Moreover, we confirmed the efficacy of CX-5461, a selective and orally bioavailable RNA polymerase I inhibitor, in inhibiting LSCC cell invasion in vitro.

2. Methods

2.1. Clinical Tissue Sample Collection

Laryngeal squamous cell carcinoma tissues, along with adjacent normal tissues, were obtained from patients diagnosed with laryngeal cancer who underwent surgical resection at the First Affiliated Hospital of Fujian Medical University. Patients with a history of chemotherapy or radiotherapy were excluded from the study. After gross examination, pathologists selectively excised non-necrotic sections from the resected tumor specimens.

Adjacent normal tissues were harvested at least 2 cm away from the tumor margin. Tumor tissues and adjacent normal tissues from the same patients were stored in liquid nitrogen and were also subjected to pathological confirmation via hematoxylin-eosin (HE) staining by pathologists. For the proteomic analysis, subsets of LSCC patients with LNM (n = 10) and without LNM (n = 10) were selected based on comparable clinical and histopathological characteristics, as well as similar age and gender distributions. The validation cohort included an additional six LSCC patients with LNM and six LSCC patients without LNM. The clinicopathological features of the 32 patients are summarized in Table 1.

Table 1. Clinical characteristics of the 32 LSCC patients.

Characteristic	Whole Cohort	Lymph Node Metastasis	
		Present	Absent
Total (cases)	32	16	16
Age [years (mean ± SD)]	64.1 ± 8.1	63.6 ± 7.5	64.6 ± 8.7
Gender [cases (%)]			
Male	32 (100)	16 (50)	16 (50)
Pathologic-T [cases (%)]			
T3	15 (50)	8 (53.3)	7 (46.7)
T4	17 (50)	8 (47.1)	9 (52.9)

Abbreviations: SD, standard deviation.

The ethical committee of Fujian Medical University granted approval for this study, and informed consent was acquired from each participant for the use of their data in this research.

2.2. Protein Extraction, Digestion, and Tandem Mass Tag (TMT) Isobaric Labeling

Twenty milligrams of tissue were homogenized in lysis buffer [8 M urea, 150 mM NaCl, 50 mM Tris-HCl (pH 8.0), and 1× protease inhibitor (Thermo Fisher Scientific, Waltham, MA, USA, 78429)] and incubated for 30 min on ice. The samples then underwent sonication to reduce lysate viscosity. After centrifugation at 16,000× g for 10 min, the soluble supernatants were collected. The protein concentration in the lysates was quantified using BCA assays.

For tryptic digestion, 500 µg of the protein samples was first reduced with 10 mM dithi-othreitol (DTT) at 37 °C for 60 min and alkylated with 50 mM iodoacetamide (IAA), in the dark, for 10 min. The proteins were precipitated with a 5-fold volume of ice-cold acetone, and the resulting pellet was collected via centrifugation at 1000× g for 10 min, followed by three washes with precooled acetone. The pellet was then redissolved in 100 mM triethylammonium bicarbonate (TEAB) and digested using trypsin at a 1:50 (w:w) trypsin-to-protein ratio and incubated at 37 °C overnight.

The peptide concentrations were determined using BCA assays. Subsequently, 100 µg of peptides from each sample were labeled with TMTpro-18plex (A52047) or TMT-11plex (A37725) isobaric tags, according to the manufacturer's protocol. The 40 samples, comprising 20 tumor-to-normal pairs, included mixed peptides that served as an internal reference across three TMT experiments (the samples' labeling details are presented in Table S1). The labeled peptides were then mixed, desalted, and vacuum-dried.

2.3. Fractionation of Peptides and LC-MS/MS Analysis

Using a high pH reversed-phase peptide fractionation kit (Thermo Fisher Scientific, Waltham, MA, USA, 84868), the labeled peptides were divided into 15 fractions and dried via vacuum centrifugation. Each peptide fraction was dissolved in 0.1% formic acid and injected into an Acclaim PepMap C18 column (75 µm × 25 cm) for LC-MS/MS analysis. A 50-min gradient was run at 200 nL/min on an EASY-nLC 1200 UPLC system (Thermo Fisher Scientific, Waltham, MA, USA); 2% to 30% of solvent B (0.1% formic acid in 98% acetonitrile) was increased to 50% within 5 min and then to 80% over a further minute, where it remained for 4 min. The peptides underwent ionization using an NSI source before a tandem MS analysis using an Orbitrap Exploris 480 MS, coupled online with the UPLC. The settings included a 2.3 kV spray voltage, a funnel RF level of 50, and a capillary temperature of 320 °C. In its data-dependent acquisition (DDA) mode, the full MS operated with a resolution of 60,000 at *m/z* 200, an AGC target of 300%, and scanned a mass range of 350–1600 *m/z*. The fragment spectra were established using a 200% AGC target, 15,000 resolution, and 50 ms injection times, using a Top12 approach. Additional parameters included an intensity threshold of 2×10^5, an isolation width of 1.6 *m/z*, and a normalized collision energy of 30%.

2.4. MS Data Processing and Data Analysis

The mass spectrometric files were processed using MaxQuant (version 2.4.2.0, Max-Planck Institute of Biochemistry, Munich, Germany). The data were searched against the Homo sapiens Uniprot database (20,597 sequences), assuming the digestion enzyme trypsin. The mass error was set to 10 ppm for precursor ions and 4.5 ppm for fragment ions. The oxidation of methionine and the protein's N-terminus acetylation were specified as variable modifications. For the TMT-labeled experiment, the carbamidomethyl of cysteine, TMT of lysine, and the N-terminus were specified as fixed modifications, while, for the TMTpro-labeled experiments, the fixed modifications were set as TMTpro lysine and the N-terminus and carbamidomethyl of cysteine. The number of max missed cleavage sites was set to 2. The enzyme was set as trypsin. The acceptance criterion for identifications was that the false discovery rate (FDR) should be less than 1% for peptides and proteins. For the quantification of proteins, the MS intensity of each protein across three TMT experiments was corrected with respect to the reference channel. The harmonized data from three TMT experiments were subsequently combined into a single expression matrix, subjected to a log2 transformation, and normalized using upper quartile normalization.

2.5. Bioinformatics Analysis

The filtered proteomic data with no missing values (n = 5545 proteins) were used as input data for the differential expression analysis. Proteins with a fold change > 1.2 and $p < 0.01$, as determined by the two-sample Student's *t*-test, were identified as differentially expressed proteins (DEPs). A functional enrichment analysis, including gene ontology (GO) and the Kyoto Encyclopedia of Genes and Genomes (KEGG), was performed using DAVID bioinformatics resources [30]. A Benjamini–Hochberg-adjusted *p*-value of less than 0.05 was considered to indicate statistical significance. A gene set enrichment analysis (GSEA) was carried out to pinpoint the predominantly enriched pathways using the "clusterProfiler" package in R software (version 4.3.2) [8], with pathways achieving a nominal q-value below 0.01 being deemed statistically significant. The Kaplan–Meier plotter, utilizing the R package "survival", was employed to compare the OS and PFS times between specific groups. The processed gene expression profiles and clinical attributes of laryngeal cancer patients were acquired from the TCGA and CPTAC databases through LinkedOmics (http://www.linkedomics.org, accessed on 10 December 2023). Any samples deficient in crucial clinicopathological or prognostic data were eliminated from the subsequent analyses.

2.6. Western Blotting

The proteins from LSCC tissues were isolated as previously described (Method 2.2). For the cell lines, we harvested and thrice washed cells with PBS. They were then lysed on ice for 30 min in RIPA buffer supplemented with phenylmethylsulfonyl fluoride (PMSF) and protease and phosphatase inhibitors. Afterwards, protein separation was conducted via SDS-PAGE, and their transfer onto a PVDF membrane followed. The mem-brane underwent blocking with 5% nonfat milk before overnight incubation with primary antibodies at 4 °C. The employed primary antibodies included GAPDH (Abclonal, Wuhan, China, AC001), β-actin (Abclonal, A17910), RPS10 (Abclonal, A6056), CDH1 (Abclonal, A24874), CDH2 (Abclonal, A19083), Snail (Abclonal, A5243), RPL29 (Immunoway, Plano, TX, USA,

YN0379), RPS28 (Immunoway, YN4647), RPL3 (Immunoway, YT4105), RPS26 (Proteintech, Wuhan, China, 14909), VIM (Proteintech, 10366), FN (Proteintech, 15613), ZO1(Proteintech, 21773), and RPL24 (Proteintech, 17082). After being rinsed with PBS and 0.1% Tween 20, the membrane was incubated with the pertinent secondary antibodies for an hour at room temperature. Protein bands were visualized using enhanced chemiluminescence (ECL) reagents and the Bio-Rad ChemiDoc MP imaging system (Hercules, CA, USA), with their quantification performed using ImageJ software (version 1.49).

2.7. RNA Isolation and Quantitative Real-Time PCR

Total RNA was isolated from the cells using TRIzol reagent and cDNA was synthesized from 1 μg of total RNA using a reverse transcription kit (YEASEN, Shanghai, China) according to the manufacturer's instructions. A quantitative mRNA analysis was performed using SYBR Green qPCR Mix (Vazyme, Najing, China). The mean Ct for each sample was normalized using GAPDH as the reference gene (for primer sequences, see Supplementary Materials, Table S2).

2.8. Immunohistochemistry

Tissue samples were fixed in 10% neutral buffered formalin for 24 h and then embedded in paraffin. Sections with a thickness of 5 μm were deparaffinized and rehydrated, with their endogenous peroxidase activity quenched using a 3% hydrogen peroxide solution. Sections were stained with anti-PRS10 or RPL24 antibodies at a 1:200 dilution ratio and incubated overnight at 4 °C. After washing with PBST, they were treated with the Elivision super HRP (Rabbit) IHC Kit (Maxim, Fuzhou, China) according to the manufacturer's protocol. For the visualization of their proteins, diaminobenzidine (DAB kit, Maxim) was applied, and the slides were counterstained with hematoxylin. Imaging was carried out using a Nikon light microscope at 200× magnification. A semiquantitative analysis of protein expression was conducted using Image Pro Plus software (version 6.0).

2.9. Cell Lines and Culture

The Tu686 and Tu212 LSCC cell lines were purchased from the Cell Center of Life Science of the Chinese Academy of Science (Shanghai, China). The cells were maintained in RPMI-1640 medium (Gibco, Carlsbad, CA, USA) supplemented with 10% fetal bovine serum and 1% penicillin–streptomycin (100 μg/mL) at 37 °C in a humidified incubator (Thermo Fisher Scientific, Waltham, MA, USA) in the presence of 5% CO_2.

2.10. Cell Viability and Invasion

Cells were seeded onto 96-well plates and left overnight, before being treated with a dose–response-determined volume of CX-5461 (MEC, Lansdale, New Jersey, USA, 13323A) for a duration of 96 h. Cell viability was assessed using a Cell Counting Kit-8 (CCK8) (YEASEN, Shanghai, China, 40203ES). For the invasion assay, cells were placed in serum-free RPMI 1640 media within Matrigelcoated chambers (8 μm pore size, Corning Inc., New York, NY, USA), and the lower chamber was filled with 600 μL of medium supplemented with 20% FBS. After a 48 h incubation at 37 °C with 5% CO_2, the cells were fixed with 4% paraformaldehyde (PFA) and stained with 0.5% crystal violet for 20 min. The invasive cells were imaged and quantified across five randomly selected fields.

2.11. Wound Healing Assay

A wound healing assay was employed for assessing cell migration. Cells were placed in a 6-well plate and left to grow overnight until they covered 80–90% of the surface. A single layer of cells was then scratched using a sterile 10 μL pipette tip and cleaned with PBS to remove any cell residue. After the scratch was made, cells were allowed to grow further in RPMI-1640 culture medium without fetal bovine serum. The movement of cells was observed and captured every 24 h using an inverted microscope.

2.12. Statistical Analysis

In the proteomic analysis, we applied a two-tailed unpaired Student's t-test to determine the statistical significance of the difference between LSCC tumor tissues with and without lymph node metastasis (LNM). For comparisons between tumor samples and their adjacent normal tissue counterparts, a two-tailed paired Student's t-test was applied. Proteins with a fold change > 1.2 and a p value < 0.01 were defined as significantly differentially expressed. In vitro experiments, such as the transwell assays, wound healing assays, cell viability measurements, and Western blot analyses of various markers, were each independently repeated at least three times. Two-tailed Student's t-tests were used to compare between groups. Data were presented as means ± SD, and $p < 0.05$ was considered significant.

3. Results

3.1. Schematic Workflow for Screening Metastasis-Specific Proteins from LSCC Patients

The survival rate of laryngeal squamous cell carcinoma (LSCC) patients is significantly affected by the tumor's high invasiveness and its tendency to spread to distant body sites, such as cervical lymph nodes and other organs. In our analysis of the clinical data from LSCC patients within the TCGA and CPTAC databases, we discovered that more than 59% of these patients experience lymph node metastasis (LNM). Those with lymph node metastasis showed lower overall survival (OS) and progression-free survival (PFS) rates, as indicated by the generated Kaplan–Meier curves, which had p values of 2.2×10^{-3} and 2.1×10^{-3}, respectively (Figure 1A,B, Supplementary Materials, Table S3).

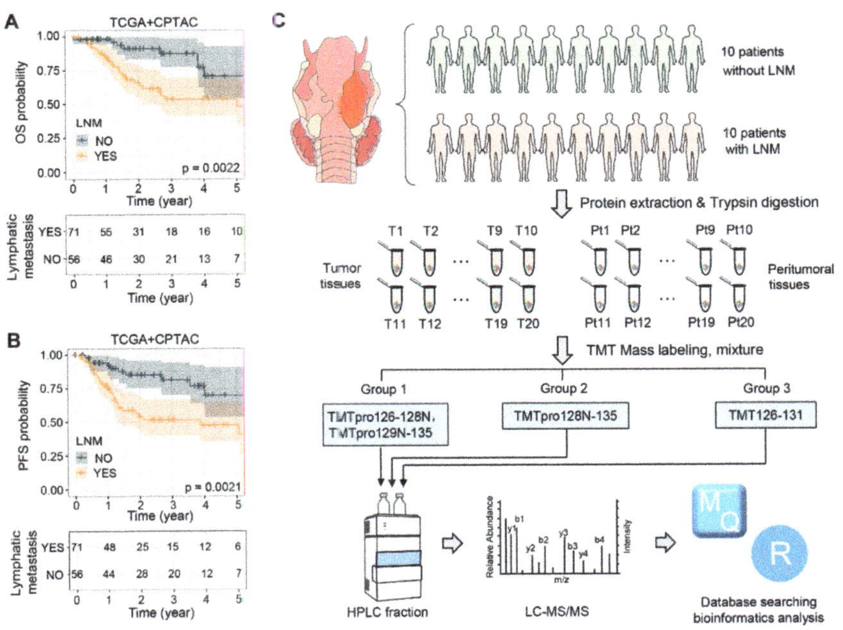

Figure 1. Study design and data analysis pipeline. (**A**,**B**) Kaplan–Meier curves illustrating the overall survival (OS) (**A**) and progression-free survival (PFS) (**B**) of patients in the CPTAC and TCGA LSCC cohorts, stratified by the presence or absence of lymphatic metastasis. (**C**) Workflow and strategy for the quantitative proteomic analysis of LSCC. Abbreviations: LNM, lymph node metastasis; T, tumor tissue; Pt, peritumoral tissue; TMT, tandem mass tag; HPRP, high-performance liquid chromatography; MS, mass spectrometry.

To gain a comprehensive understanding of LSCC patients with lymph node metastasis (LNM), we developed an efficient workflow to identify the proteins that are dysregulated specifically in relation to the LNM occurring in LSCC (Figure 1C). Paired tumor and adjacent non-tumor tissue samples from twenty LSCC patients, including ten with LNM (Patients 1–10) and ten without LNM (Patients 11–20), were collected for a global proteomic analysis utilizing a TMT-based strategy that followed stringent criteria. The clinicopathological characteristics of these 20 LSCC patients are summarized in Table 1. After protein extraction, trypsin digestion, and TMT labeling, the labeled peptides were pooled for HPLC fractionation and subsequently analyzed using LC-MS/MS. In order to avoid protein variations due to batch effects, the patients were randomly shuffled during sample preparation and MS acquisition, and the abundance of each protein was normalized, with respect to a reference channel, across three TMT groups (Groups I–III). The database search results indicated that the labeling efficiency of all three TMT groups exceeded 98% (Figure S1A) and that the overall intensities of each channel fluctuated within a small range (Figure S1B). These findings demonstrate the rigorous control we had over our experimental procedure and attest to the high quality of the proteomic data.

3.2. The Landscape of Dysregulated Proteins in LSCC Patients with LNM

For the quantitative proteomics analysis, three sets of TMT experiments identified a total of 6979, 6875, and 6692 proteins, respectively, with 6870, 6747, and 6619 of these proteins being quantified (Figure 2A). Among these proteins, 5545 were quantified across all samples and, therefore, included in subsequent analyses (Figure 2B, Table S4). Next, we compared the differentially expressed proteins between tumors with and without LNM, revealing that 126 proteins were significantly differentially expressed (fold change > 1.2, $p < 0.01$): 69 were upregulated and 57 downregulated, as shown in Figure 2C. The 69 stably upregulated proteins in tumors with LNM could serve as a potential pool for the identification of high-invasion-specific LSCC biomarkers. Furthermore, 23% of these proteins (16 out of 69) exhibited the same trend of dysregulation when comparing tumor to peritumoral tissues (Figure S2B). To better understand the biological functions of the dysregulated proteins specific to LNM, we performed Gene Ontology (GO) and Kyoto Encyclopedia of Genes and Genomes pathway (KEGG) enrichment analyses using DAVID bioinformatics resources. The most enriched pathways among the proteins positively related to LNM included ribosome ($p = 6.31 \times 10^{-20}$), spliceosome ($p = 1.96 \times 10^{-3}$), and cytoplasmic translation ($p = 5.53 \times 10^{-25}$), indicating an extraordinary activation of ribosome biogenesis and the synthesis of proteins. As expected, the proteins negatively related to LNM were significantly enriched in pathways such as complement and coagulation cascades ($p = 5.54 \times 10^{-6}$), ECM–receptor interactions ($p = 6.76 \times 10^{-6}$), and cell adhesion ($p = 5.16 \times 10^{-4}$) (Figure 2D, Table S5). This enrichment indicates a disruption of the intercellular matrix and cell–cell junctions, which, coupled with the active biosynthesis of tumor cells, collectively promotes the invasion and metastasis of LSCC.

The dysregulated proteins in T/Pt are displayed as a volcano plot (Figure S2A); a total of 848 proteins were observed to be significantly differentially expressed (a fold change > 1.2, $p < 0.01$), of which 419 were upregulated and 429 were downregulated. The most enriched pathways of the dysregulated proteins in tumor tissues are illustrated in Figure S2C. Notably, upregulated proteins were overrepresented in pathways including DNA replication ($p = 1.35 \times 10^{-4}$), spliceosome ($p = 1.18 \times 10^{-3}$), base excision repair ($p = 2.95 \times 10^{-3}$), and antigen processing and presentation ($p = 8.16 \times 10^{-3}$), while the downregulated proteins were enriched in pathways including complement and coagulation cascades ($p = 4.54 \times 10^{-12}$), thermogenesis ($p = 2.65 \times 10^{-7}$), and oxidative phosphorylation ($p = 3.23 \times 10^{-7}$). This enrichment analysis underscores the notable genomic instability and mitochondrial functional impairments in LSCC cells.

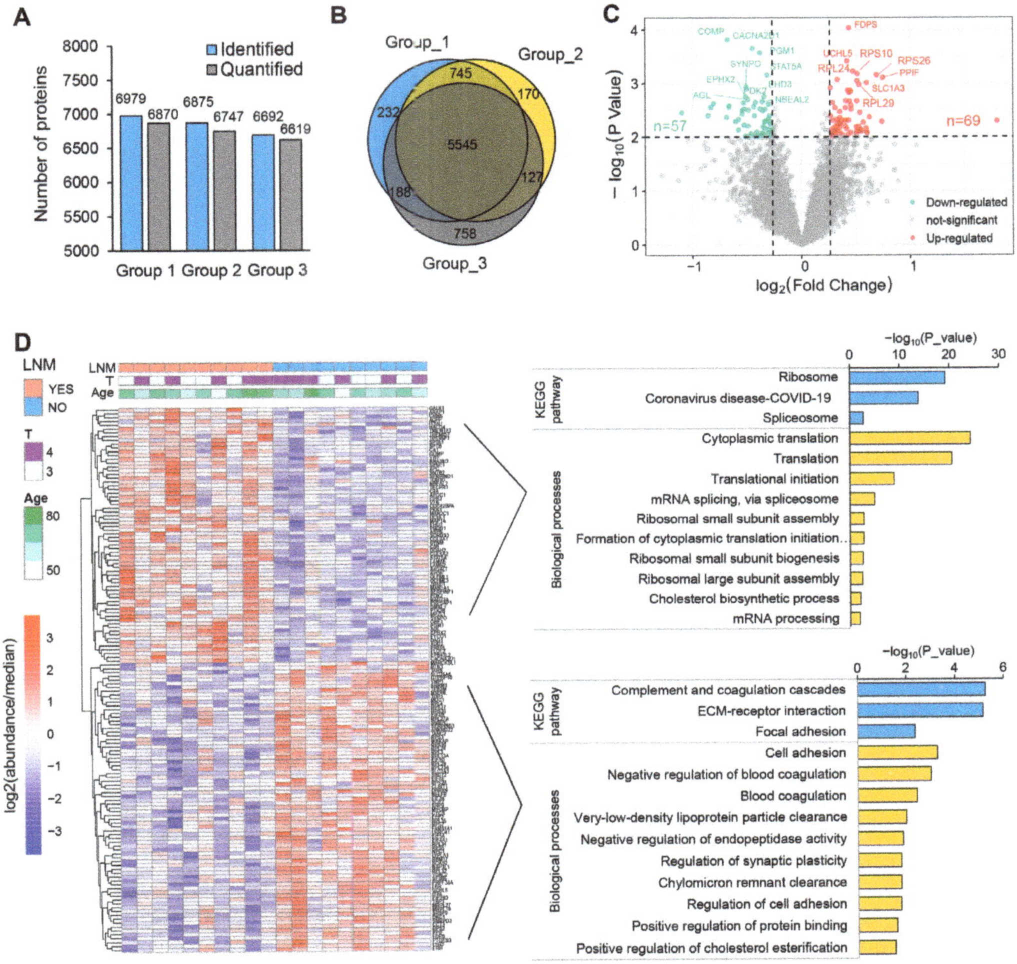

Figure 2. Quantitative profiling of whole-cell proteome in LSCC. (**A**) Summary of identified and quantified proteins in the three TMT groups. (**B**) Venn diagram of the quantified proteins of three TMT-based protein profiling: 5545 proteins were quantified across all samples. (**C**) Volcano plot indicating the differentially regulated proteins in LSCC with LNM versus LSCC without LNM. Red and blue colors represent fold changes ≥ 1.2 and a $p < 0.01$. (**D**) Heatmap showing the differently expressed proteins. Histogram showing the enrichment of KEGG and GOBP (GO biological processes) terms in upregulated (**upper right**) and downregulated (**bottom right**) proteins; this analysis was conducted using DAVID. Detailed data are available in Tables S4 and S5.

3.3. Dysregulation of Ribosomal Proteins is Closely Associated with LNM of LSCC

The aberrant growth and proliferation of tumor cells depend on increased protein synthesis, which requires an overly activated ribosomal biogenesis process. In line with this requirement, the most enriched pathways among the dysregulated proteins in LSCC with LNM are all ribosome-associated. Our gene set enrichment analysis (GSEA) reveals that most of the proteins of the ribosomal subunits, as well as those related to translation, are upregulated to various extents in LSCC with lymph node metastasis (Figure 3A). When all quantified ribosomal proteins were displayed as a heatmap, the ribosomal protein expression levels in LSCC tissues with lymph node metastasis were generally found to be higher than those in adjacent non-cancerous tissues (Figure 3B). In contrast, the fluctuations in ribosomal protein expression between cancerous and peritumoral tissues in LSCC without lymph node metastasis were found to be less pronounced.

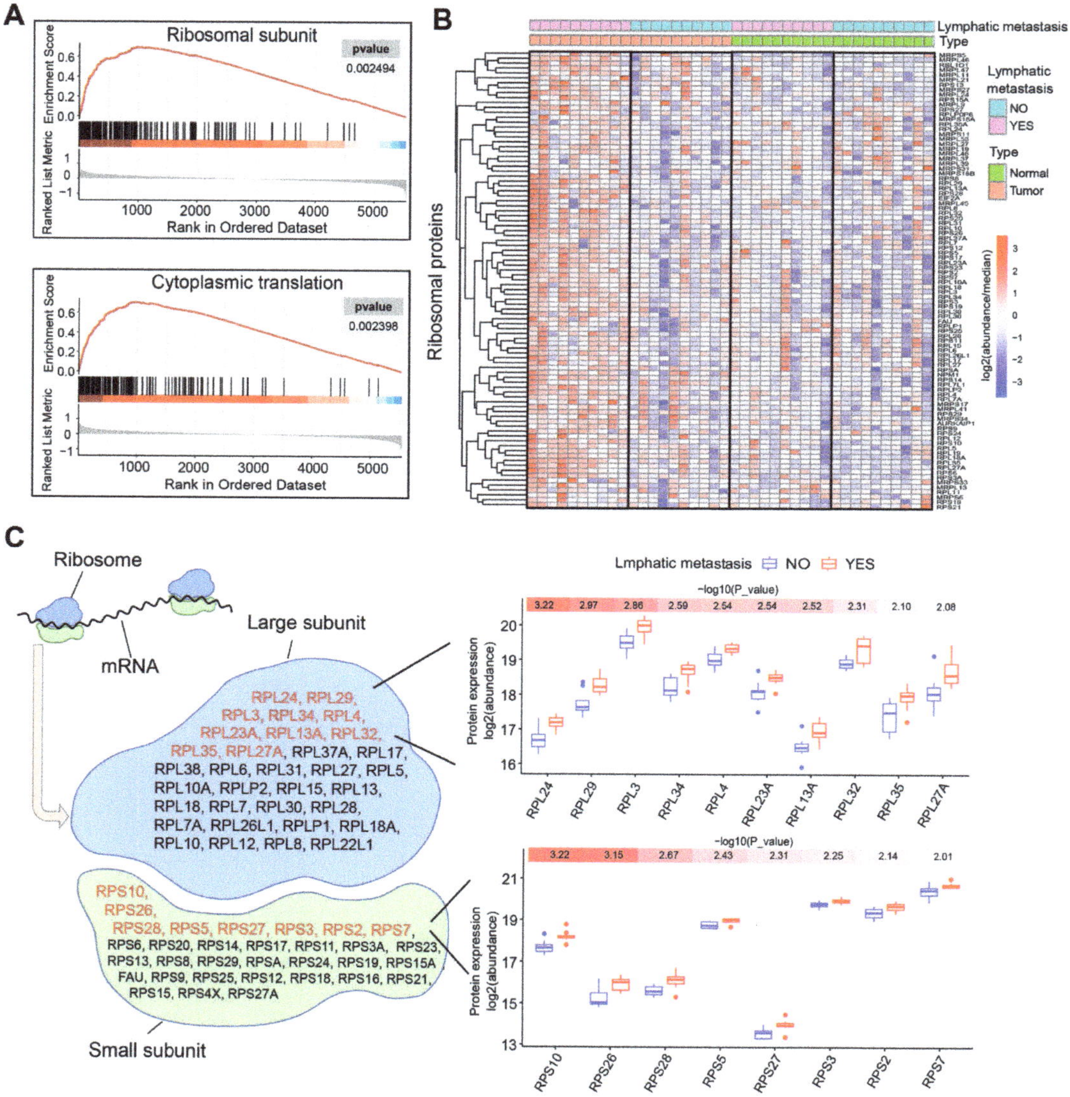

Figure 3. The ribosome is markedly activated in LSCC with LNM. (**A**) Gene set enrichment analysis (GSEA) of samples with and without LNM. (**B**) Heatmap showing the expression pattern of ribosomal proteins in LSCC with and without LNM. (**C**) The quantified ribosomal proteins have been categorized according to their presence in either the large or small subunit. Proteins specifically associated with lymph node metastasis and exhibiting a *p*-value of less than 0.01 are marked in red. To the right, box plots illustrate the expression levels of these proteins, arranged in ascending order according to their *p* values.

The ribosome consists of 60S and 40S subunits, which include a series of proteins and RNA molecules. These subunits assemble to form a specific structure that accommodates mRNA and tRNA and promotes reactions such as amino acid binding. Ten proteins, comprising up to 21% of the proteins quantified in the 60S ribosomal subunit, and eight proteins, representing 25% of those in the 40S subunit, were significantly overexpressed in LSCC with lymph node metastasis, exhibiting a *p*-value of less than 0.01, as shown in Figure 3C. These 18 stably upregulated proteins could serve as a potential resource for the identification of LSCC biomarkers specific to lymph node metastasis. Notably, RPS10 and RPL24, which are integral to the small and large ribosomal subunits, respectively, are the proteins most relevant to lymph node metastasis.

3.4. Validation of the LNM Specific Biomarkers

To validate the biomarkers identified via MS, we procured an additional 12 LSCC tissue samples, thereby extending our study beyond the initial cohort of 20 patients. Within this new subset, half the subjects exhibited lymph node metastasis, while the other half were metastasis-free. We focused on the ribosomal proteins previously identified as the most upregulated (RPS10, RPL24, RPS26, RPL29, RPL3, and RPS28). A Western blot analysis confirmed that these proteins had heightened expression specificity in LNM within this novel validation cohort (Figure 4A). To address any potential bias in protein quantification due to variations in tumor purity, we conducted immunohistochemical (IHC) analyses for RPS10 and RPL24, which were consistent with our Western blot results (Figure 4C).

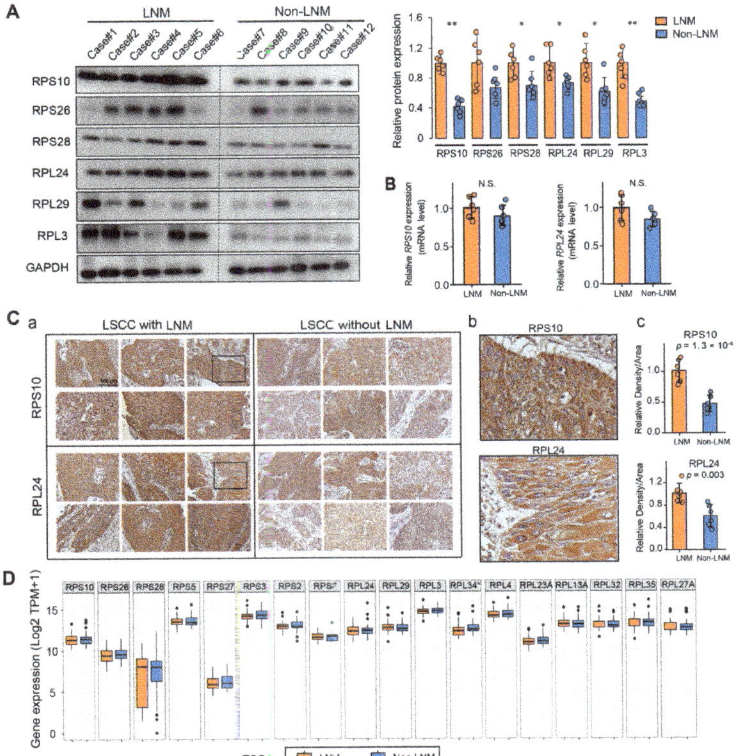

Figure 4. Validation of biomarker expression patterns in LSCC with LNM. (**A**) Western blot validation of the protein abundance of the most upregulated ribosomal proteins in LSCC with LNM ($n = 6$) compared to LSCC without LNM ($n = 6$). Densitometric quantification of Western blot signals is illustrated in the

histogram on the right. (**B**) QPCR analysis detected the expression of *rps10* and *rpl24* genes in LSCC with ($n = 6$) versus without LNM ($n = 6$). (**C**) Representative IHC staining demonstrated marked overexpression of RPS10 and RPL24 in LSCC with LNM: (**a**) Original magnification, ×20; (**b**) representative higher magnification (×40) images of the views marked by the black squares in (**a**), showing the hybridization of RPS10 and RPL24 to tumor cells; (**c**) assessment of proteins expression by relative density to area. (**D**) Gene expression of ribosomal proteins specifically associated with LNM. The mRNA expression data from LSCC cases with ($n = 53$) and without ($n = 39$) LNM were extracted from the TCGA database and compared. Abbreviations: LNM, LSCC with lymph node metastasis; NO, LSCC without lymph node metastasis; TPM, transcripts per million. Data are presented as mean ± SD. Significant differences were determined using a two-tailed *t*-test, * $p < 0.05$, ** $p < 0.01$.

To determine whether the heightened expression of these ribosomal proteins was rooted in gene expression anomalies, we performed quantitative PCR (QPCR) assays for the *rps10* and *rpl24* genes and found no significant alterations (Figure 4B). This finding implies that the overexpression of ribosomal proteins in LSCC is likely an event that occurs during translation or post-translation, rather than at the gene transcription stage. In pursuit of further evidence, we analyzed the expression of the genes encoding these ribosomal proteins in LSCC cases from The Cancer Genome Atlas (TCGA) database. In agreement with our experimental results, there were no notable disparities at the mRNA level in the identified ribosomal proteins with LNM-specific overexpression (Figure 4D). This additional analysis reinforces the notion that post-transcriptional mechanisms may account for the discrepant ribosomal protein expression observed in LSCC with lymph node metastasis.

3.5. CX-5461 Hinders Ribosome Biogenesis and Reduces the Expression of Several Ribosomal Proteins

CX-5461 is an orally available inhibitor of ribosome biogenesis capable of disrupting the production of rRNA and thereby inhibiting ribosome biogenesis within the nucleolus. Based on our previous findings of increased ribosomal activity in LSCC tissues with lymph node metastasis compared to those without metastasis, we proposed that CX-5461 could potentially inhibit the abnormal activation of ribosomes in laryngeal cancer, thereby impeding cancer cell invasion and metastatic progression. To test this hypothesis, we conducted quantitative PCR experiments to assess the effectiveness of CX-5461 in inhibiting rRNA synthesis in laryngeal cancer cells. The results showed that CX-5461 significantly reduces the production of 47S rRNA precursor in vitro at nanomolar concentrations, with a mean half-maximal inhibitory concentration (IC50) of 173 nM in the Tu686 cell line and 269 nM in the Tu212 cell line. The primary target of CX-5461 is RNA polymerase I, which is involved in rRNA transcription, rather than RNA polymerase II, which is responsible for mRNA transcription [31]. Consequently, CX-5461 does not suppress the mRNA expression levels of the genes encoding RPS10 and RPL24, as shown in Figure 5A,B.

To investigate the effects of CX-5461 on the expression of RPs at the protein level, we conducted Western blot analyses on laryngeal cancer cell lines treated with varying con-centrations of CX-5461. The results indicated that CX-5461 significantly reduced the expression levels of RPS10, RPS26, and RPL24, while not affecting RPS28, RPL29, and RPL3 (Figure 5C). The differing sensitivities of various ribosomal proteins to CX-5461 suggest that the dynamic regulation of ribosomal proteins in cells is complex and may involve multiple layers of regulatory mechanisms. Given the strong correlation of RPS10, RPL24, and RPS26 with LNM in LSCC, and as their expression is inhibited by CX-5461, we suggest that CX-5461 has the potential to be used to treat metastatic LSCC.

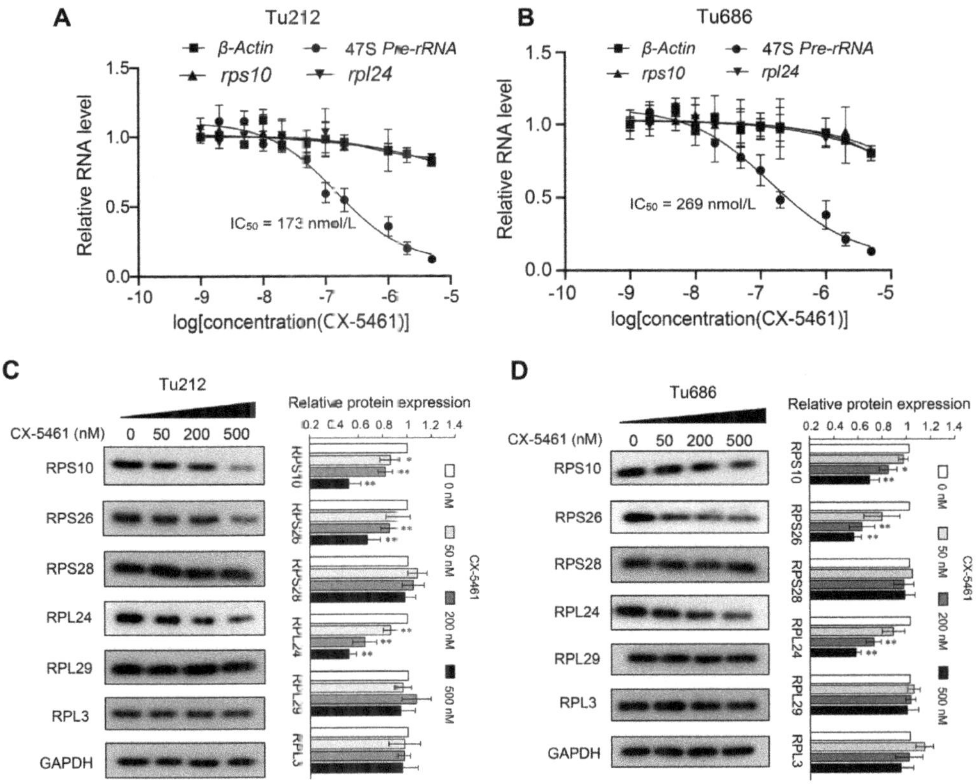

Figure 5. Inhibition of rRNA production and ribosomal protein expression by CX-5461. (**A**,**B**) qRT-PCR analyses of 47S pre-rRNA, β-actin, rps10, and rpl24 transcription after a 2 h treatment of CX-5461 in Tu686 (**A**) and Tu212 cells (**B**); (**C**,**D**) Western blot detecting the expression of six ribosomal proteins RPS10, PRS26, RPS28, RPL24, RPL29, and RPL3, after a 48 h treatment of CX-5461 in Tu686 (**C**) and Tu212 cells (**D**). Data are presented as mean ± SD, n = 3. Significant differences were determined using a two-tailed *t*-test, * $p < 0.05$, ** $p < 0.01$. Abbreviations: IC50, half-maximal inhibitory concentration.

3.6. CX-5461 More Effectively Inhibits LSCC Invasion than cell Viability

Next, we sought to investigate the anti-proliferative and anti-invasive potential of CX-5461 against laryngeal squamous cell carcinoma (LSCC). By performing the CCK-8 assay, we assessed the reduction in the cell viability of the Tu686 and Tu212 cell lines across a range of drug concentrations. Although CX-5461 indeed inhibited the viability of these laryngeal cancer cells, they displayed a relative insensitivity to it when compared to other cell lines, such as HCT116 and A375, which had IC50s in the low nanomolar range (hundreds or even tens of nM) [31]. The IC50 values of CX-5461 were notably higher for Tu686 and Tu212, at 2.13 μM and 1.71 μM, respectively (Figure 6A). Nevertheless, CX-5461 appears to have a significant inhibitory impact on the metastatic potential of laryngeal cancer cells. The results of the transwell assay show that CX-5461 concentrations of 100 nM or higher significantly reduced the invasiveness of both the Tu686 and Tu212 cell lines (Figure 6B). Interestingly, cell viability was not significantly affected by CX-5461 concentrations of 100 nM and 200 nM. Moreover, this effective concentration aligns precisely with the one required to diminish the expression levels of the ribosomal proteins RPS10 and RPL24 (Figure 5C). To further confirm the specific inhibitory ability of CX-5461 towards cell invasion and metastasis, we assessed the effects of a 200 nM CX-5461 treatment on scratch closure and the expression of epithelial–mesenchymal transition (EMT) markers in laryngeal cancer cells. The results indicated that treatment with 200 nM CX-5461 significantly inhibited cell migration (Figure 6C), promoted the expression of the epithelial cell marker E-cadherin (CDH1), and suppressed the expression of the mesenchymal cell markers N-cadherin (CDH2), vimentin (VIM), and fibronectin (FN) (Figure 6D).

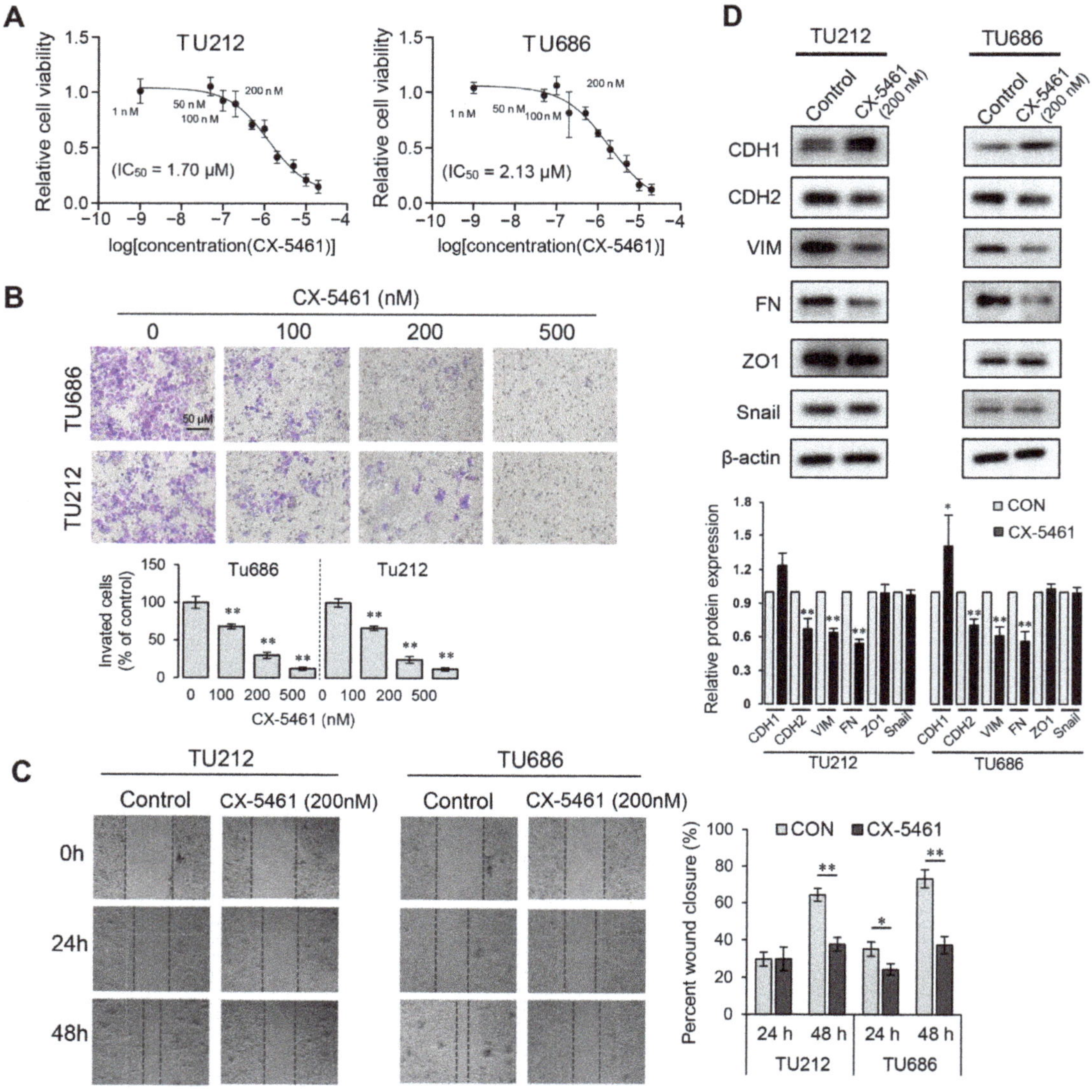

Figure 6. CX-5461's inhibition of cell viability and invasion. (**A**) Effect of CX-5461 on the cell viability of Tu686 and Tu212 cells. (**B**) Transwell invasion assays were conducted on Tu686 and Tu212 cells using various concentrations of CX-5461, as indicated. (**C**) Wound healing assay revealing the inhibition of cell migration by CX-5461. (**D**) Western blot analysis detecting the effect of CX-5461 on the expression levels of EMT markers CDH1, CDH2, VIM, FN, ZO1, and Snail. Data are presented as mean ± SD, n = 3. Significant differences were determined using a two-tailed *t*-test, * $p < 0.05$, ** $p < 0.01$.

4. Discussion

In this study, we report a comprehensive quantitative proteomic analysis of laryngeal squamous cell carcinoma, focusing on the proteome dysregulation associated with lymph node metastasis.

The potential of clinical proteomics to identify and quantify new biomarkers, as well as to distinguish patient profiles, offers remarkable promise for early molecular detection, prognostication, and tailored therapeutic strategies. However, the integration of proteomic technologies into routine clinical practice remains limited, despite the proven success of oncological identification through multi-omics research in specific cancer cohorts [32–34]. Proteogenomic data releases for common cancers, such as breast [35], lung [36], liver [37], and HNSCC [38], have deepened our understanding of tumor biology. Huang et al. contributed to this by providing an extensive proteogenomic database for HNSCC that included multi-omics data from 49 LSCC cases, focusing on distinguishing cancerous from non-cancerous tissues [38]. However, the mechanisms and biomarkers of laryngeal cancer risk, such as lymph node metastasis, vascular invasion, and tumor grading, have not yet been fully elucidated. To address this gap, our study implemented a proteomic workflow on a precisely matched cohort of 20 LSCC patients, evenly divided between those with and without lymph node metastasis and controlled for gender and age. In contrast to the proteomic data published by Huang et al., in which cancerous and non-cancerous tissues were not paired, our proteomic data include expression profiles from both cancerous and paired adjacent normal tissues. This meticulously designed proteomic analysis, which carefully considers sample selection, not only provides a refined view of metastatic laryngeal cancer but also enriches the breadth of the available data on laryngeal cancer.

Our comparative proteomic analysis identified a set of 848 proteins with marked expression differences between LSCC tissues and their normal counterparts. The enrichment analyses of these proteins highlighted several critical pathways, with DNA replication emerging as the most prominent, along with a significant overexpression of the spliceosome, cell cycle, and ribosome pathways (Figure S2). These insights reflect the tumor's proliferative vigor and align well with prior proteomic research into HNSCC [38,39]. The consistency of these findings affirms the authenticity of our proteomic data and the appropriateness of our sample selection.

A key finding of our study is the identification of 126 aberrantly expressed proteins in LSCC with lymph node metastasis. Proteins that are downregulated primarily enrich pathways related to cell adhesion (Figure 2D), corresponding to the metastatic tumor's tendency to detach from the primary site and spread distantly [40]. This pattern of protein function enrichment has also been observed in proteomic analyses of metastatic colorectal cancer [41] and lung cancer [42]. Notably, among the 69 overexpressed proteins in the lymph node metastasis group, 18 belong to ribosomal subunits. The majority of the other quantified ribosomal proteins are also overexpressed, albeit with slightly lower fold-changes than these 18 (Figure 3). Research has shown that ribosomes can modulate the rate of protein synthesis and play critical roles in cellular processes, such as proliferation, differentiation, apoptosis, and transformation [43,44]. Tumors may enhance ribosomal function to support their increased demand for active biosynthesis [45,46]. The overactivation of ribosomes in tumors is regulated by oncoproteins, noncoding RNAs, and various other factors [47]. Myc is one of the proto-oncogenes involved in abnormal ribosome biogenesis by promoting the transcription of rDNA [22,48]. Conversely, compromised ribosome function can inhibit the malignant progression of tumors [49]. Mossmann et al. have suggested that targeting abnormal ribosome biogenesis by blocking mTORC1/ribosomal protein S6 (RPS6) signaling using drugs is an effective cancer treatment strategy [50]. Our proteomic data suggest that this ribosomal overactivation may play a particularly prominent role in driving the metastasis of laryngeal cancer and could be considered a diagnostic marker for metastatic laryngeal carcinoma.

Among the aberrantly expressed ribosomal proteins in LSCC tissues with lymph node metastasis, RPS10 and RPL24 are significantly prominent and are considered biomarkers for lymph node metastasis. Mutations in RPS10 have been reported to correlate with Diamond–Blackfan anemia [51] and to have a role in regulating the mitochondrial function in plants [52]. Additionally, RPL24 may play a role in liver regeneration and could serve as a potential prognostic biomarker for cervical cancer when treated with cisplatin and concurrent chemoradiotherapy [53,54]. Both RPS10 and RPL24 have consistently shown their higher expression in the LNM group in external validation cohorts, as demonstrated by our WB and IHC assays (Figure 4). However, the qPCR and TCGA analyses identified no significant differences in their mRNA levels between the groups with and without LNM. These findings suggest that post-transcriptional regulatory mechanisms, such as translation efficiency or protein control by the ubiquitin proteasome system and autophagy, may play roles in the ribosomal hyperactivation observed in metastatic laryngeal cancer cells [55]. We noted that RPL15, a ribosomal protein well known to be overexpressed and to enhance tumor invasiveness in metastatic breast cancer [23,56], did not exhibit significant changes in our data, indicating its potential ribosomal heterogeneity across different tumor types. Recent research has proposed the concept of ribosomal heterogeneity, implying that ribosomes are not uniform entities, but rather variable complexes with components that differ across diseases and cellular states [57]. Variations can occur in rRNA modifications [58,59], ribosomal protein ratios [60], post-translational alterations [57], and their associated protein regulation, leading to the formation of "specialized ribosomes" or "onco-ribosomes" in cancer. Our findings may support this evolving viewpoint.

Given our discovery of heightened ribosomal activity in metastatic laryngeal cancer cells, we propose that inhibiting ribosome biogenesis may effectively suppress the invasion and metastasis of such cancer cells. We experimentally employed CX-5461, an inhibitor of ribosome biogenesis [31,61], and observed its potent ability to suppress ribosomal RNA transcription in laryngeal cancer cell lines. Intriguingly, it also attenuated the protein expression levels of RPS10, RPL24, and RPS26, irrespective of their mRNA expression. We speculated that this CX-5461 treatment diminishes the expression of essential rRNA, promoting the cellular proteostasis mechanisms, such as the ubiquitin–proteasome system, to degrade unincorporated ribosomal proteins [55,62]. Although CX-5461 has shown significant anti-proliferative effects on various cancer cell lines, including HCT116 and A375 [31], laryngeal cancer cells exhibit a relative resistance to it, with an IC50 value nearly 10 times higher than that of HCT116 cells.

Our in vitro experimental results demonstrate that CX-5461 preferentially inhibited the invasiveness of laryngeal cancer cells, rather than their viability (Figure 6). This suggests that CX-5461 could potentially serve as an adjunct to frontline therapies or as a prophylactic agent to prevent postoperative recurrence, rather than as the primary treatment for killing laryngeal cancer cells. This conclusion requires further validation through more extensive in vivo experiments in the future. Moreover, for CX-5461 to be applied in the treatment of laryngeal cancer, its validation through more extensive preclinical and clinical research is necessary. Considering that CX-5461 has been linked to potential DNA damage [61] and topoisomerase II poisoning [63], it is particularly essential for future studies to conduct comprehensive in vivo toxicological assessments of CX-5461 using animal models. It is noteworthy that, apart from CX-5461, other RNA polymerase I inhibitors such as BMH-22, BMH-21 [64], and POL1-IN-1 may also have promising potential applications. It is crucial to compare the efficiency of different ribosome biogenesis inhibitors at inhibiting cancer cell invasion and metastasis both in vitro and in vivo, as well as their safety profiles. There is a pressing demand for novel, safer, and more efficacious treatments targeting ribosomal biogenesis in tumors with elevated ribosomal activity to open new paths for cancer treatment.

In summary, our study characterized the comprehensive proteome of laryngeal carcinoma with lymph node metastasis and analyzed the molecular mechanisms involved. We proposed and demonstrated the value of ribosomal biogenesis as a potential therapeutic target for metastatic laryngeal cancer. We believe that this study offers valuable insights into the progression of LSCC with lymph node metastasis and facilitates advancements in the development of diagnostics and therapeutics for LSCC patients with lymph node metastasis.

5. Conclusions

Using a TMT-based proteomic workflow, we depicted the proteomic landscape of LSCC with lymph node metastasis, thereby enriching the current proteomic database of laryngeal cancer. A significant upregulation of ribosomal proteins was noted in metastatic LSCC, with the ribosomal proteins RPS10 and RPL24 identified as potential biomarkers of the condition. By employing CX-5461 as an inhibitor of ribosomal biogenesis, our preliminary in vitro experiments showcased the potential of targeting ribosomal biogenesis as a therapeutic strategy for metastatic laryngeal squamous cell carcinoma.

Supplementary Materials: The following supporting information can be downloaded at: https://www.mdpi.com/article/10.3390/toxics12050363/s1, Table S1: Labeling reagents for each sample; Table S2: List of QPCR primers; Table S3: Clinical data of patients in the TCGA-HNSC Larynx cohort and CPTAC-HNSC Larynx cohort; Table S4: The proteome data generated by this study; Table S5: Pathway enrichment analysis of proteins correlated with lymphatic metastasis. Supplementary Figures: Figure S1: Quality control of TMT-base quantitative proteomics; Figure S2: Comparison of proteins between the tumor tissues and peritumoral tissues; Supplementary images: Uncropped full-length Western blots.

Author Contributions: Conceptualization, X.L. and M.G.; methodology, T.L., M.G. and K.H.; software, M.G., X.L. and Z.L.; investigation, M.G., S.W., D.G. and T.L.; data curation, S.C. and K.H.; writing—original draft, X.L.; visualization, S.C. and M.G.; supervision, X.L.; project administration, X.L.; funding acquisition, X.L. All authors have read and agreed to the published version of the manuscript.

Funding: This work was supported by the National Natural Science Foundation of China (82203164), the Natural Science Foundation of Fujian Province (2021J05044), and the Fujian Medical University High-level Talent Research Startup Funding Project (XRCZX2020013).

Institutional Review Board Statement: The study was conducted in accordance with the Declaration of Helsinki and approved by the Medical Ethics Committee of Fujian Medical University (approval number 2022-36, 2024-38).

Informed Consent Statement: Informed consent was obtained from all subjects involved in the study.

Data Availability Statement: The data in this study are available on reasonable request from the corresponding author.

Conflicts of Interest: The authors declare that they have no competing interests.

References

1. Marur, S.; Forastiere, A.A. (Eds.) Head and neck squamous cell carcinoma: Update on epidemiology, diagnosis, and treatment. In *Mayo Clinic Proceedings*; Elsevier: Amsterdam, The Netherlands, 2016; pp. 386–396.
2. Torre, L.A.; Bray, F.; Siegel, R.L.; Ferlay, J.; Lortet-Tieulent, J.; Jemal, A. Global cancer statistics, 2012. *CA Cancer J. Clin.* **2015**, *65*, 87–108. [CrossRef]
3. Mastronikolis, N.S.; Papadas, T.A.; Goumas, P.D.; Triantaphyllidou, I.-E.; Theocharis, D.A.; Papageorgakopoulou, N.; Vynios, D.H. Head and neck: Laryngeal tumors: An overview. *Atlas Genet. Cytogenet. Oncol. Haematol.* **2009**, *13*, 888–893. [CrossRef]
4. Steuer, C.E.; El-Deiry, M.; Parks, J.R.; Higgins, K.A.; Saba, N.F. An update on larynx cancer. *CA Cancer J. Clin.* **2017**, *67*, 31–50. [CrossRef]
5. Cossu, A.M.; Mosca, L.; Zappavigna, S.; Misso, G.; Bocchetti, M.; De Micco, F.; Quagliuolo, L.; Porcelli, M.; Caraglia, M.; Boccellino, M. Long non-coding RNAs as important biomarkers in laryngeal cancer and other head and neck tumours. *Int. J. Mol. Sci.* **2019**, *20*, 3444. [CrossRef]
6. Koontongkaew, S. The tumor microenvironment contribution to development, growth, invasion and metastasis of head and neck squamous cell carcinomas. *J. Cancer* **2013**, *4*, 66–83. [CrossRef]
7. van den Bosch, S.; Dijkema, T.; Verhoef, L.C.G.; Zwijnenburg, E.M.; Janssens, G.O.; Kaanders, J.H.A.M. Patterns of Recurrence in Electively Irradiated Lymph Node Regions After Definitive Accelerated Intensity Modulated Radiation Therapy for Head and Neck Squamous Cell Carcinoma. *Int. J. Radiat. Oncol. Biol. Phys.* **2016**, *94*, 766–774. [CrossRef]
8. Wu, T.; Hu, E.; Xu, S.; Chen, M.; Guo, P.; Dai, Z.; Feng, T.; Zhou, L.; Tang, W.; Zhan, L.; et al. clusterProfiler 4.0: A universal enrichment tool for interpreting omics data. *Innovation* **2021**, *2*, 100141. [CrossRef]

9. Pantel, K.; Brakenhoff, R.H. Dissecting the metastatic cascade. *Nat. Rev. Cancer* **2004**, *4*, 448–456. [CrossRef]
10. Leemans, C.R.; Braakhuis, B.J.; Brakenhoff, R.H. The molecular biology of head and neck cancer. *Nat. Rev. Cancer* **2011**, *11*, 9–22. [CrossRef]
11. Park, B.J.; Chiosea, S.I.; Grandis, J.R. Molecular changes in the multistage pathogenesis of head and neck cancer. *Cancer Biomark.* **2011**, *9*, 325–339. [CrossRef]
12. Enepekides, D.J.; Sultanem, K.; Nguyen, C.; Shenouda, G.; Black, M.J.; Rochon, L. Occult cervical metastases: Immunoperoxidase analysis of the pathologically negative neck. *Otolaryngol. Head Neck Surg.* **1999**, *120*, 713–717. [CrossRef] [PubMed]
13. Bayram, A.; Yüce, İ.; Çağlı, S.; Canöz, Ö.; Güney, E. Predictive value of E-cadherin and Ep-CAM in cervical lymph node metastasis of supraglottic larynx carcinoma. *Am. J. Otolaryngol.* **2015**, *36*, 736–740. [CrossRef] [PubMed]
14. Karaman, S.; Detmar, M. Mechanisms of lymphatic metastasis. *J. Clin. Investig.* **2014**, *124*, 922–928. [CrossRef] [PubMed]
15. Johnson, D.E.; Burtness, B.; Leemans, C.R.; Lui, V.W.Y.; Bauman, J.E.; Grandis, J.R. Head and neck squamous cell carcinoma. *Nat. Rev. Dis. Primers* **2020**, *6*, 92. [CrossRef] [PubMed]
16. Patel, B.P.; Shah, S.V.; Shukla, S.N.; Shah, P.M.; Patel, P.S. Clinical significance of MMP-2 and MMP-9 in patients with oral cancer. *Head Neck.* **2007**, *29*, 564–572. [CrossRef] [PubMed]
17. Kessenbrock, K.; Plaks, V.; Werb, Z. Matrix metalloproteinases: Regulators of the tumor microenvironment. *Cell* **2010**, *141*, 52–67. [CrossRef] [PubMed]
18. Samanna, V.; Ma, T.; Mak, T.; Rogers, M.; Chellaiah, M.A. Actin polymerization modulates CD44 surface expression, MMP-9 activation, and osteoclast function. *J. Cell. Physiol.* **2007**, *213*, 710–720. [CrossRef] [PubMed]
19. Howell, G.M.; Grandis, J.R. Molecular mediators of metastasis in head and neck squamous cell carcinoma. *Head Neck J. Sci. Spec. Head Neck* **2005**, *27*, 710–717. [CrossRef] [PubMed]
20. Zhang, X.-W.; Liu, N.; Chen, S.; Wang, Y.; Zhang, Z.-X.; Sun, Y.-Y.; Qiu, G.-B.; Fu, W.-N. High microRNA-23a expression in laryngeal squamous cell carcinoma is associated with poor patient prognosis. *Diagn. Pathol.* **2015**, *10*, 22. [CrossRef]
21. Elhamamsy, A.R.; Metge, B.J.; Alsheikh, H.A.; Shevde, L.A.; Samant, R.S. Ribosome Biogenesis: A Central Player in Cancer Metastasis and Therapeutic Resistance. *Cancer Res.* **2022**, *82*, 2344–2353. [CrossRef]
22. van Riggelen, J.; Yetil, A.; Felsher, D.W. MYC as a regulator of ribosome biogenesis and protein synthesis. *Nat. Rev. Cancer* **2010**, *10*, 301–309. [CrossRef] [PubMed]
23. Ebright, R.Y.; Lee, S.; Wittner, B.S.; Niederhoffer, K.L.; Nicholson, B.T.; Bardia, A.; Truesdell, S.; Wiley, D.F.; Wesley, B.; Li, S.; et al. Deregulation of ribosomal protein expression and translation promotes breast cancer metastasis. *Science* **2020**, *367*, 1468–1473. [CrossRef] [PubMed]
24. Zhao, W.; Li, X.; Nian, W.; Wang, J.; Wang, X.; Sun, L.; Zhu, Y.; Tong, Z. Ribosome Proteins Represented by RPL27A Mark the Development and Metastasis of Triple-Negative Breast Cancer in Mouse and Human. *Front. Cell Dev. Biol.* **2021**, *9*, 716730. [CrossRef]
25. Dermit, M.; Dodel, M.; Lee, F.C.Y.; Azman, M.S.; Schwenzer, H.; Jones, J.L.; Blagden, S.P.; Ule, J.; Mardakheh, F.K. Subcellular mRNA Localization Regulates Ribosome Biogenesis in Migrating Cells. *Dev. Cell* **2020**, *55*, 298–313. [CrossRef]
26. Pecoraro, A.; Pagano, M.; Russo, G.; Russo, A. Ribosome biogenesis and cancer: Overview on ribosomal proteins. *Int. J. Mol. Sci.* **2021**, *22*, 5496. [CrossRef] [PubMed]
27. Wang, Z.; Li, J.; Long, X.; Jiao, L.; Zhou, M.; Wu, K. MRPS16 facilitates tumor progression via the PI3K/AKT/Snail signaling axis. *J. Cancer* **2020**, *11*, 2032–2043. [CrossRef]
28. Huang, G.; Li, H.; Zhang, H. Abnormal expression of mitochondrial ribosomal proteins and their encoding genes with cell apoptosis and diseases. *Int. J. Mol. Sci.* **2020**, *21*, 8879. [CrossRef]
29. Kim, H.-J.; Maiti, P.; Barrientos, A. Mitochondrial ribosomes in cancer. *Semin. Cancer Biol.* **2017**, *47*, 67–81. [CrossRef] [PubMed]
30. Sherman, B.T.; Hao, M.; Qiu, J.; Jiao, X.; Baseler, M.W.; Lane, H.C.; Imamichi, T.; Chang, W. DAVID: A web server for functional enrichment analysis and functional annotation of gene lists (2021 update). *Nucleic Acids Res.* **2022**, *50*, W216–W221. [CrossRef]
31. Drygin, D.; Lin, A.; Bliesath, J.; Ho, C.B.; O'Brien, S.E.; Proffitt, C.; Omori, M.; Haddach, M.; Schwaebe, M.K.; Siddiqui-Jain, A.; et al. Targeting RNA polymerase I with an oral small molecule CX-5461 inhibits ribosomal RNA synthesis and solid tumor growth. *Cancer Res.* **2011**, *71*, 1418–1430. [CrossRef]
32. Suhre, K.; McCarthy, M.I.; Schwenk, J.M. Genetics meets proteomics: Perspectives for large population-based studies. *Nat. Rev. Genet.* **2020**, *22*, 19–37. [CrossRef] [PubMed]
33. Karayel, O.; Virreira Winter, S.; Padmanabhan, S.; Kuras, Y.I.; Vu, D.T.; Tuncali, I.; Merchant, K.; Wills, A.M.; Scherzer, C.R.; Mann, M. Proteome profiling of cerebrospinal fluid reveals biomarker candidates for Parkinson's disease. *Cell Rep. Med.* **2022**, *3*, 100661. [CrossRef] [PubMed]
34. Ding, Z.; Wang, N.; Ji, N.; Chen, Z.-S. Proteomics technologies for cancer liquid biopsies. *Mol. Cancer* **2022**, *21*, 53. [CrossRef]
35. Krug, K.; Jaehnig, E.J.; Satpathy, S.; Blumenberg, L.; Karpova, A.; Anurag, M.; Miles, G.; Mertins, P.; Geffen, Y.; Tang, L.C.; et al. Proteogenomic Landscape of Breast Cancer Tumorigenesis and Targeted Therapy. *Cell* **2020**, *183*, 1436–1456. [CrossRef] [PubMed]
36. Chen, Y.J.; Roumeliotis, T.I.; Chang, Y.H.; Chen, C.T.; Han, C.L.; Lin, M.H.; Chen, H.W.; Chang, G.C.; Chang, Y.L.; Wu, C.T.; et al. Proteogenomics of Non-smoking Lung Cancer in East Asia Delineates Molecular Signatures of Pathogenesis and Progression. *Cell* **2020**, *182*, 226–244.e17. [CrossRef] [PubMed]
37. Gao, Q.; Zhu, H.; Dong, L.; Shi, W.; Chen, R.; Song, Z.; Huang, C.; Li, J.; Dong, X.; Zhou, Y.; et al. Integrated Proteogenomic Characterization of HBV-Related Hepatocellular Carcinoma. *Cell* **2019**, *179*, 561–577.e22. [CrossRef] [PubMed]

38. Huang, C.; Chen, L.; Savage, S.R.; Eguez, R.V.; Dou, Y.; Li, Y.; da Veiga Leprevost, F.; Jaehnig, E.J.; Lei, J.T.; Wen, B.; et al. Proteogenomic insights into the biology and treatment of HPV-negative head and neck squamous cell carcinoma. *Cancer Cell* **2021**, *39*, 361–379.e16. [CrossRef] [PubMed]
39. Fan, T.; Wang, X.; Zhang, S.; Deng, P.; Jiang, Y.; Liang, Y.; Jie, S.; Wang, Q.; Li, C.; Tian, G.; et al. NUPR1 promotes the proliferation and metastasis of oral squamous cell carcinoma cells by activating TFE3-dependent autophagy. *Signal Transduct. Target. Ther.* **2022**, *7*, 130. [CrossRef] [PubMed]
40. Di Martino, J.S.; Nobre, A.R.; Mondal, C.; Taha, I.; Farias, E.F.; Fertig, E.J.; Naba, A.; Aguirre-Ghiso, J.A.; Bravo-Cordero, J.J. A tumor-derived type III collagen-rich ECM niche regulates tumor cell dormancy. *Nat. Cancer* **2021**, *3*, 90–107. [CrossRef]
41. Li, C.; Sun, Y.-D.; Yu, G.-Y.; Cui, J.-R.; Lou, Z.; Zhang, H.; Huang, Y.; Bai, C.-G.; Deng, L.-L.; Liu, P.; et al. Integrated omics of metastatic colorectal cancer. *Cancer Cell* **2020**, *38*, 734–747.e9. [CrossRef]
42. Bohnenberger, H.; Kaderali, L.; Ströbel, P.; Yepes, D.; Plessmann, U.; Dharia, N.V.; Yao, S.; Heydt, C.; Merkelbach-Bruse, S.; Emmert, A.; et al. Comparative proteomics reveals a diagnostic signature for pulmonary head-and-neck cancer metastasis. *EMBO Mol. Med.* **2018**, *10*, e8428. [CrossRef] [PubMed]
43. Lv, K.; Gong, C.; Antony, C.; Han, X.; Ren, J.-G.; Donaghy, R.; Cheng, Y.; Pellegrino, S.; Warren, A.J.; Paralkar, V.R.; et al. HectD1 controls hematopoietic stem cell regeneration by coordinating ribosome assembly and protein synthesis. *Cell Stem Cell* **2021**, *28*, 1275–1290.e9. [CrossRef] [PubMed]
44. Fan, Y.; Cheng, Y.; Li, Y.; Chen, B.; Wang, Z.; Wei, T.; Zhang, H.; Guo, Y.; Wang, Q.; Wei, Y.; et al. Phosphoproteomic Analysis of Neonatal Regenerative Myocardium Revealed Important Roles of Checkpoint Kinase 1 via Activating Mammalian Target of Rapamycin C1/Ribosomal Protein S6 Kinase b-1 Pathway. *Circulation* **2020**, *141*, 1554–1569. [CrossRef] [PubMed]
45. Pelletier, J.; Thomas, G.; Volarević, S. Ribosome biogenesis in cancer: New players and therapeutic avenues. *Nat. Rev. Cancer* **2017**, *18*, 51–63. [CrossRef] [PubMed]
46. Zhuang, A.; Zhuang, A.; Chen, Y.; Qin, Z.; Zhu, D.; Ren, L.; Wei, Y.; Zhou, P.; Yue, X.; He, F.; et al. Proteomic characteristics reveal the signatures and the risks of T1 colorectal cancer metastasis to lymph nodes. *eLife* **2023**, *12*, e82959. [CrossRef] [PubMed]
47. Jiao, L.; Liu, Y.; Yu, X.Y.; Pan, X.; Zhang, Y.; Tu, J.; Song, Y.H.; Li, Y. Ribosome biogenesis in disease: New players and therapeutic targets. *Signal Transduct. Target. Ther.* **2023**, *8*, 15. [CrossRef] [PubMed]
48. White, R.J. RNA polymerases I and III, growth control and cancer. *Nat. Rev. Mol. Cell Biol.* **2005**, *6*, 69–78. [CrossRef] [PubMed]
49. Zhou, L.H.; Zhu, X.P.; Xiao, H.F.; Xin, P.L.; Li, C.T. Effects of mTOR Inhibitor Rapamycin on Burkitt's Lymphoma Cells. *Zhongguo Shi Yan Xue Ye Xue Za Zhi* **2017**, *25*, 1397–1405. [PubMed]
50. Mossmann, D.; Park, S.; Hall, M.N. mTOR signalling and cellular metabolism are mutual determinants in cancer. *Nat. Rev. Cancer* **2018**, *18*, 744–757. [CrossRef]
51. Doherty, L.; Sheen, M.R.; Vlachos, A.; Choesmel, V.; O'Donohue, M.F.; Clinton, C.; Schneider, H.E.; Sieff, C.A.; Newburger, P.E.; Ball, S.E.; et al. Ribosomal protein genes RPS10 and RPS26 are commonly mutated in Diamond-Blackfan anemia. *Am. J. Hum. Genet.* **2010**, *86*, 222–228. [CrossRef]
52. Choury, D.; Farre, J.C.; Jordana, X.; Araya, A. Gene expression studies in isolated mitochondria: Solanum tuberosum rps10 is recognized by cognate potato but not by the transcription, splicing and editing machinery of wheat mitochondria. *Nucleic Acids Res.* **2005**, *33*, 7058–7065. [CrossRef]
53. Ming, C.; Bai, X.; Zhao, L.; Yu, D.; Wang, X.; Wu, Y. RPL24 as a potential prognostic biomarker for cervical cancer treated by Cisplatin and concurrent chemoradiotherapy. *Front. Oncol.* **2023**, *13*, 1131803. [CrossRef] [PubMed]
54. Jia, Y.; Li, L.; Lin, Y.H.; Gopal, P.; Shen, S.; Zhou, K.; Yu, X.; Sharma, T.; Zhang, Y.; Siegwart, D.J.; et al. In vivo CRISPR screening identifies BAZ2 chromatin remodelers as druggable regulators of mammalian liver regeneration. *Cell Stem Cell* **2022**, *29*, 372–385.e8. [CrossRef] [PubMed]
55. An, H.; Harper, J.W. Ribosome Abundance Control Via the Ubiquitin-Proteasome System and Autophagy. *J. Mol. Biol.* **2020**, *432*, 170–184. [CrossRef]
56. Wu, Z.; Sun, H.; Liu, W.; Zhu, H.; Fu, J.; Yang, C.; Fan, L.; Wang, L.; Liu, Y.; Xu, W.; et al. Circ-RPL15: A plasma circular RNA as novel oncogenic driver to promote progression of chronic lymphocytic leukemia. *Leukemia* **2019**, *34*, 919–923. [CrossRef] [PubMed]
57. Li, D.; Wang, J. Ribosome heterogeneity in stem cells and development. *J. Cell Biol.* **2020**, *219*, e202001108. [CrossRef] [PubMed]
58. Babaian, A.; Rothe, K.; Girodat, D.; Minia, I.; Djondovic, S.; Milek, M.; Spencer Miko, S.E.; Wieden, H.J.; Landthaler, M.; Morin, G.B.; et al. Loss of $m^1acp^3\Psi$ Ribosomal RNA Modification Is a Major Feature of Cancer. *Cell Rep.* **2020**, *31*, 107611. [CrossRef] [PubMed]
59. Marcel, V.; Kielbassa, J.; Marchand, V.; Natchiar, K.S.; Paraqindes, H.; Nguyen Van Long, F.; Ayadi, L.; Bourguignon-Igel, V.; Lo Monaco, P.; Monchiet, D.; et al. Ribosomal RNA 2′O-methylation as a novel layer of inter-tumour heterogeneity in breast cancer. *NAR Cancer* **2020**, *2*, zcaa036. [CrossRef] [PubMed]
60. Bee, A.; Ke, Y.; Forootan, S.; Lin, K.; Beesley, C.; Forrest, S.E.; Foster, C.S. Ribosomal protein l19 is a prognostic marker for human prostate cancer. *Clin. Cancer Res.* **2006**, *12*, 2061–2065. [CrossRef]
61. Sanij, E.; Hannan, K.M.; Xuan, J.; Yan, S.; Ahern, J.E.; Trigos, A.S.; Brajanovski, N.; Son, J.; Chan, K.T.; Kondrashova, O.; et al. CX-5461 activates the DNA damage response and demonstrates therapeutic efficacy in high-grade serous ovarian cancer. *Nat. Commun.* **2020**, *11*, 2641. [CrossRef]

62. Filbeck, S.; Cerullo, F.; Pfeffer, S.; Joazeiro, C.A.P. Ribosome-associated quality-control mechanisms from bacteria to humans. *Mol. Cell* **2022**, *82*, 1451–1466. [CrossRef] [PubMed]
63. Bruno, P.M.; Lu, M.; Dennis, K.A.; Inam, H.; Moore, C.J.; Sheehe, J.; Elledge, S.J.; Hemann, M.T.; Pritchard, J.R. The primary mechanism of cytotoxicity of the chemotherapeutic agent CX-5461 is topoisomerase II poisoning. *Proc. Natl. Acad. Sci. USA* **2020**, *117*, 4053–4060. [CrossRef] [PubMed]
64. Peltonen, K.; Colis, L.; Liu, H.; Jäämaa, S.; Zhang, Z.; Hällström, T.A.; Moore, H.M.; Sirajuddin, P.; Laiho, M. Small molecule BMH-compounds that inhibit RNA polymerase I and cause nucleolar stress. *Mol. Cancer Ther.* **2014**, *13*, 2537–2546. [CrossRef] [PubMed]

Disclaimer/Publisher's Note: The statements, opinions and data contained in all publications are solely those of the individual author(s) and contributor(s) and not of MDPI and/or the editor(s). MDPI and/or the editor(s) disclaim responsibility for any injury to people or property resulting from any ideas, methods, instructions or products referred to in the content.

toxics

MDPI

Article

Integrating Epigenetics, Proteomics, and Metabolomics to Reveal the Involvement of Wnt/β-Catenin Signaling Pathway in Oridonin-Induced Reproductive Toxicity

Qibin Wu [1,2,†], Xinyue Gao [3,†], Yifan Lin [3,†], Caijin Wu [1,2,†], Jian Zhang [3,4], Mengting Chen [3], Jiaxin Wen [3], Yajiao Wu [3], Kun Tian [3], Wenqiang Bao [3], Pengming Sun [1,2,*] and An Zhu [1,3,4,*]

1 Laboratory of Gynecologic Oncology, Department of Gynecology, Fujian Maternity and Child Health Hospital, College of Clinical Medicine for Obstetrics & Gynecology and Pediatrics, Fujian Medical University, Fuzhou 350108, China
2 Fujian Key Laboratory of Women and Children's Critical Diseases Research, Fujian Clinical Research Center for Gynecological Oncology, Fujian Maternity and Child Health Hospital (Fujian Women and Children's Hospital), Fuzhou 350108, China
3 Key Laboratory of Ministry of Education for Gastrointestinal Cancer, School of Basic Medical Sciences, Fujian Medical University, Fuzhou 350108, China
4 School of Public Health, Fujian Medical University, Fuzhou 350108, China
* Correspondence: sunfemy@hotmail.com (P.S.); zhuan@fjmu.edu.cn (A.Z.)
† These authors contributed equally to this work.

Abstract: Oridonin is the primary active component in the traditional Chinese medicine *Rabdosia rubescens*, displaying anti-inflammatory, anti-tumor, and antibacterial effects. It is widely employed in clinical therapy for acute and chronic pharyngitis, tonsillitis, as well as bronchitis. Nevertheless, the clinical application of oridonin is significantly restricted due to its reproductive toxicity, with the exact mechanism remaining unclear. The aim of this study was to investigate the mechanism of oridonin-induced damage to HTR-8/SVneo cells. Through the integration of epigenetics, proteomics, and metabolomics methodologies, the mechanisms of oridonin-induced reproductive toxicity were discovered and confirmed through fluorescence imaging, RT-qPCR, and Western blotting. Experimental findings indicated that oridonin altered m6A levels, gene and protein expression levels, along with metabolite levels within the cells. Additionally, oridonin triggered oxidative stress and mitochondrial damage, leading to a notable decrease in WNT6, β-catenin, CLDN1, CCND1, and ZO-1 protein levels. This implied that the inhibition of the Wnt/β-catenin signaling pathway and disruption of tight junction might be attributed to the cytotoxicity induced by oridonin and mitochondrial dysfunction, ultimately resulting in damage to HTR-8/SVneo cells.

Keywords: oridonin; reproductive toxicity; Wnt/β-catenin signaling pathway; tight junction; mitochondrial dysfunction

1. Introduction

Oridonin, characterized by a tetracyclic diterpenoid structure with isoprene as its core framework, is recognized as the primary bioactive constituent of the traditional Chinese medicine *Rabdosia rubescens* [1]. Studies have demonstrated the potent pharmacological properties of oridonin, including anti-inflammatory, anti-tumor, and antibacterial effects [2,3]. It is frequently prescribed for treating pharyngitis, tonsillitis, and bronchitis in clinical practice [4]. Conversely, an increasing amount of research has been dedicated to exploring the adverse reactions associated with oridonin. After 21 days of continuous injection of 10 mg/kg of oridonin in healthy nude mice, it led to hepatic sinusoidal constriction and a significant increase in alanine aminotransferase level [5]. Treatment with 10 μM of oridonin for 24 h resulted in DNA damage and cellular accumulation of reactive oxygen species (ROS), promoting H460 human lung epithelial cell apoptosis [6]. Notably, after treating ovarian granulosa cells with 15 μg/mL of oridonin for 24 h, it was observed that cell proliferation was inhibited, SOD activity decreased, and the levels of malondialdehyde and ROS increased, resulting in oxidative damage to the ovarian granulosa cells [7]. However, few studies have been conducted on the reproductive toxicity of oridonin, and its potential toxicity mechanism remains unclear, which hinders its clinical application.

The mitochondria serve as the central hub for cellular energy synthesis and represent the primary source of ROS. Given the intricate structure and diverse functions of mitochondria, numerous mechanisms can contribute to mitochondrial toxicity triggered by drugs and other chemical compounds [8]. Previous research has demonstrated that the combination of AG1478 and oridonin enhances ROS generation. Cells treated with n-acetylcysteine during incubation mitigated apoptosis and prevented disruption of mitochondrial membrane potential (MMP) caused by the combined treatment of AG1478 and oridonin, implying that ROS are crucial in mediating cell death triggered by oridonin [9]. Furthermore, given the limited protective system against oxidative stress, mitochondria are anticipated to be prone to oxidative damage [10]. It has been firmly established that an excess of ROS is responsible for impeding the respiratory chain complexes, particularly complex I, as well as ATP synthesis. Additionally, ROS causes the oxidation of lipid peroxidation, and protein oxidation. These consequences ultimately trigger the initiation of the mitochondrial permeability transition pore (mPTP) and a subsequent reduction in MMP [11,12]. During embryogenesis, WNTs act as signaling molecules that regulate essential processes such as cell division, tissue morphogenesis, and cell development. By binding to specific receptors on neighboring cells, WNTs activate intracellular signaling pathways, leading to changes in gene expression and cellular homeostasis [13]. The Wnt signaling pathway primarily refers to mediation by the activation of target genes and the nuclear translocation of β-catenin [14]. Regulation of the cytoskeleton, adhesion, and migration involves the Wnt signaling via the Wnt/Ca^{2+} and Wnt/PCP pathways [15]. By modulating the β-catenin stability, a crucial constituent of the adherens junction, canonical Wnt signaling significantly impacts the regulation of cell adhesion [16]. The upregulation of Wnt-5a led to enhanced cell–substrate adhesion, cell migration, and focal adhesion kinase activation dependent on adhesion in cancer cells [17]. The tumor suppressor protein APC plays a crucial role in the Wnt signaling pathway by coordinating cytoskeletal networks. By binding to the plasma membrane in an actin-dependent fashion, APC modulates the actin cytoskeleton, which is necessary for cell polarization and directed migration [18]. Overexpression of CLDN1, which serves as a primary element within tight junction complexes governing the permeability of epithelial barriers in the colorectal cancer mouse model, led to decreased survival. Transcriptome analysis supported an upregulation in the Wnt signaling pathway [19]. However, the exact mechanism behind oridonin-induced reproductive toxicity is not thoroughly elucidated and there is no evidence of a relationship between its toxicity to mitochondria and Wnt/β-catenin signaling pathway.

The advancement of omics methodologies in recent years has been crucial in driving progress in the field of biology, with the ultimate goal of unraveling intricate mechanisms underlying complex phenomena. Instead of employing conventional biochemical methods to analyze individual components of an organism, the omics approach encompasses a comprehensive examination of all components and their intricate interconnections throughout the entire system. Omics technology is commonly used in traditional Chinese medicine and other ethnomedical practices. Genomics, transcriptomics, proteomics, and metabolomics are increasingly integral to pharmaceutical research, often used individually or in combination. The application of omics technologies is becoming more prevalent, with its effectiveness acknowledged in target discovery, toxicology studies, and traditional Chinese medicine research [20]. Epigenetics primarily encompasses the investigation of heritable variations in cell phenotype or gene expression that occur without alterations to the nucleotide sequence. Based on the extent of modification, it can be divided into transcriptional, post-transcriptional, and post-translational modifications [21,22]. RNA modifications also exert regulatory functions at the post-transcriptional level. More than 170 RNA modifications have been discovered [23], with N6-methyladenosine (m6A) being widely acknowledged as the most prevalent and abundant modification [24,25]. With the advancement of our comprehension regarding regulatory mechanisms, it has become evident that m6A methylation is critical in various stages of RNA metabolism [26]. Recent research has emphasized the crucial role of m6A methylation modifications in orchestrating diverse cellular processes, encompassing the regulation of cell proliferation and differentiation [27], DNA damage response regulation [28], and cellular autophagy modulation [29]. For instance, the collaborative involvement of methyltransferase 3, N6-adenosine-methyltransferase complex catalytic subunit (METTL3), and fat mass and obesity (FTO)-mediated m6A modifications is observed in the cadmium sulfate-induced oxidative stress process, leading to cellular apoptosis [30]. The downregulation of METTL3 modulates the response to oxidative stress in mouse renal tubular epithelial cell models when exposed to colistin [31]. In addition, advancements in proteomics have significantly broadened its applications in the field of biomedicine, enabling specific identification and quantification of proteins within organisms [32]. The utilization of proteomics shows great potential in the realm of drug development, particularly in identifying drug targets, exploring drug mechanisms, and conducting toxicology research. Gambogic acid and gambogenic acid, two derivatives of Gamboge, have been discovered to be capable of inhibiting the target protein stathmin 1 in HepG2 cell proliferation [33]. Metabolomics, an emerging omics technology that follows transcriptomics and proteomics, investigates endogenous metabolites of small molecules within organisms to explore organismal metabolic states and enhance the comprehensive understanding of the entire system when integrated with other omics approaches [34]. Metabolites serve as the ultimate products of biological processes, enabling metabolomic findings to depict prior toxicological events. In a metabolomic investigation, nephrotoxicity induced by aristolochic acid was characterized by the significant acceleration of specific metabolic pathways such as the folate cycle and homocysteine synthesis, alongside a decrease in activity in pathways such as arachidonic acid biosynthesis [35]. By integrating assessments of the epigenetic transcriptome, proteome, and metabolome, potential biomarkers within crucial signaling pathways can be effectively discerned.

In the present study, the reproductive toxicity of oridonin was evaluated on HTR-8/SVneo cells and potential molecular mechanisms were demonstrated. It was found that there is a dose-dependent inhibition of viability in HTR-8/SVneo cells by oridonin. Moreover, oridonin demonstrated damage to mitochondria and disruption of tight junction. Mechanistically, our study suggested that oridonin might mediate its reproductive toxicity by suppressing the activation of the Wnt/β-catenin signaling pathway.

2. Materials and Methods

2.1. Chemical Reagent and Cell Culture

Oridonin, provided by Chengdu Must Bio-Technology Co., Ltd. (Chengdu, China), boasted a purity of 99.64% (Figure 1D). The purity and chemical structure (Figure 1A) of oridonin were verified through high-performance liquid chromatography (HPLC) and 400 MHz ^{13}C (Figure 1B) and ^{1}H (Figure 1C) nuclear magnetic resonance spectroscopy, respectively. The human trophoblast cell line HTR-8/SVneo was sourced from the American Type Culture Collection and cultured in DMEM supplemented with 100 μg/mL streptomycin, 100 U/mL penicillin G sodium salt, and 10% fetal bovine serum. The maintenance conditions included a temperature of 37 °C and 5% CO_2. To treat HTR-8/SVneo cells, it was dissolved in DMSO at concentrations of 12.5, 25, and 37.5 μM in well plates for 24 h. The concentration of DMSO in the cell culture was maintained at 1%.

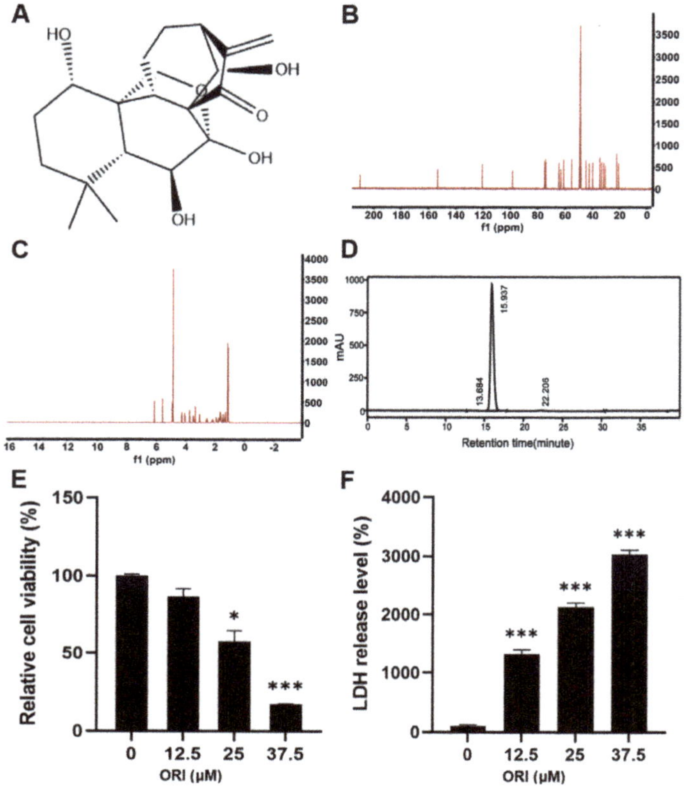

Figure 1. (**A**) The chemical structure of oridonin. (**B**) 400 MHz ^{13}C NMR spectra of oridonin. (**C**) 400 MHz ^{1}H NMR spectra of oridonin. (**D**) Purity analysis of oridonin by HPLC. The viability (**E**) and LDH release level (**F**) of HTR-8/SVneo cells following treatment with 0, 12.5, 25, and 37.5 μM oridonin for 24 h. * $p < 0.05$, *** $p < 0.001$, n = 3.

2.2. MTT and LDH Release Assay for Determining Cytotoxic Effects

The evaluation of HTR-8/SVneo cell viability following exposure to oridonin was carried out through the MTT cytotoxicity assay. Briefly, 4 × 10^3 cells were plated in individual wells of 96-well plates and exposed to 0, 12.5, 25, and 37.5 μM oridonin for 24 h. Subsequently, each well received 10% MTT solution and was then incubated in a 37 °C cell culture incubator for 4 h. Post-medium removal, 100 μL DMSO was added to each well to dissolve the intracellular formazan product. The absorbance of formazan was determined at 490 nm with a microplate reader (BioTek, Santa Clara, CA, USA).

The assessment of cell membrane integrity included quantifying the release of LDH. Following a 24 h treatment with 0, 12.5, 25, and 37.5 μM oridonin, the 96-well plate was centrifuged at 400× *g* for 5 min. Subsequently, a volume of 120 μL supernatant was transferred to a new 96-well culture plate and incubated with LDH detection reagent for 30 min. The release level of LDH was assessed using a microplate reader (BioTek) at a wavelength of 490 nm.

2.3. RNA Extraction and High-Throughput Sequence

The HTR-8/SVneo cells were exposed to 25 μM oridonin for 24 h, followed by washing with PBS. Subsequently, total RNA was isolated using Trizol reagent (Invitrogen, Carlsbad, CA, USA), followed by DNaseI treatment to remove DNA. The quality of samples was evaluated by a Nanodrop One C spectrophotometer (Thermo Fisher, Waltham, MA, USA), while the integrity was assessed using agarose gel electrophoresis. A total of 50 μg eligible RNA was used for high-throughput sequence, including m6A MeRIP-seq and mRNA-seq, conducted by Seqhealth (Wuhan, China). To address the issue of duplication bias during RNA library establishment, the KC-Digital Stranded mRNA Library Prep Kit for Illumina (Seqhealth) was applied. The resulting library fragments, ranging from 200 to 500 bps, were enriched and quantified. The comparison between the oridonin group and the control group was conducted using fold change and *p*-value. To obtain RIP-Seq peaks, motifs, and data analysis of Kyoto Encyclopedia of Genes and Genomes (KEGG) and Gene Ontology (GO), the data were inputted into exomePeak (Suzhou, China), Homer (San Diego, CA, USA), and DAVID (Frederick, MD, USA). Each group was sequenced with three independent samples.

Quality control of mRNA-seq data is shown in Table S1. The control groups obtained average quantities of 75.1 million raw reads of mRNA, with 68.1 million clean reads. Meanwhile, the oridonin groups obtained average quantities of 71.0 million raw reads of mRNA, with 64.1 million clean reads. The Q20 was 99.4% and Q30 was 97.0% in all samples. The above results suggest that our mRNA-seq was of high quality.

2.4. Molecular Docking and Molecular Dynamics (MD) Simulation

The interaction between oridonin and m6A regulators was explored through SYBYL software (Tripos, St Louis, MO, USA). The structure of oridonin was obtained from PubChem, subjected to energy minimization, and converted into 3D structures using Chem3D (Waltham, MA, USA) [36]. The crystalline structure of docking proteins was acquired from PDB. Then, the high-precision and semi-flexible docking was performed in SYBYL-X 2.0. A stable binding between proteins and molecules was considered if the total score surpassed 5 [37].

To investigate protein–ligand interactions, we employed the Simulation Package tOward Next GEneration (SPONGE, Beijing, China) [38]. Throughout the simulation study, the FF14SB united-atom force field was utilized [39]. The resolution of complex systems involved the utilization of the SPC/E water model within cubic boxes [40], keeping a minimum distance of 1.2 nm from the box edges. Neutralization was achieved by introducing potassium and chloride ions, while periodic boundary conditions were imposed. Energy minimizations were computed utilizing the steepest descent algorithm with a tolerance of 5.0 kJ/mol. Subsequently, a 100 ps NVT equilibration was executed at 300 K employing Langevin thermostat temperature coupling, with relaxation time constants set at 1.0 ps. This was followed by a 100 ps NPT simulation at 1 bar, performed utilizing Andersen barostat in conjunction with Nosé–Hoover thermostat to maintain constant pressure. Subsequently, 50 ns MD simulations were conducted for each system. Various MD trajectory analyses were employed to evaluate binding stability under dynamic conditions.

2.5. Proteomics Sample Processing and LC-MS/MS Analysis

After exposure to 25 μM oridonin for 24 h, cells were lysed using a lysis buffer comprising 100 mM triethyl-ammonium bicarbonate and 1% SDS. After centrifugation at 12,000× *g* for 10 min, the supernatant was subjected to protein concentration measurement using bicinchoninic acid (BCA) assays. A total of 150 μg protein underwent reduction and alkylation with 200 mM Tris (2-carboxyethyl) phosphine hydrochloride and 375 mM iodoacetamide, respectively. After pre-cooled acetone treatment, the precipitate was accumulated through a 5 min centrifugation and then dried in air. Following mixing with a 200 mM triethylammonium bicarbonate buffer, the samples were incubated with trypsin overnight at 37 °C.

After labeling, blending, desalting, and vacuum-drying, the peptides were partitioned into 15 fractions employing the high-pH reversed-phase peptide fractionation kit (Thermo Fisher). The 0.1% formic acid was used for dissolution processing, loaded directly onto a C18, 75 μm × 25 cm reversed-phase analytical column (Thermo Fisher) for LC-MS/MS analysis. The output data underwent processing in Proteome Discoverer version 3.0, where it was matched against the mus musculus Uniprot database. Methionine oxidation and protein N-terminus acetylation were considered as the variable modification, while fixed modifications were specified as carbamidomethyl for cysteine and TMTpro for lysine and the N-terminus.

2.6. Sample Preparation and Analysis for Metabolomics

HTR-8/SVneo cells, exposed to 25 μM oridonin for 24 h, were washed with PBS and flash-frozen in liquid nitrogen before being prepared for UPLC-MS/MS analysis performed by Metware (Wuhan, China). The cells were then treated with 300 μL methanol extract containing 20% acetonitrile and vortexed. After centrifugation at 12,000 rpm for 10 min to separate the supernatant, the samples were incubated at −20 °C for 30 min. A further centrifugation under the same conditions was performed to collect supernatant.

Metabolites were separated using a 1.8 μm, 2.1 mm × 100 mm ACQUITY UPLC HSS T3 C18 column (Waters, Milford, MA, USA), under the conditions of an injection volume of 2 μL, flow rate of 0.4 mL/min, and a column temperature maintained at 40 °C. The solvent setup comprised water containing 0.1% formic acid (mobile phase A) and acetonitrile with 0.1% formic acid (mobile phase B). The linear gradient began at 5% to 90% mobile phase B over an 11 min period, followed by holding it for an additional minute before returning to the initial composition within just 0.1 min and maintaining it for another 1.9 min. After separation, the nanoparticles were ionized and analyzed using a Triple TOF-6600 mass spectrometer (AB Sciex, Foster City, CA, USA). The resulting data were cross-referenced with the NIST Chemistry WebBook, the Human Metabolome Database, as well as various personal and public databases. Statistical algorithms were then employed to process the data for missing value supplementation and fold change calculation of metabolites. Subsequently, significantly different metabolites were identified for further multi-level bioinformatics and functional analysis.

2.7. ROS Measurement

Cellular ROS levels were quantified utilizing an ROS assay kit (Solarbio, Beijing, China) following the provided guideline. In brief, cells were treated with oridonin at concentrations of 0, 12.5, 25, and 37.5 μM and subsequently exposed to DCFH-DA (10 μM) at 37 °C for 30 min, followed by rinsing with PBS. Afterwards, visualization of intracellular fluorescence was accomplished utilizing a fluorescence microscope (Zeiss, Oberko-chen, Germany), and quantification of fluorescence intensity was analyzed using ImageJ software (Bio-Rad, Hercules, CA, USA).

2.8. DNA Damage Assay by γ-H2AX Immunofluorescence

The DNA damage assay kit (Beyotime, Shanghai, China) was utilized to assess the immunofluorescence of γ-H2AX. HTR-8/SVneo cells were exposed to oridonin at concentrations of 0, 12.5, 25, and 37.5 μM for 24 h. Cells were fixed and blocked at room temperature for 15 min. The cells underwent incubation with a rabbit anti-γ-H2AX primary antibody and corresponding secondary antibody for 1 h. Subsequently, nuclear staining was conducted using 4′,6-diamidino-2-phenylindole (DAPI). Ultimately, the green fluorescence images were captured by a microscope (Zeiss) at 519 nm.

2.9. Detection of Calcium by Fluo-4 AM

Intracellular Ca^{2+} levels in HTR-8/SVneo cells were detected using Fluo-4 AM (Beyotime), a fluorescence probe that can penetrate cell membranes. Cells were cultured with 0, 12.5, 25, and 37.5 μM oridonin for 24 h and washed thrice in PBS. Fluo-4 AM was diluted to 1 μM working solution with PBS and used to incubate cells at 37 °C for 1 h. Following a single wash, the fluorescence of Ca^{2+} was observed using a fluorescence microscope (Zeiss).

2.10. Detection of MMP and mPTP

The MMP was assessed using the JC-10 probe (Solarbio). In general, the MMP is in a relatively high state. Within the mitochondria matrix, the JC-10 probe forms polymers that result in red fluorescence. When the mitochondria are damaged, the membrane potential decreases. At this point, JC-10 cannot aggregate in the matrix and exists as monomers, producing green fluorescence. This shift from red to green fluorescence with the JC-10 probe enables easy detection of MMP reduction. The HTR-8/SVneo cells were exposed to concentrations of 0, 12.5, 25, and 37 5 μM oridonin for 24 h. Subsequently, the cells were incubated with the JC-10 probe under dark conditions at 37 °C for 20 min. Finally, red and green fluorescence were analyzed using a microscope (Zeiss).

The mPTP opening of HTR-8/SVneo cells in each group was evaluated using Calcein AM probe (Beyotime). The mPTP is a non-selective channel formed by both the inner and outer mitochondrial membranes and plays a role in substance release from the mitochondria during cell death. The Calcein AM probe can passively enter the cell and accumulate in cellular components, including the cytoplasm and mitochondria. Within the cell, the nearly non-fluorescent Calcein AM undergoes hydrolysis by intracellular esterases to remove the acetyl methyl ester, leading to the generation of the membrane-impermeable polar fluorescent dye calcein This allows Calcein to be retained within the cell, emitting intense green fluorescence. Calcein is also utilized as a metal chelating agent. When the opening degree of the mPTP increases, it complexes with metal ions such as Co^{2+}, causing fluorescence signal quenching. Therefore, $CoCl_2$ serves as a positive control for mPTP detection. The HTR-8/SVneo cells were exposed to oridonin (0, 12.5, 25, and 37.5 μM) for 24 h. Afterward, they were incubated with the Calcein AM probe at 37 °C in the dark for 40 min. The staining solution was then substituted with warm culture medium, and the cells were cultured for an additional 30 min. Subsequently, Hoechst 33342 was used to stain the nuclei for 10 min, and the fluorescence was observed under a fluorescence microscope (Zeiss).

2.11. RT-qPCR

The HTR-8/Svneo cells were exposed to concentrations of 0, 12.5, 25, and 37.5 μM oridonin for 24 h. As previously specified, the RNA extraction was subsequently executed, quantified to 1 μg. Then, the RNA underwent reverse transcription into cDNA using Evo M-MLV reverse transcription premixed kit (Accurate Biology, Changsha, China) for RT-qPCR. The reaction took place in a 20 μL volume, with 10 μL SYBR Green qPCR Mix, 2 μL template, and 10 μM primers (Monad, Suzhou, China). The relative gene expression under oridonin treatment was determined utilizing the $2^{-\Delta\Delta Ct}$ method [41], with the fold change compared to the control group. Table 1 displays the RT-qPCR primer sequences employed in this investigation. *GAPDH* was designated as the endogenous control for the remaining target genes.

Table 1. The RT-qPCR primer sequences employed in this study.

Gene	Forward Primer (5′→3′)	Reverse Primer (5′→3′)
GSK3B	GCACTCTTCAACTTCACCACTCAAG (F)	CTGTCCACGGTCTCCAGTATTAGC (R)
β-catenin	ATAGAGGCTCTTGTGCGTACTGTC (F)	TTGGTGTCGGCTGGTCAGATG (R)
WNT-6	TGCCAGTTCCACTTCCGCTTC (F)	CCGTCTCCCGAATGTCCTGTTG (R)
CLDN1	AGCCAAGGTGTTGACTCAGACTC (F)	AGCCTCCGCATTAGTTCCATAGC (R)
TCF7L1	GGAGCCGAGCAGCGATAGC (F)	CCTCTCCGCCTCCGAGTCC (R)
ZO-1	GCGGATGGTGCTACAAGTGATG (F)	GCCTTCTGTGTCTGTGTCTTCATAG (R)
CCND1	CGCCCTCGGTGTCCTACTTC (F)	GACCTCCTCCTCGCACTTCTG (R)
OCLN	ACTTCGCCTGTGGATGACTTCAG (F)	TTCTCTTTGACCTTCCTGCTCTTCC (R)
GAPDH	TGACATCAAGAAGGTGGTGAAGCAG (F)	GTGTCGCTGTTGAAGTCAGAGGAG (R)

2.12. Western Blotting Assay

Cells exposed to oridonin with 0, 12.5, 25, and 37.5 μM for 24 h were collected and lysed using RIPA buffer (Beyotime) containing a phosphatase inhibitor cocktail (Beyotime) and PMSF for protein extraction. The BCA protein assay kit (Vazyme, Nanjing, China) was used to quantify total protein concentration. Protein samples were separated through electrophoresis on 10% sodium dodecyl sulphate–polyacrylamide gel and subsequently transferred onto polyvinylidene fluoride (PVDF) membranes (Millipore, Billerica, MA, USA) for 90 min. The membranes were then blocked by 5% skimmed milk at room temperature for 90 min and then incubated with primary antibodies, including WNT6 (Proteintech, Wuhan, China), β-catenin (Proteintech), GSK3B (Proteintech), CCND1 (Proteintech), CLDN1 (Proteintech), ZO-1 (Proteintech), and TCF7L1 (Proteintech), which were used at a dilution of 1:1000, 1:10,000, 1:4500, 1:10,000, 1:4500, 1:10,000, and 1:1000, respectively. GAPDH (ABclonal, Wuhan, China) was used as internal control at a dilution of 1:10,000. Following primary antibody incubation, PVDF membranes were incubated with either goat anti-mouse IgG secondary antibody or horseradish peroxidase-conjugated goat anti-rabbit IgG secondary antibody (both at a dilution of 1:10,000; Proteintech) at room temperature for 90 min. Visualization of protein bands was carried out using the Amersham Imager 680 (GE Healthcare Bio-Sciences AB, Uppsala, Sweden). The Image J software (Bio-Rad) was utilized for quantitative analysis of the target bands.

2.13. Statistical Analysis

SPSS 26 (IBM, New York, NY, USA) was used for conducting the data analysis. The test of homogeneity of variances and one-way analysis of variance (ANOVA) were employed to assess variance consistency and group differences, respectively. Data were presented as mean ± standard error of the mean (SEM). Statistically significant ANOVA results were determined by p-values < 0.05.

3. Results

3.1. The Cytotoxic Effect of Oridonin on HTR-8/SVneo Cells

Cell viability of HTR-8/SVneo cells was examined through the MTT assay. A concentration-dependent inhibition of cell viability was observed for oridonin, as illustrated in Figure 1E. Exposure to 37.5 μM oridonin for 24 h resulted in a cell viability of 17% for HTR-8/SVneo cells. Moreover, at concentrations of 12.5 and 25 μM, cell viability decreased to 86.4% and 57.7%, respectively.

LDH level serves as a crucial indicator for assessing the integrity of cell membranes. Quantitative analysis of cytotoxicity can be carried out by measuring the amount of LDH released into the supernatant due to membrane rupture. As depicted in Figure 1F, treatment with oridonin resulted in an elevation in the LDH release, suggesting that oridonin compromised cell integrity and caused cellular damage.

3.2. Transcriptome-Wide Assessment of m6A Modification Post-Oridonin Treatment in HTR-8/SVneo Cells

RNA epigenetic modifications, particularly m6A, have been reported to be involved in gene expression regulation. We performed MeRIP-seq on both oridonin-treated cells and control cells that were untreated to analyze the changes in m6A modification following oridonin treatment. The analysis revealed 22,329 peaks across 8074 genes in the control group, while 20,209 m6A peaks were identified in 7564 m6A genes in the oridonin group (Figure 2A,B). STREME analysis revealed that the mammalian m6A conserved modification motif RRACH was enriched in both the control and oridonin groups, with R representing adenine or guanine and H representing adenine, uracil, or cytosine (Figure 2C). Transcripts containing m6A modifications were classified based on the quantity of modification peaks observed in each transcript. The analysis revealed that over 3000 genes displayed 1–2 m6A modification peaks in every group, while a relatively limited number of transcripts showed an increased occurrence of more than 4 m6A modification peaks (Figure 2D). m6A modification on transcripts was not randomly distributed. Figure 2E shows that m6A modifications were primarily concentrated in the coding region sequence and the 3′ untranslated region of mRNA, and were highly enriched in the stop codon region. Interestingly, m6A modifications were also abundant in non-coding RNA (Figure 2F).

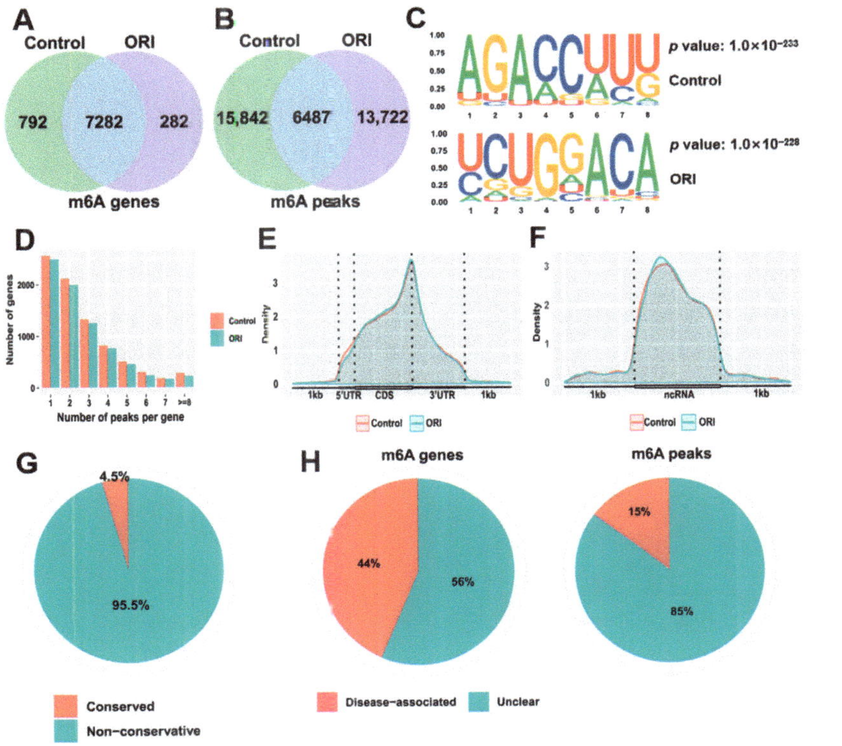

Figure 2. Illustration in a Venn diagram depicting the overlap of m6A-modified genes (**A**) and peaks (**B**) between oridonin and control groups. (**C**) Analysis of m6A motifs in the oridonin and control groups. (**D**) Distribution pattern of m6A modification peaks per gene. Comparing the difference in density of m6A-modified peaks in mRNA (**E**) and ncRNA (**F**). Identification of conserved m6A sites (**G**), m6A genes and peaks related to the disease (**H**) in differentially modified m6A-mRNAs.

By conducting ConsRM and RMDisease analyses, we explored the conservation of m6A and its association with diseases. The ConsRM analysis showed that 95.5% of m6A-modified sites exhibited non-conservative characteristics in differentially modified m6A and differentially expressed genes (DEGs) (Figure 2G). Additionally, the RMDisease analysis indicated that 15% of m6A peaks and 44% of m6A genes were linked to various diseases (Figure 2H).

3.3. Combined Analysis of RNA-seq and MeRIP-seq

To demonstrate the regulatory effect of m6A modification on the Wnt signaling pathway, this study combined RNA-seq and MeRIP-seq data analysis to identify genes with notable changes at both mRNA expression and m6A modification. The PCA results demonstrated marked distinctions among samples from the oridonin and control groups, with well-clustered samples within each group indicating that gene expression levels were significantly altered after oridonin treatment of HTR-8/SVneo cells, and also confirmed the reliability of the sequencing data (Figure 3A). The screening criteria for DEGs and differentially modified m6A genes were set as fold change > 1.2 or <0.83, with $p < 0.05$. A total of 2296 DEGs were detected by mRNA-seq, with 1437 genes upregulated and 1559 genes downregulated. MeRIP-seq identified a total of 4039 differentially modified m6A genes, including 2741 genes with enhanced m6A modification and 1298 genes with weakened m6A modification (Figure 3C,D). Notably, 829 genes showed significant changes at both levels (Figure 3B). The 4039 differentially modified m6A genes, along with their *p*-values and fold changes, as well as the 2296 DEGs with their corresponding *p*-values and fold changes, are listed in Table S2 and Table S3, respectively.

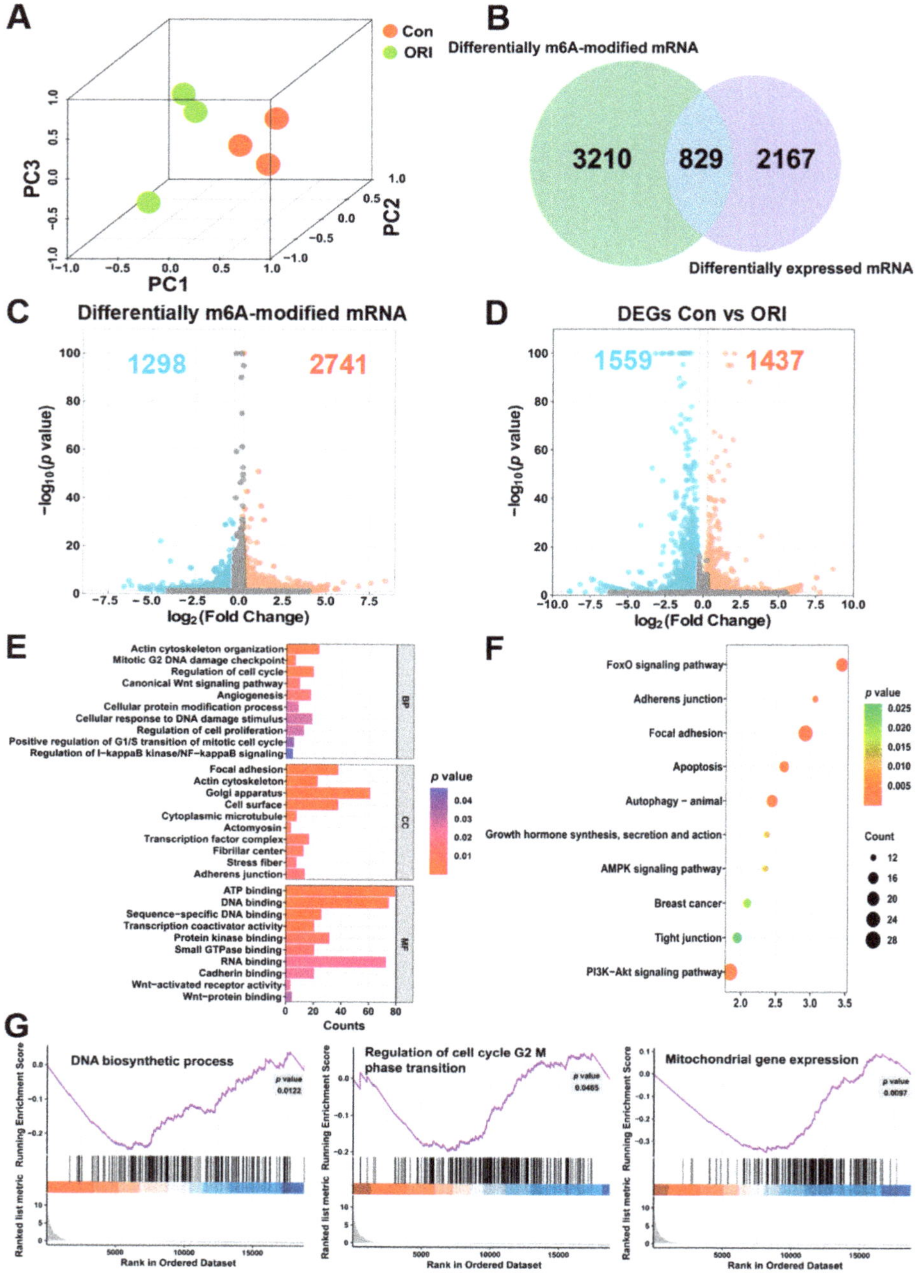

Figure 3. Molecular diversity of HTR-8/SVneo cells post-treatment with oridonin. (**A**) PCA for the mRNA expression between the oridonin and control groups. (**B**) Venn plot illustrating the intersection between differentially modified m6A genes and DEGs. (**C**) Volcano plot depicting genes m6A methylation downregulated (in blue) or upregulated (in red). (**D**) Volcano plot depicting genes expression downregulated (in blue) or upregulated (in red). The GO (**E**) and KEGG (**F**) enrichment of 829 overlapped genes among DEGs and differentially m6A-methylated mRNAs. (**G**) GSEA revealed that genes in oridonin group were enriched for DNA biosynthetic process, regulation of cell cycle G2/M phase transition, and mitochondrial gene expression.

Subsequently, 829 overlapping genes were analyzed for KEGG and GO enrichment. GO enrichment analysis revealed that these genes were mainly enriched in regulation of cell cycle, cellular response to DNA damage stimulus, regulation of cell proliferation, adherens junction, focal adhesion, Wnt-activated receptor activity, and Wnt-protein binding (Figure 3E). KEGG enrichment results mainly included focal adhesion, adherens junction, growth hormone synthesis, secretion and action, and tight junction (Figure 3F). We conducted gene set enrichment analysis (GSEA) to further clarify the signaling pathways linked to oridonin treatment. Comparative GSEA analysis between the oridonin and control groups indicated that regulation of cell cycle G2/M phase transition, DNA biosynthetic process, and mitochondrial gene expression were inhibited (Figure 3G).

3.4. Potential Regulators of RNA m6A Methylation

An analysis of mRNA expression levels for 22 RNA m6A methylation regulators was conducted to identify potential regulators using mRNA-seq data. As shown in Table 2, writers *RBM15*, *RBM15B*, *WTAP*, and reader *IGF2BP2* were significantly downregulated, while readers *FMR1*, *HNRNPA2B1*, and *YTHDF2* were significantly upregulated.

Table 2. The mRNA expression levels of m6A regulators in oridonin-treated HTR-8/SVneo cells.

Genes	Regulation	Base Mean	log_2Fold Change	*p* Value
IGF2BP2	reader	12,299	−0.42	6.2×10^{-16}
FMR1	reader	5256	0.44	1.2×10^{-5}
HNRNPA2B1	reader	190,433	0.27	1.4×10^{-4}
RBM15B	writer	4641	−0.15	3.2×10^{-3}
WTAP	writer	4354	−0.19	1.2×10^{-2}
RBM15	writer	810	−0.68	2.3×10^{-2}
YTHDF2	reader	1870	0.17	3.2×10^{-2}
IGF2BP1	reader	8764	−0.22	5.6×10^{-2}
HNRNPC	reader	82,291	−0.09	7.4×10^{-2}
YTHDF3	reader	883	1.15	1.1×10^{-1}
ZC3H13	writer	47,093	0.12	1.3×10^{-1}
IGF2BP3	reader	2040	−0.12	1.6×10^{-1}
FTO	eraser	1580	0.14	1.7×10^{-1}
ALKBH5	eraser	16,193	0.08	2.4×10^{-1}
YTHDC2	reader	1778	−0.09	2.4×10^{-1}
METTL14	writer	5153	−0.06	3.5×10^{-1}
METTL5	writer	2978	−0.06	3.7×10^{-1}
YTHDF1	reader	3137	0.04	4.6×10^{-1}
CBLL1	writer	1580	0.03	7.7×10^{-1}
YTHDC1	reader	18,686	−0.08	8.0×10^{-1}
VIRMA	writer	10,151	0.01	8.3×10^{-1}
METTL3	writer	1885	0.01	9.4×10^{-1}

We collected genes related to the Wnt signaling pathway, regulation of cell cycle, cellular response to DNA damage, and tight junction from GO and KEGG enrichment results. Subsequently, we utilized STRING to investigate the regulatory connections between these genes and m6A regulators, thereby conducting network analysis for protein–protein interactions. In Figure 4A–D, the top five genes in Wnt signaling pathway term were *SFRP1*, *FZD2*, *TCF7*, *FZD3*, and *FZD1*, with the degrees of 10, 8, 7, 7, and 7 (Figure 4A); the top five genes in cellular response to DNA damage term were *CCND1*, *BCL2*, *CDKN1A*, *SETD7*, and *SFPQ*, with the degrees of 15, 15, 10, 10, and 7 (Figure 4B); in regulation of cell cycle term, the top-ranking genes included *FOXM1*, *ACTB*, *JUN*, *PLK1*, and *CDKN1A*, with the degrees of 20, 20, 17,16, and 15 (Figure 4C); the top five genes in tight junction term were *CCND1*, *ACTB*. *JUN*, *TJP1*, and *ACTN4*, with the degrees of 18, 18, 17, 13, and 10 (Figure 4D).

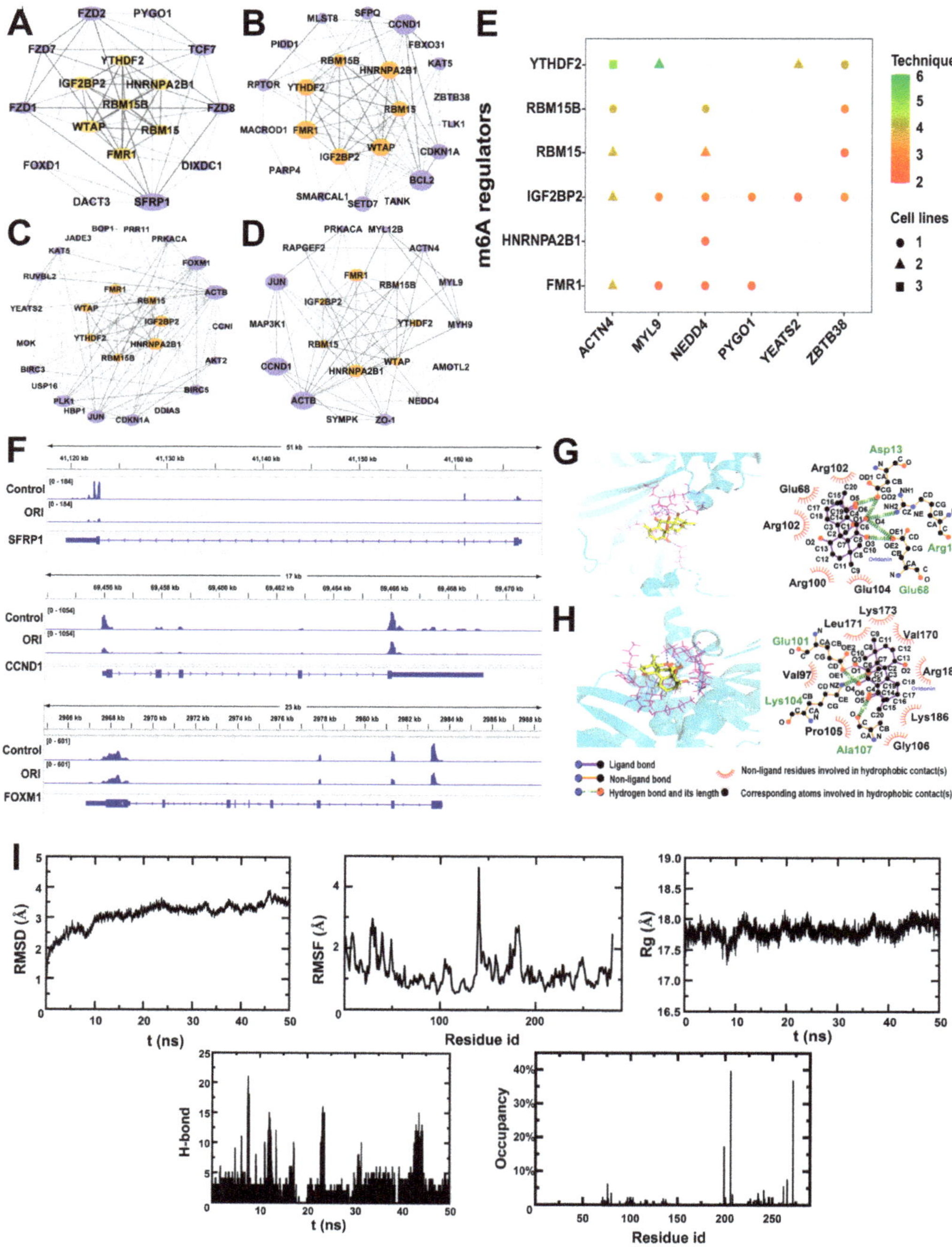

Figure 4. The associations between m6A regulators and the genes of Wnt signaling pathway (**A**), cellular response to DNA damage (**B**), regulation of cell cycle (**C**), and tight junction (**D**). (**E**) The impact of m6A regulators on the DEGs within Wnt signaling pathway, regulation of cell cycle, cellular response to DNA damage, and tight junction. (**F**) The level of m6A modification on *SFRP1*, *CCND1*, and *FOXM1* mRNA transcripts visualized by IGV. The interactions of oridonin with m6A regulators of FMR1 protein (**G**) and HNRNPA2B1 protein (**H**). (**I**) Molecular dynamics simulation between FMR1 protein and oridonin.

To explore substrates targeted by RNA m6A methylation regulators, the writers RBM15, RBM15B, WTAP, and readers IGF2BP2, FMR1, HNRNPA2B1, and YTHDF2 were selected, along with genes related to the Wnt signaling pathway, regulation of the cell cycle, cellular response to DNA damage, and tight junction. The results indicated that IGF2BP2 and FMR1 were extensively involved in regulating the majority of genes within these four terms (Figure 4E). Utilizing IGV, the m6A methylation patterns of transcripts were visualized. After treatment with oridonin, the m6A methylation levels of the Wnt signaling pathway-related gene *SFRP1*, regulation of cell cycle-related gene *FOXM1*, and cellular response to DNA damage-related gene *CCND1* decreased (Figure 4F).

3.5. Molecular Interactions and Molecular Dynamics between Oridonin and m6A Regulatory Proteins

Predictions of the interactions between oridonin and m6A regulatory proteins are presented in Table 3, Figure 4G,H. Oridonin formed hydrogen bonds with Arg11, Asp13, Arg102, and Glu68 in FMR1 protein, as well as with Glu101, Lys104, and Ala107 in HNRNPA2B1 protein. In Arg100 and Glu104 sites, FMR1 made hydrophobic contacts with oridonin, while in Pro105, Gly106, Lys186, Arg185, Val170, Lys173, Leu171, and Val197 sites, HNRNPA2B1 made hydrophobic contacts with oridonin. The total scores of the above two proteins exceeded 5, suggesting that the proteins were the most likely to bind to oridonin.

Table 3. The interactions between oridonin and m6A regulatory proteins.

Protein	PDB ID	Total Score	Crash	Polar	H-Bond Number	Residues Involve in H-Bond Formation	Hydrophobic Contact Number	Residues Involve in Hydrophobic Contacts
FMR1	2QND	6.5681	−0.9503	6.7019	5	Arg11, Asp13, Glu68 (3 H-bonds)	2	Arg100, Glu104
HNRNPA2B1	5WWG	5.9849	−4.3987	3.4371	3	Glu101, Lys104, Ala107	8	Pro105, Gly106, Lys186, Arg185, Val170, Lys173, Leu171, Val197
IGF2BP2	6ROL	4.432	−0.8333	3.5298	4	Lys509 (3 H-bonds), Asn503	5	Phe502, Leu510, Glu511, Ile562, Gol604
RBM15	7Z27	4.1057	−0.6563	3.4976	4	Lys9, Lys51, Leu12 (2 H-bonds)	2	Ala13, Gln15
WTAP	7YFJ	3.6498	−0.9403	2.5236	3	Gln61 (3 H-bonds)	3	Tyr64, Leu68, Ser65
YTHDF2	4WQN	3.1273	−0.587	2.3001	2	Arg425, Lys428	2	Asp421, His424

In evaluating the binding stability and conformational variability of the FMR1 protein and oridonin complex throughout MD simulation, RMSD, RMSF, Rg, H-bound, and occupancy analyses were performed (Figure 4I). The complex demonstrated average RMSD values spanning from 0.6 to 3.9 Å, with Rg values showing fluctuations within a 1 Å range. The residue-wise fluctuations of FMR1 protein and oridonin were plotted. Analysis of RMSF indicated that no amino acid residues exhibited conformational fluctuations exceeding 4.7 Å relative to their mean structure, highlighting the significant stability of backbone atoms within this complex system. The quantity of hydrogen bonds established throughout the simulation was recorded. Noteworthy is the observation that among the 280 amino acid residues, aspartic acid at position 206 exhibited the highest hydrogen bond occupancy at 40%.

3.6. Results of the Analysis of Differentially Expressed Proteins (DEPs)

The PCA plot between the oridonin and control groups (Figure 5A) shows a significant difference. The volcano plot illustrates the distribution of all proteins identified through the LC-MS/MS approach. Proteins that were significantly downregulated and upregulated (FDR < 0.05, fold change > 1.2 or <0.83) are highlighted in blue and red, while proteins showing non-significant distinctions between the oridonin and control groups are depicted in grey. A total of 62 differentially expressed proteins (DEPs) were screened, with 26 downregulated and 36 upregulated (Figure 5B). The clustering analysis of DEPs is presented in the heatmap (Figure 5C). The 62 DEPs, along with their corresponding FDR and fold changes, are listed in Table S4.

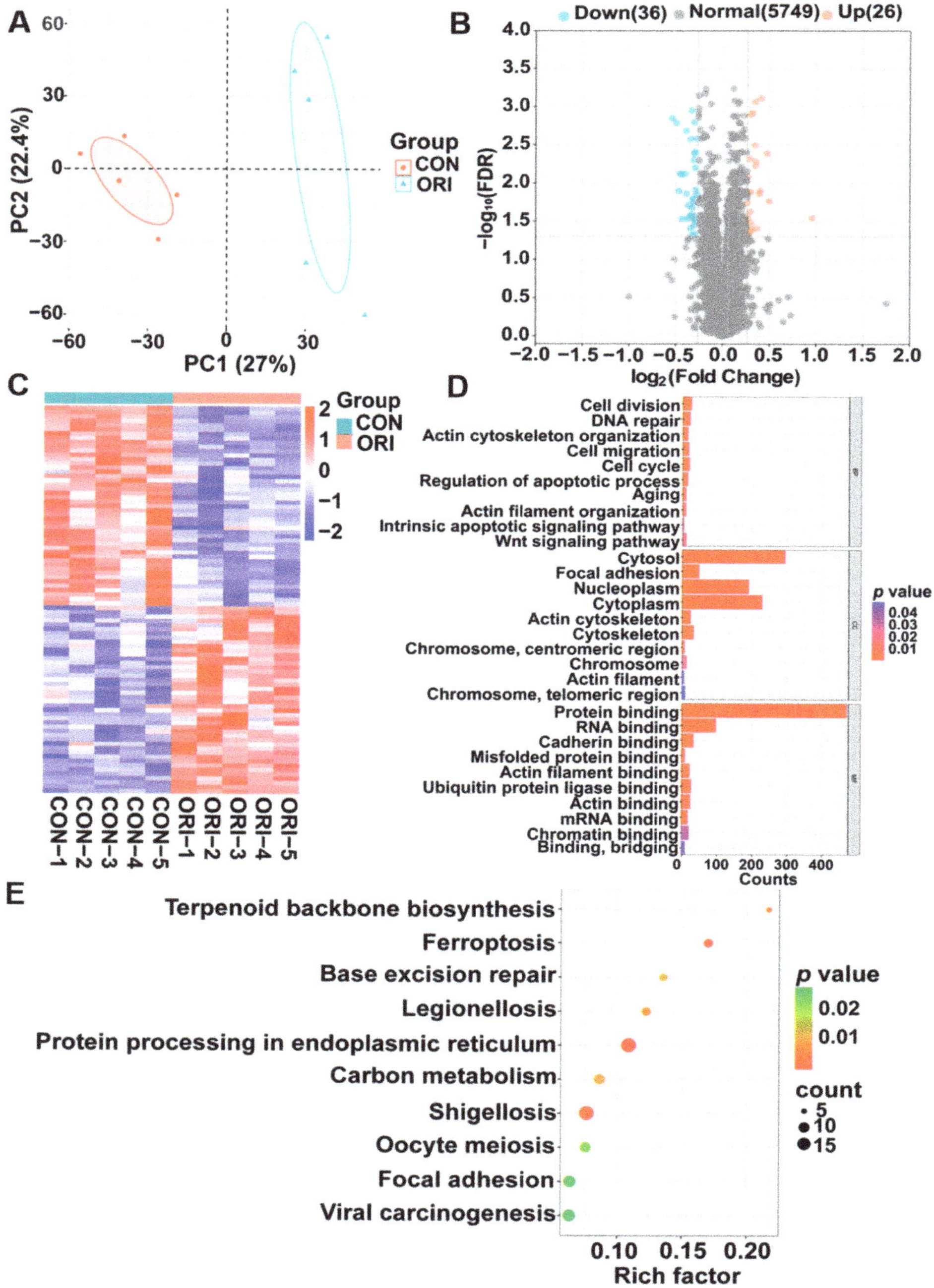

Figure 5. (**A**) PCA for the protein expression in the oridonin and control groups. (**B**) The volcano plot showed the DEPs in the oridonin and control groups. (**C**) Heatmap of DEPs in the oridonin and control groups. Enrichment analysis for GO terms (**D**) and KEGG pathway (**E**) related to DEPs.

3.7. Analysis Results from GO Annotation and Enrichment of KEGG Pathways

Supplementary analyses using GO and KEGG pathways were carried out to examine potential significant enrichment trends of DEPs (FDR < 0.05) in distinct functional categories. The DEPs associated with biological processes (BPs) were mainly enriched in functions associated with cell division, cytoskeleton organization, cell cycle regulation, the Wnt signaling pathway, and apoptosis. In terms of cellular components (CC), the DEPs were significantly enriched in terms such as focal adhesion, actin cytoskeleton, and chromosome. For molecular functions (MFs), terms showed predominant enrichment in actin binding, RNA binding, and cadherin binding, as illustrated in Figure 5D. The KEGG pathway is associated with the terpenoid backbone biosynthesis, ferroptosis, and focal adhesion (Figure 5E).

In comparison to the control group, GSEA of oridonin-treated samples revealed inhibition in cytoskeletal protein binding, positive regulation of cell differentiation, regulation of cytoskeleton organization, and cadherin binding, while the DNA templated transcription initiation and mRNA binding were activated (Figure 6A–F).

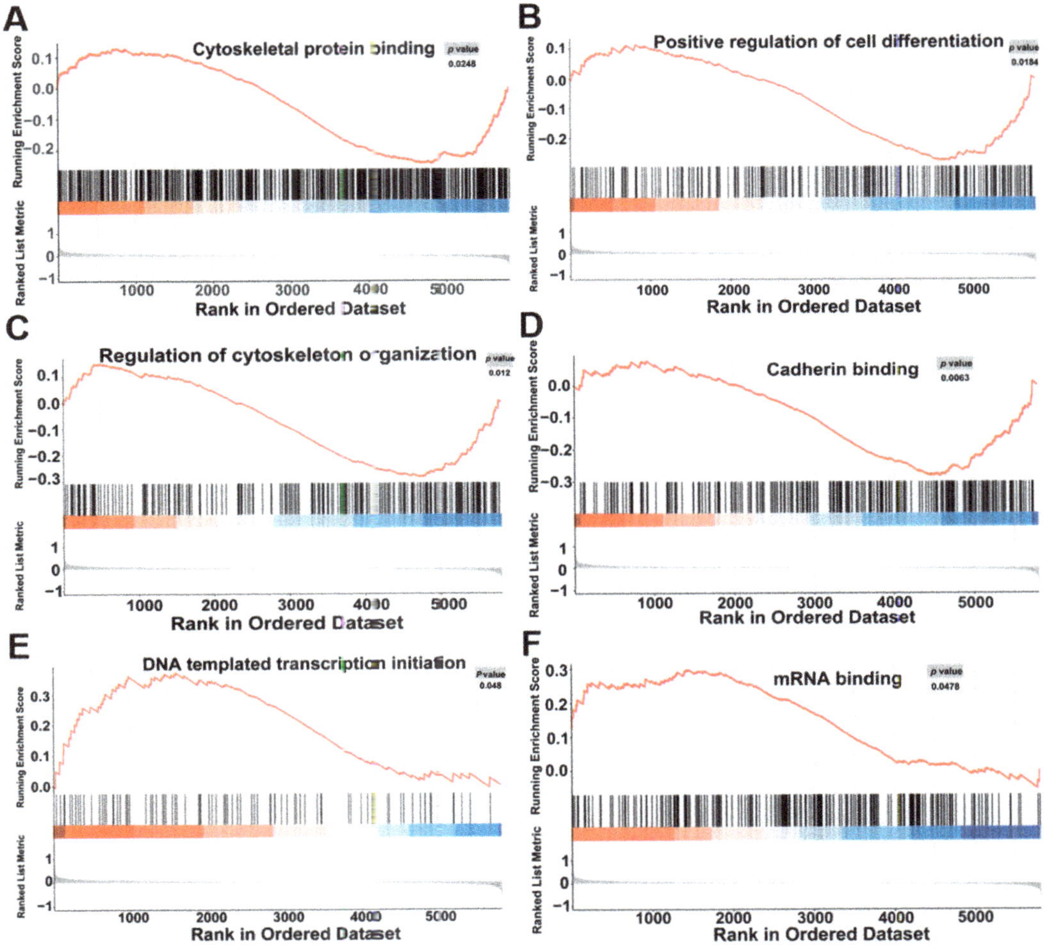

Figure 6. GSEA results between the oridonin and control groups. Cytoskeletal protein binding (**A**), positive regulation of cell differentiation (**B**), regulation of cytoskeleton organization (**C**), cadherin binding (**D**), DNA templated transcription initiation (**E**), and mRNA binding (**F**).

3.8. Analysis of Metabolomics Data between Oridonin-Treated and Control Groups

Metabolites in the samples were detected using LC-MS/MS, with PCA plots (Figure 7A) showing substantial variances in metabolite compositions between the two groups. Moreover, the OPLS-DA analysis demonstrated effective differentiation of the oridonin group from the control group. Results of the permutation test showed $R^2X = 0.389$, $R^2Y = 0.995$, and $Q^2 = 0.79$, confirming the reliability of the predictive ability of the OPLS-DA model (Figure 7B,C).

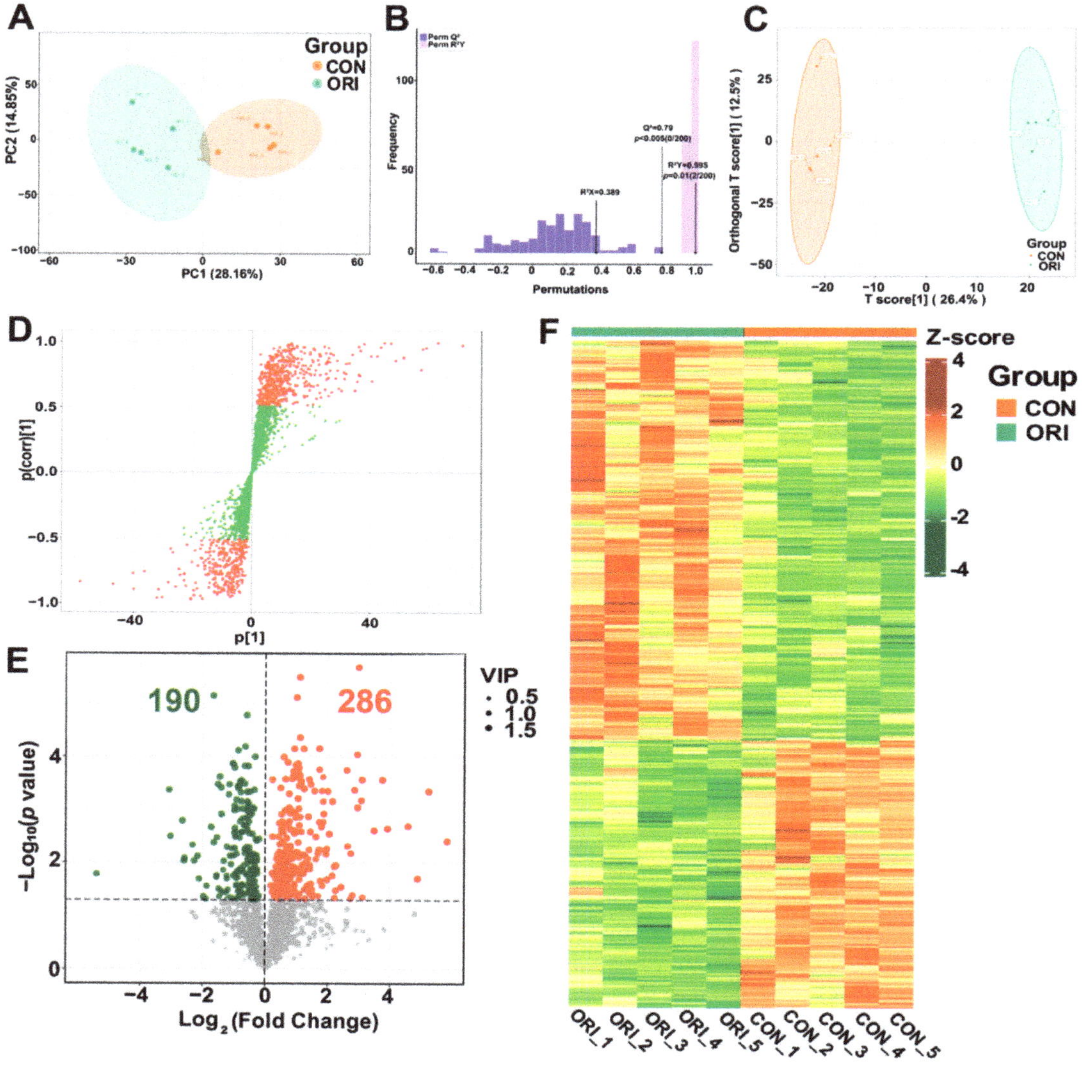

Figure 7. (**A**) PCA plots between the oridonin and control groups. (**B**) The predictive ability of the OPLS-DA model is reliable. (**C**) The OPLS-DA model was able to clearly separate the oridonin group from the control group. (**D**) OPLS-DA S-plot. Red dots indicate metabolites with VIP values greater than 1, while green dots indicate metabolites with VIP values less than or equal to 1. (**E**) Volcano plots showing upregulated and downregulated metabolites. (**F**) Correlation heatmap of DEMs.

The OPLS-DA S-plot displays metabolites with significant differences based on VIP values (Figure 7D). Metabolites positioned closer to the upper right and lower left corners indicate more pronounced variances. In this plot, red dots represent metabolites with VIP > 1, while green dots represent those with VIP ≤ 1. According to the VIP values in the OPLS-DA model variables, where $p < 0.05$ and VIP > 1, 476 differentially expressed metabolites (DEMs) were identified, comprising 190 downregulated and 286 upregulated metabolites (Figure 7E). As shown in the volcano diagram, green represents downregulated changes and red represents upregulated changes. In order to express the clustering relationships between the two groups, 476 DEMs were selected to construct a heatmap (Figure 7F). The information of 476 DEMs is listed in Table S5.

Among the differentially accumulated metabolites, 2,3-bis-0-(geranylgeranyl)-sn-glycerol 1-phosphate had the highest $|\log_2$Fold Change$|$ values (Figure 8A). The analysis of the differential metabolites identified in the previous screening was conducted using KEGG metabolic database; the primary pathways in these differential metabolites were cholinergic synapse, thiamine metabolism, longevity regulating pathways, and valine, leucine, and isoleucine degradation pathways (Figure 8B). Figure 8C illustrates a differential metabolite correlation network diagram, showing the top 20 metabolites with the largest VIP values. In this diagram, pink lines represent positive correlations, while blue lines indicated negative correlations. The thickness of the lines reflects the absolute value of the correlation coefficient; thicker lines denote stronger correlations. A violin plot (Figure 8D) displays the top 20 metabolites with the greatest differential multiplicity, with red indicating upregulated and green indicating downregulated. The names of the 20 metabolites corresponding to their IDs are listed in Table S6.

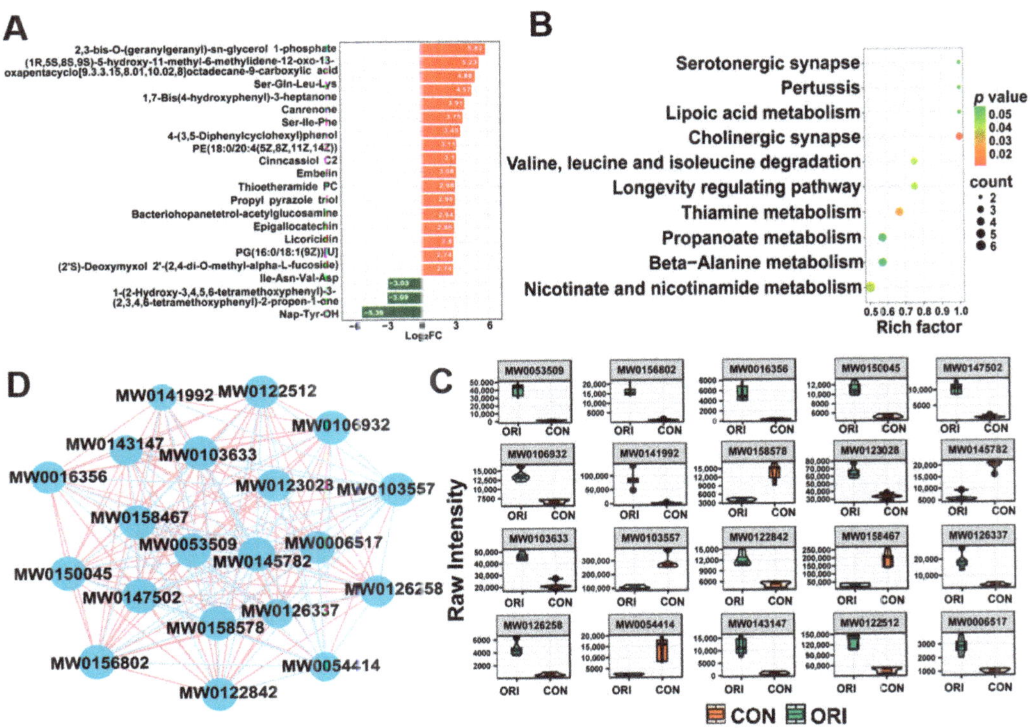

Figure 8. (**A**) Bar graph of DEM multiplicity, presenting the top 20 metabolites with the highest difference in multiplicity. (**B**) The top 10 enriched KEGG pathways of DEMs displayed by *p*-value in the oridonin and control groups ($p < 0.05$, VIP > 1). (**C**) Correlation analysis among samples. The top 20 differential metabolites with the highest VIP values are included. (**D**) Violin plot showing the top 20 DEMs based on VIP values.

3.9. Oxidative Stress and DNA Damage Induced by Oridonin

Oridonin-induced oxidative damage in HTR-8/SVneo cells was evaluated by measuring the level of intracellular ROS. After a 24 h exposure, the fluorescence intensity of DCF, which indicates the level of ROS production, exhibited a significant rise from 100% in the control group to 123.6%, 165.2%, and 382.7% in the 12.5, 25, and 37.5 μM oridonin groups (Figure 9A,B). The excessive accumulation of intracellular ROS is considered detrimental to the cells.

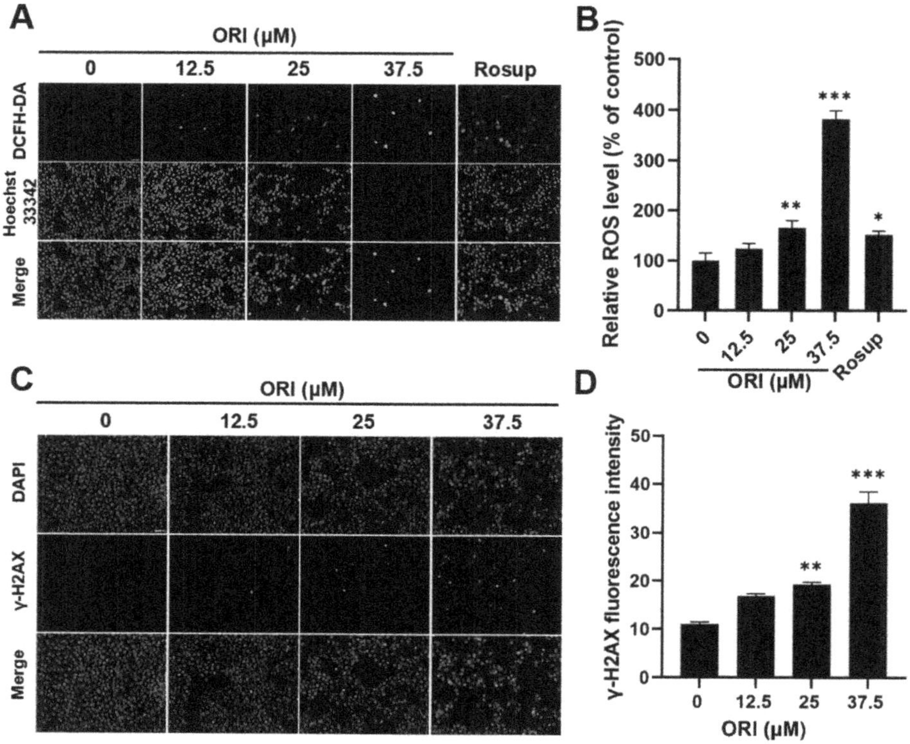

Figure 9. (**A**) Representative images showing the intracellular ROS production. (**B**) Analysis of the relative fluorescence intensity of DCF in the oridonin group and the control group. Immunofluorescence analysis (**C**) and quantitative analysis (**D**) of phosphorylated γ-H2AX induced by 0, 12.5, 25, and 37.5 μM oridonin. * $p < 0.05$, ** $p < 0.01$, and *** $p < 0.001$, n = 3. Scale bar = 100 μm.

γ-H2AX acts as a highly sensitive marker for detecting DNA damage that leads to double-strand breaks. Figure 9C,D demonstrate that treatment with oridonin resulted in intensified green fluorescence and a notable increase in the level of γ-H2AX, indicating DNA damage occurred in HTR-8/SVneo cells.

3.10. The Adverse Impacts of Oridonin Therapy on Mitochondrial Function

In this study, intracellular Ca^{2+} levels were measured by fluorescence probe Fluo-4 AM. Compared with the control group, exposure of HTR-8/SVneo cells to oridonin increased intracellular Ca^{2+} levels (Figure 10A,B), and revealed the overload of intracellular calcium ions. Figure 10C,D illustrate a decreasing trend in the red–green fluorescence ratio, which was measured in the 12.5, 25, and 37.5 μM groups compared to the control group ($p < 0.05$), with values of 1.53 ± 0.07, 1.03 ± 0.04, and 0.83 ± 0.01, respectively. This indicated that oridonin treatment leads to a decrease in MMP in HTR-8/SVneo cells. The fluorescence intensities of Calcein were measured in different groups in Figure 10E,F. The obtained results demonstrated that the fluorescence intensities of Calcein were 136.14 ± 2.85, 105.16 ± 1.85, 36.58 ± 3.14, and 24.73 ± 1.85 in the 0, 12.5, 25, and 37.5 μM oridonin groups, respectively. This result indicated that oridonin treatment led to a dose-dependent reduction in the green fluorescence intensity of Calcein, suggesting a notable induction of mPTP opening.

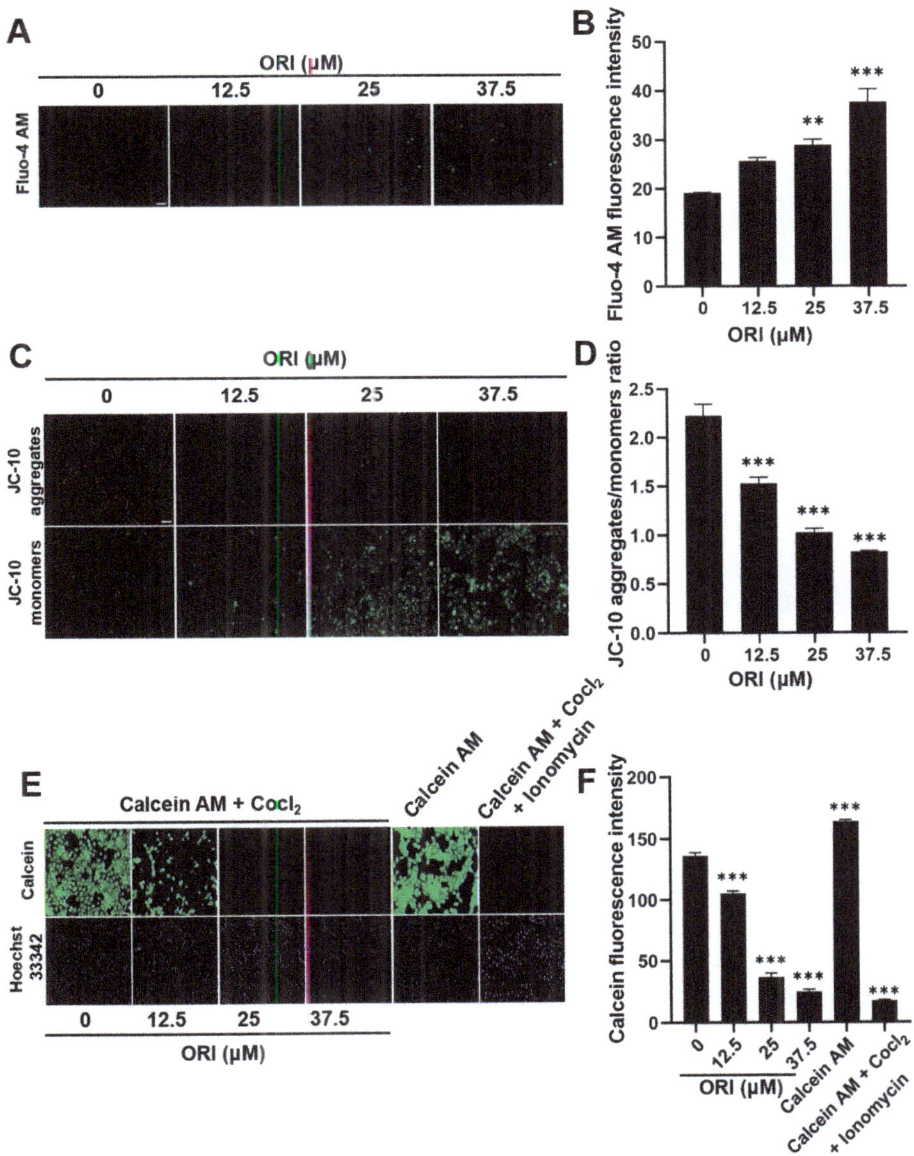

Figure 10. (**A**) Intracellular Ca^{2-} was visualized using Fluo-4 AM in fluorescence microscopy images. (**B**) Statistics of intracellular Ca^{2+} level Oridonin induced mitochondrial damage in HTR-8/SVneo cells. JC-10 (**C**) and Calcein AM (**E**) probes were used to detect the MMP and mPTP in oridonin-treated HTR-8/SVneo cells, respectively. Quantitative results of the JC-10 probe (**D**) and Calcein AM probe (**F**) in oridonin-treated HTR-8/SVneo cells. ** $p < 0.01$, *** $p < 0.001$, n = 3. Scale bar = 100 μm.

3.11. Expression Levels of mRNA and Proteins

In order to demonstrate the high correlation of Wnt signaling pathway, cell cycle, and tight junction with the reproductive toxicity of oridonin, we selected pivotal genes and proteins associated with these terms for experimental validation. RT-qPCR was employed to evaluate the mRNA expression levels of these pivotal genes. The results depicted in Figure 11A demonstrate that oridonin led to a decrease in the expression of *β-catenin*, *CLDN1*, and *OCLN* in HTR-8/SVneo cells, while increasing expression of *GSK3B*, *TCF7L1*, *WNT-6*, *CCND1*, and *ZO-1*.

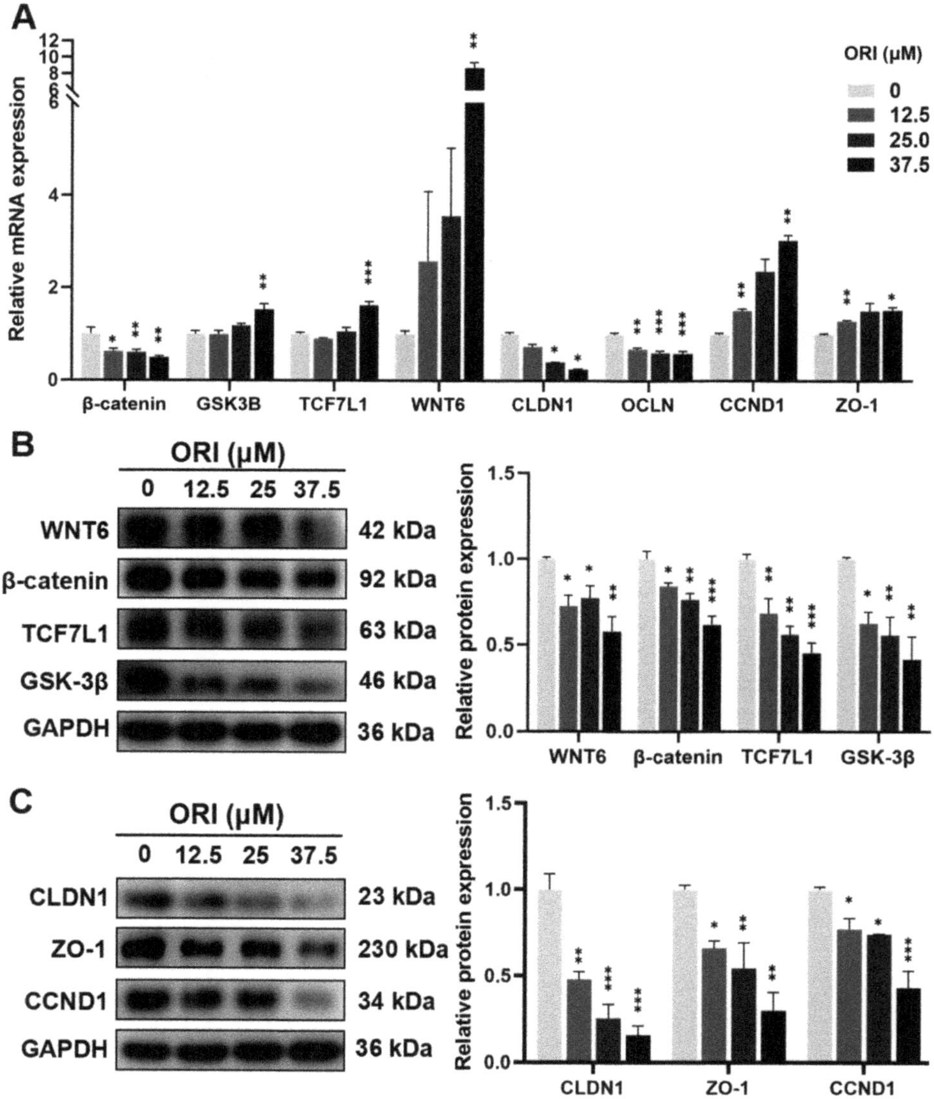

Figure 11. (**A**) The mRNA levels were measured through RT-qPCR analysis. (**B**) Expression levels of WNT6, β-catenin, TCF7L1, and GSK-3β proteins in 0, 12.5, 25, and 37.5 μM oridonin-treated HTR-8/SVneo cells. (**C**) Protein expression levels of CLDIN1, ZO-1, and CCND1 in 0, 12.5, 25, and 37.5 μM oridonin-treated HTR-8/SVneo cells. * $p < 0.05$, ** $p < 0.01$, and *** $p < 0.001$, n = 3.

As shown in Figure 11B,C, results of Western blotting indicated a significant reduction in the expression level of WNT6, β-catenin, TCF7L1, and GSK-3β in the oridonin group compared to the control group. Additionally, the levels of CLDN1, ZO-1, and CCND1 also decreased in response to oridonin.

4. Discussion

Traditional Chinese medicine has long been recognized for its safety. However, there have been frequent reports of adverse reactions in recent years. Oridonin is a tetracyclic diterpene compound extracted from *Rabdosia rubescens*, which exhibits anti-inflammatory [42] and anti-tumor effects [43]. However, studies have shown that oridonin promotes apoptosis by inhibiting nuclear factor-κB activation and causing G2/M phase arrest [44–47]. Furthermore, oridonin inhibits caspase-9 and activates TP53-related and PI3K/Akt pathways to promote ROS accumulation, resulting in cell death [48,49]. Therefore, these reports suggest that attention should be paid to the safety problems associated with oridonin in clinical practice. Although the toxic effects of oridonin have been reported, the exact toxicity mechanisms remain incompletely understood.

The combination of multiple omics methods has been utilized to investigate the mechanisms and potential biomarkers of reproductive toxicity induced by Chinese medicine components. In a study on testicular injury induced by *Tripterygium wilfordii* polyglycoside tablet (TWP) in rats, it was observed that TWP significantly reduced the protein levels of ZO-1, OCT4, CLDN11, and PLZF, indicating dysfunction of the blood–testis barrier and impairment of spermatogenesis. Furthermore, levels of ferroptosis-related proteins NRF2, SLC7A11, and GPX4 were notably decreased, while the expression level of 4-HNE was elevated. Additionally, the integrated analysis of DEGs and altered metabolites revealed the crucial roles of ferroptosis and glutathione metabolism in testicular injury [50]. Our study successfully constructed a comprehensive multiomics map of oridonin and identified the signaling pathways and biomarkers. Utilizing epigenetic transcriptome and proteome data, we uncovered key signaling pathways including the Wnt signaling pathway, tight junction, and focal adhesion. m6A regulators confer biological functions to m6A in RNA, precisely regulating balance under stimulation to maintain proper cellular metabolism. Defects in m6A methylation or demethylation may lead to severe physiological consequences, such as abnormal reproductive development in mammals. The study indicated that treatment with oridonin increased the expression of FRM1, a ribosome-associated RNA-binding protein involved in follicular genesis. The expression of FRM1 was notably upregulated in patients with premature ovarian insufficiency [51]. Metabolomics analysis indicated that differential metabolites mainly participated in thiamine metabolism, longevity regulating pathway, and valine, leucine, and isoleucine degradation pathway. Adequate thiamine levels help sustain maternal and fetal mitochondrial function, ensuring normal cell division and growth progression, particularly in germ cell maturation [52].

Oridonin has been found to exert effects across multiple cellular levels [43,53,54]. Numerous investigations have associated oridonin toxicity with the modification of essential biomolecule structure and function through involvement in ROS generation [43,44,55]. Ca^{2+} ions serve as multifunctional second messengers, and participate in various intracellular processes, including signal transduction, muscle contraction, and oxidative stress. Treatment of HTR-8/SVneo cells with oridonin increased Ca^{2+} levels and demonstrated the presence of mitochondrial dysfunction and oxidative stress. Free radicals and oxidative molecules produced during oxidative stress can trigger DNA damage. Exposure of human colorectal cancer cells SW1116 and SW480 to alantolactone caused a substantial increase in ROS level, leading to profound oxidative DNA damage [56]. The results indicated that oridonin triggered HTR-8/SVneo cell ROS accumulation and DNA damage. The study demonstrated that reproductive toxicity was mediated by oridonin, as shown by increased ROS levels, elevated LDH leakage, reduced MMP, and changes in WNT6, β-catenin, TCF7L1, GSK-3β, CLDN1, ZO-1, and CCND1 mRNA and protein expression. We confirmed through RT-qPCR and Western blotting that these factors associated with the

Wnt signaling pathway, cell cycle, and tight junctions were highly correlated with the reproductive toxicity of oridonin. However, the observed mRNA and protein expression levels in our experimental results were inconsistent with those obtained from transcriptomics and proteomics analysis, possibly due to differences in technical sensitivity between omics approaches and experimental methods. Oxidative damage leads to mitochondrial dysfunction, which is characterized by alterations in mitochondrial morphology and impaired mitochondrial function. Pathological conditions often give rise to structural changes in mitochondria, including swelling and fragmentation, with increased mitochondrial fission. A significant indicator of mitochondrial dysfunction is the disruption of the MMP. Loss of MMP leads to dysfunction in the mitochondrial electron transport chain, diminished oxygen consumption for metabolism, ATP depletion, and compromised energy metabolism. More specifically, the opening of the mPTP leads to the liberation of cytochrome c from mitochondria into the cytoplasm, thereby activating pro-apoptotic caspases. Mitochondrial dysfunction is frequently associated with disruptions in calcium homeostasis and mutations in mitochondrial DNA [57]. The Wnt/β-catenin signaling pathway serves as a crucial controller of cell proliferation and maintains the pluripotent state in embryonic stem cells (ESCs). Dysregulation of the Wnt signaling pathway during early development stages gives rise to a range of hereditary diseases that result in abnormalities in embryonic development [58]. To further understand the mechanism of reproductive toxicity induced by oridonin, the status of the Wnt signaling pathway was examined. The Wnt/β-catenin signaling pathway is crucial and highly conserved in embryonic development and is also implicated in carcinogenesis due to its involvement in regulating cell differentiation, proliferation, and migration [59]. Berberine antagonized the increase in FITC-dextran permeability in rat intestinal microvascular endothelial cells caused by LPS and upregulated the expression levels of VE-cadherin, β-catenin, and claudin-12 [60]. Furthermore, the upregulation of Wnt1 expression in C57MG mammary tumor-derived cell line results in elevated levels of Connexin43 protein expression [61]. In this study, the downregulation of tight junction-associated proteins CLDN1 and ZO1 led to damage in HTR-8/SVneo cell junctions caused by oridonin. This damage may have resulted in injury to the epithelial barrier, restricting embryo growth and development. According to the transcriptomics, proteomics, and metabolomics analysis, the Wnt/β-catenin signaling pathway is one of the most relevant pathways involved in the adverse reproductive effects of oridonin. In the current study, a notable decrease in the expression of Wnt6 and β-catenin proteins was observed in HTR-8/SVneo cells following treatment with oridonin, as compared to the control group. This discovery aligns with a recent investigation that demonstrated the persistent activation of the Wnt signaling pathway during oridonin-induced reproductive toxicity injury. These results indicate that inhibiting the Wnt/β-catenin signaling pathway and disruption of tight junction are associated with oridonin-induced cytotoxicity and mitochondrial dysfunction.

5. Conclusions

The study identified that oridonin can induce reproductive toxicity by eliciting oxidative stress, DNA damage, and mitochondrial dysfunction. The integration of multi-omics approaches revealed the participation of the Wnt/β-catenin signaling pathway and tight junction in the damage caused by oridonin to HTR-8/SVneo cells. The mechanism uncovered in this study may provide new strategies to mitigate oridonin-induced reproductive toxicity.

Supplementary Materials: The following supporting information can be downloaded at: https://www.mdpi.com/article/10.3390/toxics12050339/s1, Table S1: Summary of mRNA sequence reads from HTR-8/SVneo cells with or without oridonin treatment. Table S2: 4039 differentially modified m6A genes were obtained after treating with 25 μM oridonin for 24 h in HTR-8/SVneo cells. Table S3: 2996 DEGs were obtained after treating with 25 μM oridonin for 24 h in HTR-8/SVneo cells. Table S4: 62 DEPs were obtained after treating with 25 μM oridonin for 24 h in HTR-8/SVneo cells. Table S5: 476 DEMs were obtained after treating with 25 μM oridonin for 24 h in HTR-8/SVneo cells. Table S6: The names of 20 metabolites corresponding to the IDs.

Author Contributions: Conceptualization, Q.W. and A.Z.; methodology, Q.W. and A.Z.; software, M.C. and K.T.; formal analysis, Q.W., X.G., Y.L. and C.W.; investigation, Q.W., X.G., Y.L. and C.W.; data curation, J.Z., J.W. and W.B.; writing—original draft preparation, Q.W., X.G., Y.L., J.Z., M.C., J.W., Y.W. and C.W.; writing—review and editing, A.Z. and P.S.; funding acquisition, Q.W. and A.Z. All authors have read and agreed to the published version of the manuscript.

Funding: This research was funded by the Natural Science Foundation of Fujian Province (2021J01409, 2021J05045), Science and Technology Plan Project of Fujian Provincial Health Commission (2021CXA033), Fujian Provincial Science and Technology Innovation Joint Fund Project (2020Y9155), National Natural Science Foundation of China (82104520), Fujian Medical University High-level Talent Research Startup Funding Project (XRCZX2020014), Open Research Fund of Fujian Key Laboratory of Tumor Microbiology, Fujian Medical University (FMUTM-202301).

Institutional Review Board Statement: Not applicable.

Informed Consent Statement: Not applicable.

Data Availability Statement: Data are contained within the article and Supplementary Materials.

Conflicts of Interest: The authors declare no conflicts of interest.

References

1. Zhang, Y.; Wang, L.; Zi, Y.; Zhang, L.; Guo, Y.; Huang, Y. Oridonin effectively reverses the drug resistance of cisplatin involving induction of cell apoptosis and inhibition of MMP expression in human acute myeloid leukemia cells. *Saudi J. Biol. Sci.* **2017**, *24*, 678–686. [CrossRef] [PubMed]
2. Ding, Y.; Ding, C.; Ye, N.; Liu, Z.; Wold, E.A. Chen, H.; Wild, C.; Shen, Q.; Zhou, J. Discovery and development of natural product oridonin-inspired anticancer agents. *Eur. J. Med. Chem.* **2016**, *122*, 102–117. [CrossRef]
3. Li, X.; Zhang, C.T.; Ma, W.; Xie, X.; Huang Q. Oridonin: A review of its pharmacology, pharmacokinetics and toxicity. *Front. Pharmacol.* **2021**, *12*, 645824. [CrossRef]
4. Zhang, Y.; Wang, S.; Dai, M.; Nai, J.; Zhu L.; Sheng, H. Solubility and bioavailability enhancement of oridonin: A review. *Molecules* **2020**, *25*, 332. [CrossRef]
5. Xu, L.; Bi, Y.; Xu, Y.; Zhang, Z.; Xu, W.; Zhang, S.; Chen, J. Oridonin inhibits the migration and epithelial-to-mesenchymal transition of small cell lung cancer cells by suppressing FAK-ERK1/2 signalling pathway. *J. Cell. Mol. Med.* **2020**, *24*, 4480–4493. [CrossRef]
6. Park, H.; Jeong, Y.J.; Han, N.K.; Kim, J.S.; Lee, H.J. Oridonin enhances radiation-induced cell death by promoting DNA damage in non-small cell lung cancer cells. *Int. J. Mol. Sci.* **2018**, *19*, 2378. [CrossRef]
7. Ying, Y. Effects of Oridonin on Estrogen and Antioxidative Function of Ovarian Granulosa Cells. Master's Thesis, Beijing University of Agriculture, Beijing, China, 2017.
8. Rosell-Hidalgo, A.; Moore, A.L.; Ghafourian, T. Prediction of drug-induced mitochondrial dysfunction using succinate-cytochrome c reductase activity, QSAR and molecular docking. *Toxicology* **2023**, *485*, 153412. [CrossRef]
9. Kang, N.; Zhang, J.H.; Qiu, F.; Tashiro, S.; Onodera, S.; Ikejima, T. Inhibition of EGFR signaling augments oridonin-induced apoptosis in human laryngeal cancer cells via enhancing oxidative stress coincident with activation of both the intrinsic and extrinsic apoptotic pathways. *Cancer Lett.* **2010**, *294*, 147–158. [CrossRef]
10. Quinlan, C.L.; Orr, A.L.; Perevoshchikova, I.V.; Treberg, J.R.; Ackrell, B.A.; Brand, M.D. Mitochondrial complex II can generate reactive oxygen species at high rates in both the forward and reverse reactions. *J. Biol. Chem.* **2012**, *287*, 27255–27264. [CrossRef]
11. Takeyama, N.; Matsuo, N.; Tanaka, T. Oxidative damage to mitochondria is mediated by the Ca^{2+}-dependent inner-membrane permeability transition. *Biochem. J.* **1993**, *294*, 719–725. [CrossRef]
12. Dykens, J.A.; Marroquin, L.D.; Will, Y. Strategies to reduce late-stage drug attrition due to mitochondrial toxicity. *Expert Rev. Mol. Diagn.* **2007**, *7*, 161–175. [CrossRef]
13. Nusse, R.; Clevers, H. Wnt/β-catenin signaling, disease, and emerging therapeutic modalities. *Cell* **2017**, *169*, 985–999. [CrossRef] [PubMed]
14. Xu, X.; Zhang, M.; Xu, F.; Jiang, S. Wnt signaling in breast cancer: Biological mechanisms, challenges and opportunities. *Mol. Cancer* **2020**, *19*, 165. [CrossRef]
15. Jati, S.; Sarraf, T.R.; Naskar, D.; Sen, M. Wnt signaling: Pathogen incursion and immune defense. *Front. Immunol.* **2019**, *10*, 2551. [CrossRef] [PubMed]
16. Amin, N.; Vincan, E. The Wnt signaling pathways and cell adhesion. *Front. Biosci.* **2012**, *17*, 784–804. [CrossRef] [PubMed]
17. Preda, V.; Larkin, S.J.; Karavitaki, N.; Ansorge, O.; Grossman, A.B. The Wnt signalling cascade and the adherens junction complex in craniopharyngioma tumorigenesis. *Endocr. Pathol.* **2015**, *26*, 1–8. [CrossRef] [PubMed]
18. May-Simera, H.L.; Kelley, M.W. Cilia, Wnt signaling, and the cytoskeleton. *Cilia* **2012**, *1*, 7. [CrossRef] [PubMed]

19. Pope, J.L.; Ahmad, R.; Bhat, A.A.; Washington, M.K.; Singh, A.B.; Dhawan, P. Claudin-1 overexpression in intestinal epithelial cells enhances susceptibility to adenamatous polyposis coli-mediated colon tumorigenesis. *Mol. Cancer* **2014**, *13*, 167. [CrossRef] [PubMed]
20. Yan, S.K.; Liu, R.H.; Jin, H.Z.; Liu, X.R.; Ye, J.; Shan, L.; Zhang, W.D. "Omics" in pharmaceutical research: Overview, applications, challenges, and future perspectives. *Chin. J. Nat. Med.* **2015**, *13*, 3–21. [CrossRef]
21. Zhang, Y.; Jiang, J.; Ma, J.; Wei, Z.; Wang, Y.; Song, B.; Meng, J.; Jia, G.; de Magalhães, J.P.; Rigden, D.J.; et al. DirectRMDB: A database of post-transcriptional RNA modifications unveiled from direct RNA sequencing technology. *Nucleic Acids Res.* **2023**, *51*, D106–D116. [CrossRef]
22. Wu, Y.; Chen, X.; Bao, W.; Hong, X.; Li, C.; Lu, J.; Zhang, D.; Zhu, A. Effect of humantenine on mRNA m6A modification and expression in human colon cancer cell line HCT116. *Genes* **2022**, *13*, 781. [CrossRef]
23. Ma, J.; Song, B.; Wei, Z.; Huang, D.; Zhang, Y.; Su, J.; de Magalhães, J.P.; Rigden, D.J.; Meng, J.; Chen, K. m5C-Atlas: A comprehensive database for decoding and annotating the 5-methylcytosine (m5C) epitranscriptome. *Nucleic Acids Res.* **2022**, *50*, D196–D203. [CrossRef] [PubMed]
24. Meyer, K.D.; Saletore, Y.; Zumbo, P.; Elemento, O.; Mason, C.E.; Jaffrey, S.R. Comprehensive analysis of mRNA methylation reveals enrichment in 3′ UTRs and near stop codons. *Cell* **2012**, *149*, 1635–1646. [CrossRef]
25. Shen, X.; Chen, M.; Zhang, J.; Lin, Y.; Gao, X.; Tu, J.; Chen, K.; Zhu, A.; Xu, S. Unveiling the impact of ApoF deficiency on liver and lipid metabolism: Insights from transcriptome-wide m6A methylome analysis in mice. *Genes* **2024**, *15*, 347. [CrossRef]
26. Shi, H.; Wei, J.; He, C. Where, When, and How: Context-dependent functions of RNA methylation writers, readers, and erasers. *Mol. Cell* **2019**, *74*, 640–650. [CrossRef]
27. Klungland, A.; Dahl, J.A.; Greggains, G.; Fedorcsak, P.; Filipczyk, A. Reversible RNA modifications in meiosis and pluripotency. *Nat. Methods* **2016**, *14*, 18–22. [CrossRef]
28. Xiang, Y.; Laurent, B.; Hsu, C.H.; Nachtergaele, S.; Lu, Z.; Sheng, W.; Xu, C.; Chen, H.; Ouyang, J.; Wang, S.; et al. RNA m^6A methylation regulates the ultraviolet-induced DNA damage response. *Nature* **2017**, *543*, 573–576. [CrossRef]
29. Wu, Y.; Bao, W.; Ren, J.; Li, C.; Chen, M.; Zhang, D.; Zhu, A. Integrated profiles of transcriptome and mRNA m6A modification reveal the intestinal cytotoxicity of Aflatoxin B1 on HCT116 cells. *Genes* **2022**, *14*, 79. [CrossRef]
30. Reyfman, P.A.; Walter, J.M.; Joshi, N.; Anekalla, K.R.; McQuattie-Pimentel, A.C.; Chiu, S.; Fernandez, R.; Akbarpour, M.; Chen, C.I.; Ren, Z.; et al. Single-cell transcriptomic analysis of human lung provides insights into the pathobiology of pulmonary fibrosis. *Am. J. Respir. Crit. Care Med.* **2019**, *199*, 1517–1536. [CrossRef] [PubMed]
31. Wang, J.; Ishfaq, M.; Xu, L.; Xia, C.; Chen, C.; Li, J. METTL3/m^6A/miRNA-873-5p attenuated oxidative stress and apoptosis in colistin-induced kidney injury by modulating Keap1/Nrf2 pathway. *Front. Pharmacol.* **2019**, *10*, 517. [CrossRef] [PubMed]
32. Budayeva, H.G.; Kirkpatrick, D.S. Monitoring protein communities and their responses to therapeutics. *Nat. Rev. Drug Discov.* **2020**, *19*, 414–426. [CrossRef] [PubMed]
33. Wang, X.; Chen, Y.; Han, Q.B.; Chan, C.Y.; Wang, H.; Liu, Z.; Cheng, C.H.; Yew, D.T.; Lin, M.C.; He, M.L.; et al. Proteomic identification of molecular targets of gambogic acid: Role of stathmin in hepatocellular carcinoma. *Proteomics* **2009**, *9*, 242–253. [CrossRef] [PubMed]
34. Rochfort, S. Metabolomics reviewed: A new "omics" platform technology for systems biology and implications for natural products research. *J. Nat. Prod.* **2005**, *68*, 1813–1820. [CrossRef] [PubMed]
35. Chen, M.; Su, M.; Zhao, L.; Jiang, J.; Liu, P.; Cheng, J.; Lai, Y.; Liu, Y.; Jia, W. Metabonomic study of aristolochic acid-induced nephrotoxicity in rats. *J. Proteome Res.* **2006**, *5*, 995–1002. [CrossRef] [PubMed]
36. Sun, Y.; Zhang, X.; Shen, X.; Wang, S.; Wang, Q.; Yang, X. Computational and experimental characterization of isomers of escin-induced renal cytotoxicity by inhibiting heat shock proteins. *Eur. J. Pharmacol.* **2021**, *908*, 174372. [CrossRef] [PubMed]
37. Zhu, A.; Sun, Y.; Zhong, Q.; Yang, J.; Zhang, T.; Zhao, J.; Wang, Q. Effect of euphorbia factor L1 on oxidative stress, apoptosis, and autophagy in human gastric epithelial cells. *Phytomedicine* **2019**, *64*, 152929. [CrossRef] [PubMed]
38. Huang, Y.-P.; Xia, Y.; Yang, L.; Wei, J.; Yang, Y.I.; Gao, Y.Q. SPONGE: A GPU-accelerated molecular dynamics package with enhanced sampling and AI-driven algorithms. *Chin. J. Chem.* **2022**, *40*, 160–168. [CrossRef]
39. Maier, J.A.; Martinez, C.; Kasavajhala, K.; Wickstrom, L.; Hauser, K.E.; Simmerling, C. ff14SB: Improving the accuracy of protein side chain and backbone parameters from ff99SB. *J. Chem. Theory Comput.* **2015**, *11*, 3696–3713. [CrossRef] [PubMed]
40. Chatterjee, S.; Debenedetti, P.G.; Stillinger, F.H.; Lynden-Bell, R.M. A computational investigation of thermodynamics, structure, dynamics and solvation behavior in modified water models. *J. Chem. Phys.* **2008**, *128*, 124511. [CrossRef] [PubMed]
41. Schmittgen, T.D.; Livak, K.J. Analyzing real-time PCR data by the comparative C_T method. *Nat. Protoc.* **2008**, *3*, 1101–1108. [CrossRef]
42. He, H.; Jiang, H.; Chen, Y.; Ye, J.; Wang, A.; Wang, C.; Liu, Q.; Liang, G.; Deng, X.; Jiang, W.; et al. Oridonin is a covalent NLRP3 inhibitor with strong anti-inflammasome activity. *Nat. Commun.* **2018**, *9*, 2550. [CrossRef] [PubMed]
43. Zhou, F.; Gao, H.; Shang, L.; Li, J.; Zhang, M.; Wang, S.; Li, R.; Ye, L.; Yang, S. Oridonin promotes endoplasmic reticulum stress via TP53-repressed TCF4 transactivation in colorectal cancer. *J. Exp. Clin. Cancer Res.* **2023**, *42*, 150. [CrossRef] [PubMed]
44. Cao, Y.; Wei, W.; Zhang, N.; Yu, Q.; Xu, W.B.; Yu, W.J.; Chen, G.Q.; Wu, Y.L.; Yan, H. Oridonin stabilizes retinoic acid receptor alpha through ROS-activated NF-κB signaling. *BMC Cancer* **2015**, *15*, 248. [CrossRef] [PubMed]
45. Zhang, T.; Tan, Y.; Zhao, R.; Liu, Z. DNA damage induced by oridonin involves cell cycle arrest at G2/M phase in human MCF-7 cells. *Contemp. Oncol.* **2013**, *17*, 38–44. [CrossRef] [PubMed]

46. Liu, Z.; Ouyang, L.; Peng, H.; Zhang, W.Z. Oridonin: Targeting programmed cell death pathways as an anti-tumour agent. *Cell Prolif.* **2012**, *45*, 499–507. [CrossRef] [PubMed]
47. Shi, M.; Lu, X.J.; Zhang, J.; Diao, H.; Li, G.; Xu, L.; Wang, T.; Wei, J.; Meng, W.; Ma, J.L.; et al. Oridonin, a novel lysine acetyltransferases inhibitor, inhibits proliferation and induces apoptosis in gastric cancer cells through p53- and caspase-3-mediated mechanisms. *Oncotarget* **2016**, *7*, 22623–22631. [CrossRef] [PubMed]
48. Kang, N.; Cao, S.J.; Zhou, Y.; He, H.; Tashiro, S.; Onodera, S.; Qiu, F.; Ikejima, T. Inhibition of caspase-9 by oridonin, a diterpenoid isolated from Rabdosia rubescens, augments apoptosis in human laryngeal cancer cells. *Int. J. Oncol.* **2015**, *47*, 2045–2056. [CrossRef] [PubMed]
49. Lu, J.; Chen, X.; Qu, S.; Yao, B.; Xu, Y.; Wu, J.; Jin, Y.; Ma, C. Oridonin induces G2/M cell cycle arrest and apoptosis via the PI3K/Akt signaling pathway in hormone-independent prostate cancer cells. *Oncol. Lett.* **2017**, *13*, 2838–2846. [CrossRef] [PubMed]
50. Qin, Z.; Zhang, G.; Jiang, S.; Ning, F.; Zhao, Z.; Huang, M.; Jin, J. Integration of metabolomics and transcriptomics to reveal ferroptosis is involved in Tripterygium wilfordii polyglycoside tablet-induced testicular injury. *J. Ethnopharmacol.* **2023**, *304*, 116055. [CrossRef] [PubMed]
51. Rehnitz, J.; Messmer, B.; Bender, U.; Nguyen, X.P.; Germeyer, A.; Hinderhofer, K.; Strowitzki, T.; Capp, E. Activation of AKT/mammalian target of rapamycin signaling in the peripheral blood of women with premature ovarian insufficiency and its correlation with FMR1 expression. *Reprod. Biol. Endocrinol.* **2022**, *20*, 44. [CrossRef]
52. Liu, W.X.; Liu, H.N.; Weng, Z.P.; Geng, Q.; Zhang, Y.; Li, Y.F.; Shen, W.; Zhou, Y.; Zhang, T. Maternal vitamin B1 is a determinant for the fate of primordial follicle formation in offspring. *Nat. Commun.* **2023**, *14*, 7403. [CrossRef]
53. Yang, H.; Lv, H.; Li, H.; Ci, X.; Peng, L. Oridonin protects LPS-induced acute lung injury by modulating Nrf2-mediated oxidative stress and Nrf2-independent NLRP3 and NF-κB pathways. *Cell Commun. Signal.* **2019**, *17*, 62. [CrossRef]
54. Yu, D.; Li, J.; Wang, Y.; Guo, D.; Zhang, X.; Chen, M.; Zhou, Z. Oridonin ameliorates acetaminophen-induced acute liver injury through ATF4/PGC-1α pathway. *Drug Dev. Res.* **2023**, *84*, 211–225. [CrossRef]
55. Pi, J.; Cai, H.; Jin, H.; Yang, F.; Jiang, J.; Wu, A.; Zhu, H.; Liu, J.; Su, X.; Yang, P.; et al. Qualitative and quantitative analysis of ROS-mediated oridonin-induced oesophageal cancer KYSE-150 cell apoptosis by atomic force microscopy. *PLoS ONE* **2015**, *10*, e0140935. [CrossRef]
56. Ding, Y.; Wang, H.; Niu, J.; Luo, M.; Gou, Y.; Miao, L.; Zou, Z.; Cheng, Y. Induction of ROS overload by alantolactone prompts oxidative DNA damage and apoptosis in colorectal cancer cells. *Int. J. Mol. Sci.* **2016**, *17*, 558. [CrossRef]
57. Siemen, D.; Ziemer, M. What is the nature of the mitochondrial permeability transition pore and what is it not? *IUBMB Life* **2013**, *65*, 255–262. [CrossRef]
58. Sidrat, T.; Rehman, Z.U.; Joo, M.D.; Lee, K.L.; Kong, I.K. Wnt/β-catenin pathway-mediated PPARδ expression during embryonic development differentiation and disease. *Int. J. Mol. Sci.* **2021**, *22*, 1854. [CrossRef]
59. Zhan, T.; Rindtorff, N.; Boutros, M. Wnt signaling in cancer. *Oncogene* **2017**, *36*, 1461–1473. [CrossRef]
60. He, Y.; Yuan, X.; Zuo, H.; Sun, Y.; Feng, A. Berberine exerts a protective effect on gut-vascular barrier via the modulation of the Wnt/Beta-catenin signaling pathway during depsis. *Cell. Physiol. Biochem.* **2018**, *49*, 1342–1351. [CrossRef]
61. van der Heyden, M.A.; Rook, M.B.; Hermans, M.M.; Rijksen, G.; Boonstra, J.; Defize, L.H.; Destrée, O.H. Identification of connexin43 as a functional target for Wnt signalling. *J. Cell Sci.* **1998**, *111 Pt 12*, 1741–1749. [CrossRef]

Disclaimer/Publisher's Note: The statements, opinions and data contained in all publications are solely those of the individual author(s) and contributor(s) and not of MDPI and/or the editor(s). MDPI and/or the editor(s) disclaim responsibility for any injury to people or property resulting from any ideas, methods, instructions or products referred to in the content.

toxics

Article

Biochemical Toxicological Study of Insulin Overdose in Rats: A Forensic Perspective

Cunhao Bian [1,2,3,†], Xin He [1,2,3,†], Qi Wang [1,2,3], Zhe Zheng [1,2,3], Yongtai Zhang [1,2,3], Hongli Xiong [1,2,3], Yongguo Li [1,2,3], Mingzhu Zhao [1,2,3] and Jianbo Li [1,2,3,*]

1 Department of Forensic Medicine, Faculty of Basic Medical Sciences, Chongqing Medical University, Chongqing 400016, China; 2022320004@stu.cqmu.edu.cn (C.B.); hx_isabella@163.com (X.H.); forensic.wangqi@cqmu.edu.cn (Q.W.); forensiczheng@sina.com (Z.Z.); zyongtai1536@163.com (Y.Z.); 15023159916@163.com (H.X.); 100399@cqmu.edu.cn (Y.L.); 102870@cqmu.edu.cn (M.Z.)
2 Chongqing Engineering Research Center of Criminal Investigation Technology, Chongqing 400016, China
3 Chongqing Key Laboratory of Forensic Medicine, Chongqing 400016, China
* Correspondence: 100390@cqmu.edu.cn
† These authors contributed equally.

Abstract: Due to nonspecific pathological changes and the rapid degradation of insulin in postmortem blood samples, the identification of the cause of death during insulin overdose has always been a difficulty in forensic medicine. At present, there is a lack of studies on the toxicological changes and related mechanisms of an insulin overdose, and the specific molecular markers of insulin overdose are still unclear. In this study, an animal model of insulin overdose was established, and 24 SD rats were randomly divided into a control group, insulin overdose group, and a recovery group ($n = 8$). We detected the biochemical changes and analyzed the toxicological mechanism of an insulin overdose. The results showed that after insulin overdose, the rats developed irregular convulsions, Eclampsia, Opisthotonos, and other symptoms. The levels of glucose, glycogen, and C-peptide in the body decreased significantly, while the levels of lactate, insulin, and glucagon increased significantly. The decrease in plasma K^+ was accompanied by the increase in skeletal muscle K^+. The PI3K-AKT signaling pathway was significantly activated in skeletal muscle, and the translocation of GLUT4/Na^+-K^+-ATPase to sarcolemma was significantly increased. Rare glycogenic hepatopathy occurred in the recovery group after insulin overdose. Our study showed that insulin overdose also plays a role in skeletal muscle cells, mainly through the PI3K-Akt signaling pathway. Therefore, the detection of signaling pathway proteins of the skeletal muscle cell membrane GLUT4 and Na^+-K^+-ATPase has a certain auxiliary diagnostic value for forensic insulin overdose identification. Glycogen detection in the liver and skeletal muscle is important for the diagnosis of insulin overdose, but it still needs to be differentiated from other causes of death. Skeletal muscle has great potential for insulin detection, and the ratio of insulin to the C-peptide (I:C) can determine whether an exogenous insulin overdose is present.

Keywords: insulin overdose; forensic medicine; hypoglycemia; toxicology

1. Introduction

Insulin is an anabolic hormone produced by pancreatic β-cells and consists of two polypeptide chains, A and B, linked by disulfide bonds [1,2]. The main functions of insulin include regulating blood glucose levels and promoting glucose uptake by peripheral cells [1–3]. Insulin biosynthesis is performed by the cleavage and processing of the precursor single-chain molecule proinsulin to secrete equimolar masses of mature insulin and C-peptide into the blood [2–4]. The blood glucose level is the only major physiological stimulus of insulin secretion, and insulin and C-peptide secretion almost ceases when the blood glucose level stabilizes between 2.5 and 3.33 mmol/L [2,3].

Insulin is the most common drug used in the clinical treatment of diabetes [3], so insulin overdose is mostly an accidental treatment for diabetic patients, including the miscalculation of dosage and incorrect use of insulin specifications [1,5–7]. An insulin overdose can lead to hypoglycemia, with blood glucose levels below 3.9 mmol/L (70 mg/dL) defined as clinical hypoglycemia and blood glucose levels below 3 mmol/L (54 mg/dL) defined as clinically important hypoglycemia [7–9]. The clinical symptoms of hypoglycemia can be summarized into the following two aspects: sympathetic hyperactivity, including sweating, hunger, palpitation, and brain dysfunction, including confusion, drowsiness, impaired coordination, visual impairment, paresthesia, serious convulsions, coma, and even death [5,6,8–10]. The exact mechanism by which hypoglycemia leads to sudden death is unknown, but arrhythmias and cerebral epilepsy appear to play a major role [8,11–13].

Insulin overdose also appears in forensic cases, especially among medical personnel and families of diabetic patients, who can easily obtain insulin to commit suicide or murder [7,14–17]. In 1958, BIRKINSHAW reported the first insulin murder in history [18]. Since then, the number of insulin homicides has gradually increased, and some novelists have described insulin as "the perfect murder method" [17,19–23]. The identification of the cause of death after an insulin overdose has always been difficult in forensic medicine due to the lack of evidence left at the crime scene, the difficulty in finding insulin injection needle marks on the corpse's surface, the lack of obvious pathological characteristics in autopsy, the rapid degradation of insulin caused by postmortem hemolysis, and the significant difference in postmortem blood biochemistry compared with antemortem conditions [14,15,17,20,21,23]. At present, the studies of insulin overdose are mostly limited to case reports and reviews of the literature [7,14,17,18,23], and there is a lack of research on the biochemical and toxicological mechanism of insulin overdose death, molecular markers related to insulin overdose, and alternative samples for insulin forensic determination.

The purpose of this experiment was to study the biochemical changes and toxicological mechanisms of insulin overdose through animal models and to search for specific molecular markers after insulin overdose so as to provide a reference for the clinical treatment of insulin overdose and theoretical support for the forensic diagnosis of insulin.

2. Materials and Methods

2.1. Experimental Animals

A total of 24 SPF male SD rats (8 weeks, 310 g ± 20 g) were purchased from Chongqing Medical University Laboratory Animal Center. All rats were maintained at 22–24 °C (12 h light/dark cycle) with sterile rat chow and water ad libitum. All rats were sacrificed or died under intraperitoneal sodic pentobarbital anesthesia (100 mg/kg, ip). All animal procedures were performed in accordance with animal care ethics, and all animal experiments for this study were approved by the Experimental Animal Care and Use Committee of Chongqing Medical University.

2.2. Experimental Design

All rats fasted overnight before the experiment and were provided with pure water only. In total, 24 SD rats were randomly divided into the control group, insulin overdose group, and insulin overdose recovery group (n = 8). The rats in the insulin overdose group were intraperitoneally injected with 20 IU/kg of insulin (insulin aspart injection, Novonordisk A/S, Copenhagen, Denmark). Their blood glucose levels were measured every 30 min from the end of their tail veins using a glucometer (Accu-Chek-performa, Roche, Mannheim, Germany) until they died, and their physical signs were recorded throughout the experiment. The rats in the recovery group were intraperitoneally injected with 20 IU/kg of insulin; a 0.3 mL mixture of 50% glucose and bicarbonate buffer (1:1) was injected intraperitoneally when blood glucose dropped to 1.5 mmol/L (27 mg/dL); 5 mL of a 50% glucose solution (H50020071, TaiJi, Chongqing, China) was injected intraperitoneally for resuscitation if the rats developed convulsions or opisthotonos; they were fed in cages after their blood glucose levels rose above 3.9 mmol/L (70 mg/dL) and were sacrificed

3 days later. The rats in the control group were injected intraperitoneally with the same volume of sterile normal saline (BL158 A, Biosharp, Hefei, China) only; blood glucose levels were measured every 30 min, and the rats were sacrificed 3 h later. Plasma, the quadriceps femoris muscle, and the liver were collected from all rats and stored at −80 °C for further analysis. The experimental protocol is shown in Figure 1A.

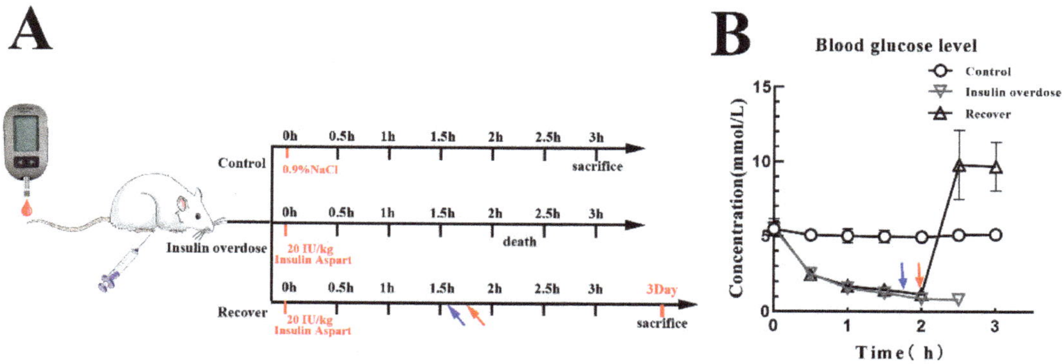

Figure 1. (**A**) Experimental protocol. Rats were divided into three groups: Control (*n* = 8), Insulin overdose (*n* = 8), Recovery (*n* = 8). Blood glucose was measured per 30 min in all rats. Control group rats were injected with normal saline (ip). Insulin overdose group rats were injected with insulin (20 IU/kg,ip). Recovery group rats were injected with insulin (20 IU/kg,ip) injected with a 0.3 mL mixture (50%-glucose: bicarbonate buffer = 1:1, ip) after blood glucose dropped to 1.5 mmol/L (27 mg/dL) (blue arrow), and intraperitoneally injected with 5 mL of 50%-glucose (red arrow). (**B**) Blood glucose in all rats was recorded within 3 h.

2.3. Biochemical Index

The glucose content in liver and skeletal muscle tissue was determined using the glucose colorimetric method kit (E-BC-K234-M, Elabscience, Wuhan, China) according to the manufacturer's instructions. Lactate levels in plasma and the skeletal muscle, potassium levels in plasma and the skeletal muscle, and ALT and AST levels in plasma were determined using kits (A019-2-1, C001-2-1, C009-2-1, C010-2-1, NanJing Jiancheng Bioengineering Institute, NanJing, China) according to the manufacturer's instructions. The plasma total ketone body content was determined via ultraviolet spectrophotometry according to the manufacturer's instructions (BC5060, Solarbio, Beijing, China). All tissue homogenates were obtained using a Cryogenic freezing grinder (JXFSTPRP-CL, JINXIN, Shanghai, China).

2.4. ELISA for Hormone Levels

Insulin in plasma and the skeletal muscle were determined using the Iso-Insulin ELISA kit (10-1128-01, Mercodia, Uppsala, Sweden) with standardized cross-reaction validation. Glucagon (MM-21295R1, MEIMIAN, Yancheng, China) and C-peptide (MM-0588R1, MEIMIAN, Yancheng, China) levels in the plasma were determined using reagent vendors standardized ELISA kits according to the manufacturer's protocol.

2.5. Liver Pathology

Liver weights were determined by analytical balance. Liver tissues were fixed in Carnoy's solution, embedded in paraffin, sectioned at 4 µm, and stained using H&E to observe pathological changes in the liver.

2.6. Glycogen Determination

The absolute glycogen content in fresh liver and skeletal muscle was determined using an anthrone method kit (A043-1-1, NanJing Jiancheng Bioengineering Institute, NanJing,

China) according to the manufacturer's instructions. Parts of the liver and skeletal muscle from the same site were fixed in Carnoy's solution, embedded in paraffin, sectioned at 4 μm, and stained with PAS. Image J was used to analyze the degree of PAS staining.

2.7. Western Blotting Analysis

Skeletal muscle samples were ground and homogenized in a RIPA lysis buffer containing protease inhibitors and phosphatase inhibitors (P0013B, Beyotime, Shanghai, China), and total protein supernatants were obtained after centrifugation and protein concentrations were determined using the BCA protein assay kit (P0010, Beyotime, Shanghai, China). The protein supernatant was mixed with bromophenol blue and boiled at 95 °C for 10 min. Total proteins (20 ug) were separated via 10% SDS-PAGE gel electrophoresis and transferred onto PVDF membranes (PR05505, Immobilon, Darmstadt, Germany). After blocking with 5% free-fat milk for 2 h at room temperature, membranes were incubated with the primary antibodies against GSK3 (1:5000, ab185141, abcam, Cambridge, UK), Phosphorylated-GSK3-Ser9 (1:5000, ab75814, abcam, Cambridge, UK), AKT (1:1000, T55561F, Abmart, Shanghai, China), Phosphorylated-AKT-Ser473 (1:1000, T40067F, Abmart, Shanghai, China), Phosphorylated-AKT-Thr308 (1:1000, T40068F, Abmart, Shanghai, China), PI3K (1:5000, 60225-1-lg, proteintech, Wuhan, China), Phosphorylated-PI3K (1:1000, bs-3332R, Bioss, Beijing, China), GLUT4 (1:1000, 66846-1-lg, proteintech, Wuhan, China), Na^+/K^+-ATPase (1:5000, 14418-1-AP, proteintech, Wuhan, China), and β-actin (1:5000, 66009-1-lg, proteintech, Wuhan, China) overnight at 4 °C, then incubated with HRP secondary antibodies(1:2000, proteintech, Wuhan, China), detected using ECL(BL520B, Biosharp, Hefei, China), and visualized using the ChemiDoc imaging system(Bio-Rad, California, USA). Total protein normalization was performed using 10% acryl-amide TGX Stain-free^{TM} gels(Bio-Rad, California, USA). Protein levels were quantified using Image Lab 5.2.1 software. The mean density of protein bands was normalized to β-actin and control data, expressed as fold changes relative to the control.

2.8. Confocal Immunofluorescent Staining

Skeletal muscles were fixed in a 4% formaldehyde solution, embedded in paraffin, and sectioned at 4 μm for immunofluorescence staining to detect the expression and subcellular localization of GLUT4 and Na^+/K^+-ATPase. Sections were deparaffinized, antigen-repaired, blocked, and incubated with the anti-GLUT4 antibody (1:200, 66846-1-lg, proteintech, Wuhan, China) and anti-Na^+/K^+-ATPase antibody (1:400, 14418-1-AP, proteintech, Wuhan, China) overnight at 4 °C. After washing with PBS, sections were incubated with the fluorescent secondary antibody CoraLite594/CoraLite488 (1:100, proteintech, Wuhan, China) for 2 h at room temperature, washed again with PBS, stained with nuclei and sealed with the DAPI-containing anti-fluorescence-quenching agent (P0131, Beyotime, Shanghai, China). Imaging was performed using the Leica confocal microscope (STELLARIS, Leica, Hessen, Germany) and analyzed using Leica LAS X software.

2.9. Statistical Analysis

The results are expressed as the mean ± SEM. GraphPad Prism version 8.0.2 was used for statistical analysis and graphs. One-way ANOVA was used to compare multiple groups. Tukey's post hoc test was performed only if F reached $p < 0.05$ with homogeneity of variance. p-values < 0.05 were considered statistically significant.

3. Results

3.1. Blood Glucose Levels and Corresponding Symptoms after Insulin Overdose

Following the insulin overdose injection, blood glucose levels decreased significantly over time, and various symptoms appeared, as shown in Figure 1B and Table 1. When blood glucose dropped below 1.5 mmol/L (27 mg/dL), severe symptoms were observed, including irregular convulsions, hypermyotonia, eclampsia, opisthotonos, etc. The blood glucose levels in the insulin overdose group decreased further until death. By contrast, after the injection of glucose, the blood glucose levels in the recovery group increased rapidly to more than 3.9 mmol/L (70 mg/dL); the symptoms gradually disappeared, and all the rats survived.

Table 1. Blood glucose levels and corresponding symptoms in rats. Data are expressed as the mean ± SEM.

Time	Blood Glucose		Symptoms
	mmol/L $\overline{X}\pm$ SEM	mg/dL $\overline{X}\pm$SEM	
0 h	5.5 ± 0.4	99.0 ± 7.2	Normal behavior
0.5 h	2.5 ± 0.4	45.0 ± 7.2	Blunted response; hypodynamia; hypotonia
1 h	1.5 ± 0.3	27.0 ± 5.4	Irregular convulsions; hypermyotonia
1.5 h	1.2 ± 0.2	21.6 ± 3.6	Eclampsia; opisthotonos
2 h	0.9 ± 0.2	16.2 ± 3.6	Collapse; uroclepsia; near-death
2.5 h	0.8 ± 0.1	14.4 ± 1.8	Death

3.2. Effects of Insulin Overdose on Biochemical Indexes

As shown in Figure 2A–C, compared with the control group, glucose levels in plasma, liver, and muscle tissue were significantly decreased in the insulin overdose group ($p < 0.0001$). After 3 days of recovering from an insulin overdose, glucose levels in the blood, liver, and muscle tissue returned to normal. As shown in Figure 2D,E, lactate levels in the skeletal muscle and plasma were significantly increased in the insulin overdose group compared with the control group (muscle $p < 0.0001$, plasma $p < 0.001$). In the recovery group, lactate levels in skeletal muscle and plasma returned to normal. The glucose consumption and lactate accumulation indicated that glycolysis increased after the insulin overdose. In addition, the plasma total ketone body level in the recovery group was slightly increased, but there was no significant difference compared with the other groups ($p > 0.05$), Figure 2F.

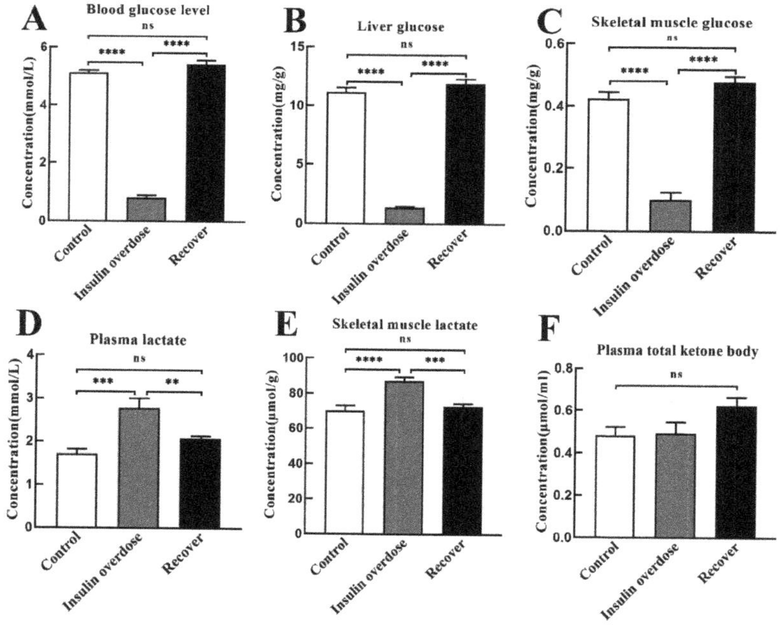

Figure 2. Energy index determination. **(A–C)** Glucose levels in plasma, liver, and skeletal muscle of each group; **(D,E)** Lactate levels in plasma and skeletal muscle of each group; **(F)** Plasma ketone body levels of each group. Data are expressed as mean ± SEM, ns $p > 0.05$, ** $p < 0.01$, *** $p < 0.001$, **** $p < 0.0001$, One-way ANOVA.

As shown in Figure 3A,B, compared with the other groups, the plasma potassium level decreased in the insulin overdose group ($p < 0.01$), while the potassium level in skeletal muscle was increased in the insulin overdose group ($p < 0.05$). These data indicate that insulin overdose alters potassium distribution in plasma and the skeletal muscle.

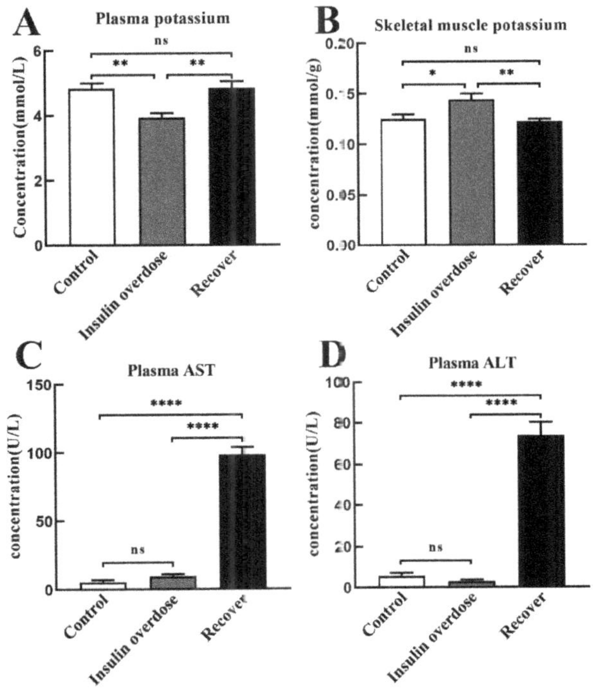

Figure 3. Other biochemical indexes. (**A**,**B**) Potassium levels in plasma and skeletal muscle of each group; (**C**,**D**) Plasma AST and ALT levels in each group. AST, Aspartate aminotransferase; ALT, alanine aminotransferase. Data are expressed as mean ± SEM, ns $p > 0.05$, * $p < 0.05$, ** $p < 0.01$, **** $p < 0.0001$, One-way ANOVA.

As shown in Figure 3C,D, compared with the other groups, plasma alanine aminotransferase (ALT) and aspartate transaminase (AST) in the recovery group were significantly increased ($p < 0.0001$), indicating that liver function was damaged after insulin overdose and glucose resuscitation.

3.3. *Effects of Insulin Overdose on Glucose Metabolic Hormones*

As shown in Figure 4A,B, compared with the other groups, the insulin levels of plasma and skeletal muscle in the insulin overdose group significantly increased ($p < 0.0001$). After recovery, the insulin levels in plasma and skeletal muscle decreased to the control level ($p > 0.05$). Plasma C-peptide levels in the insulin overdose group decreased significantly compared with the control group ($p < 0.0001$); after recovery, plasma C-peptide levels to returned to the control group ($p > 0.05$), as shown in Figure 4C. In addition, plasma glucagon levels in the insulin overdose group were significantly increased compared with the control group ($p < 0.0001$), but plasma glucagon levels in the recovery group decreased to the control level ($p > 0.05$), as shown in Figure 4D. These hormone levels indicate that after insulin overdose, endogenous insulin secretion is suppressed, while glucagon secretion is stimulated sharply.

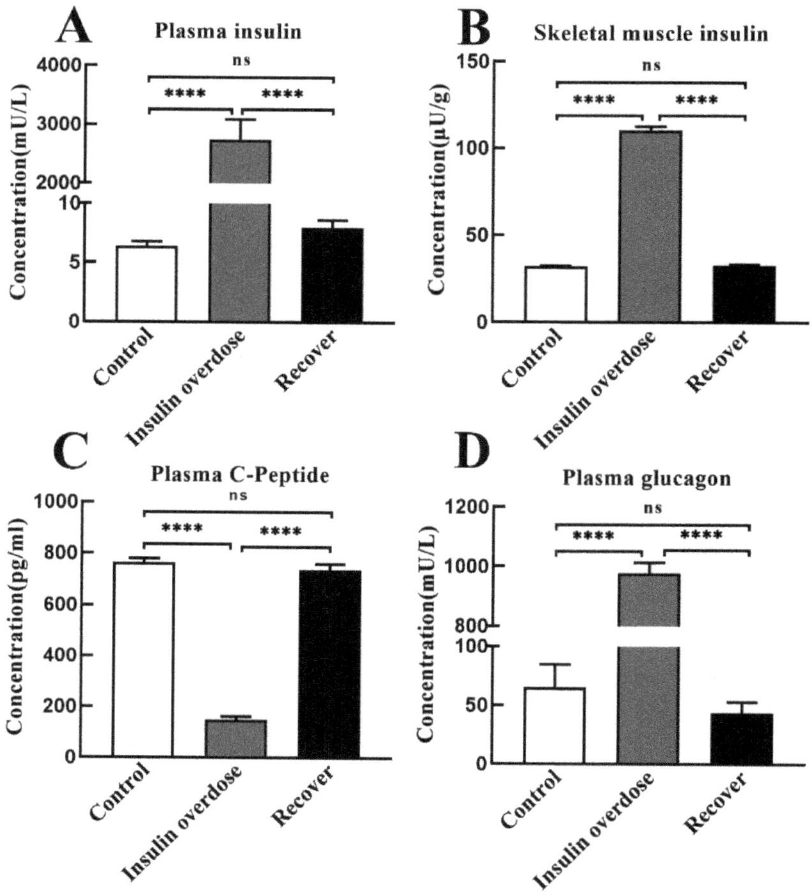

Figure 4. Hormone Levels. (**A**,**B**) Insulin levels in plasma and skeletal muscle of each group; (**C**) Plasma C-peptide levels in each group; (**D**) Plasma glucagon levels in each group. Data are expressed as mean ± SEM, ns $p > 0.05$, **** $p < 0.0001$, One-way ANOVA.

3.4. Glycogen Deposition after Insulin Overdose and Glucose Recovery

Liver H&E staining, as shown in Figure 5A, resulted in the congestion of the central hepatic vein and hepatic sinuses in the insulin overdose group, including swelling and balloon-like changes in hepatocytes in the recovery group. As shown in Figure 5B,C, there was no significant change in the liver mass and liver coefficient in the insulin overdose group compared with the control group ($p > 0.05$), while the liver mass and liver coefficient were significantly increased in the recovery group ($p < 0.0001$). Compared with the control group, as shown in Figure 6A–C, liver glycogen in the insulin overdose group decreased significantly (PAS staining $p < 0.0001$, glycogen quantification $p < 0.01$), while liver glycogen in the recovery group increased significantly (PAS staining $p < 0.05$, glycogen quantification $p < 0.0001$). Compared with the control group, as shown in Figure 7A–C, skeletal muscle glycogen in the insulin overdose group decreased significantly (PAS staining $p < 0.0001$, glycogen quantification $p < 0.05$), while skeletal muscle glycogen in the recovery group increased significantly (PAS staining $p < 0.05$, glycogen quantification $p < 0.05$). These data indicate that glycogen in both the liver and skeletal muscle decreased after an insulin overdose. However, the glycogen of the liver and skeletal muscle increased after insulin overdose and glucose resuscitation, and hepatocyte degeneration and balloon-like changes, resulting in glycogenic hepatopathy.

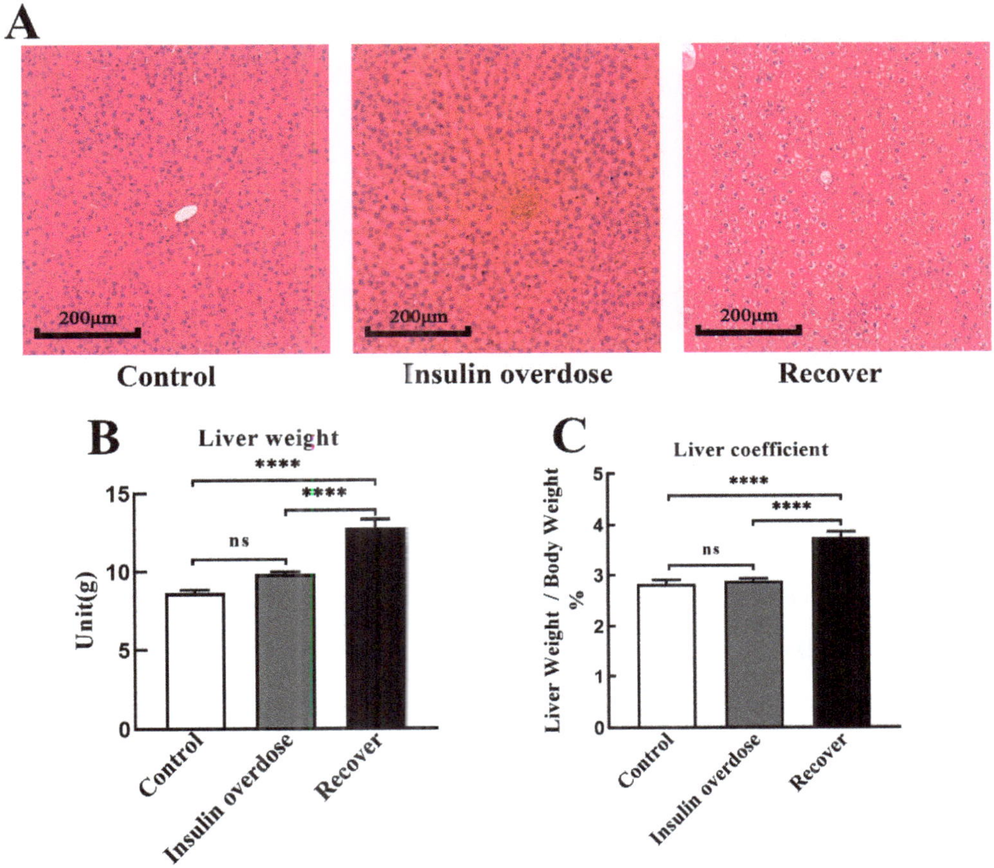

Figure 5. Liver weight and HE staining. (**A**) Representative images of liver HE staining in each group, scale 200 μm; (**B**,**C**) Liver weight and liver coefficient in each group. Data are expressed as mean ± SEM, ns $p > 0.05$, **** $p < 0.0001$, One-way ANOVA.

3.5. Insulin Overdose Activates the PI3K-AKT Signaling Pathway in Skeletal Muscle

AKT is a key protein that regulates cellular metabolism. As shown in Figure 8A–C, there were no significant changes in the total protein loading amount and the expression of the reference β-actin in each group. As shown in Figure 8B,D, compared with the other groups, the ratio of P-PI3K to total PI3K in the insulin overdose group was significantly increased ($p < 0.01$ VS control group, $p < 0.05$ VS recover group). As shown in Figure 8B,E, compared with the other groups, the ratio of P-AKT-Ser473 to total AKT was significantly increased in the insulin overdose group ($p < 0.0001$ VS control group, $p < 0.0001$ VS recover group), while the ratio of P-AKT-Thr308 to the total AKT was not significantly changed in the hypoglycemia group ($p > 0.05$). As shown in Figure 8B,F, compared with the other groups, the ratio of P-GSK3-Ser9 to total GSK3 was significantly increased in the insulin overdose group ($p < 0.0001$ VS control group, $p < 0.0001$ VS recover group). These data indicate that insulin overdose significantly activates the PI3K-AKT signaling pathway in skeletal muscle and stimulates the ability of glycogen synthesis.

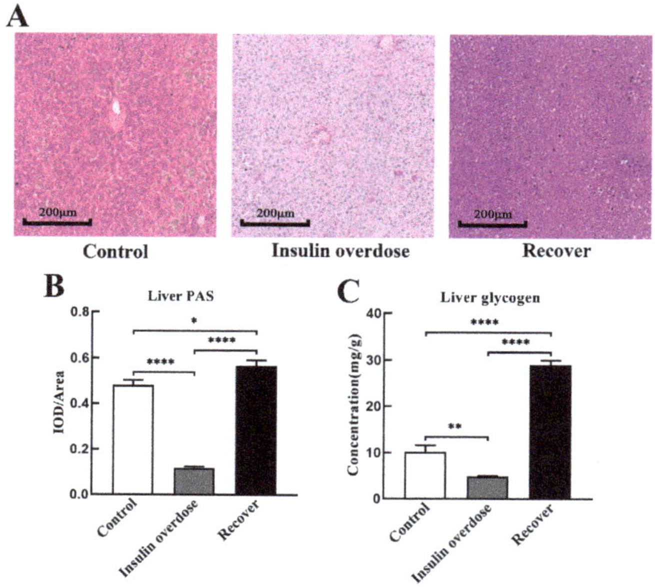

Figure 6. Liver PAS staining and glycogen quantification. (**A**) Representative images of liver PAS staining in each group, scale 200 μm; (**B**) The ratio of IOD and the distribution area of liver PAS staining were calculated using Image J software in each group; (**C**) Liver glycogen was quantitatively detected in each group. Data are expressed as mean ± SEM, * $p < 0.05$, ** $p < 0.01$, **** $p < 0.0001$, One-way ANOVA.

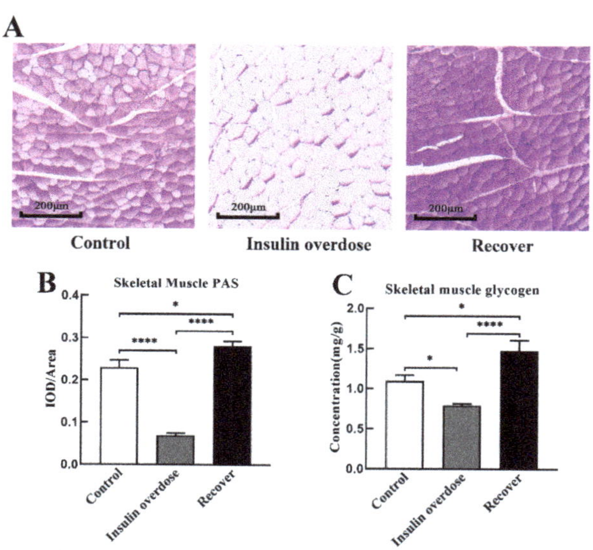

Figure 7. Skeletal muscle PAS staining and glycogen quantification. (**A**) Representative images of skeletal muscle PAS staining in each group, scale 200 μm; (**B**) The ratio of IOD and the distribution area of skeletal muscle PAS staining was calculated using Image J software in each group; (**C**) Skeletal muscle glycogen was quantitatively detected in each group. Data are expressed as mean ± SEM, * $p < 0.05$, **** $p < 0.0001$, One-way ANOVA.

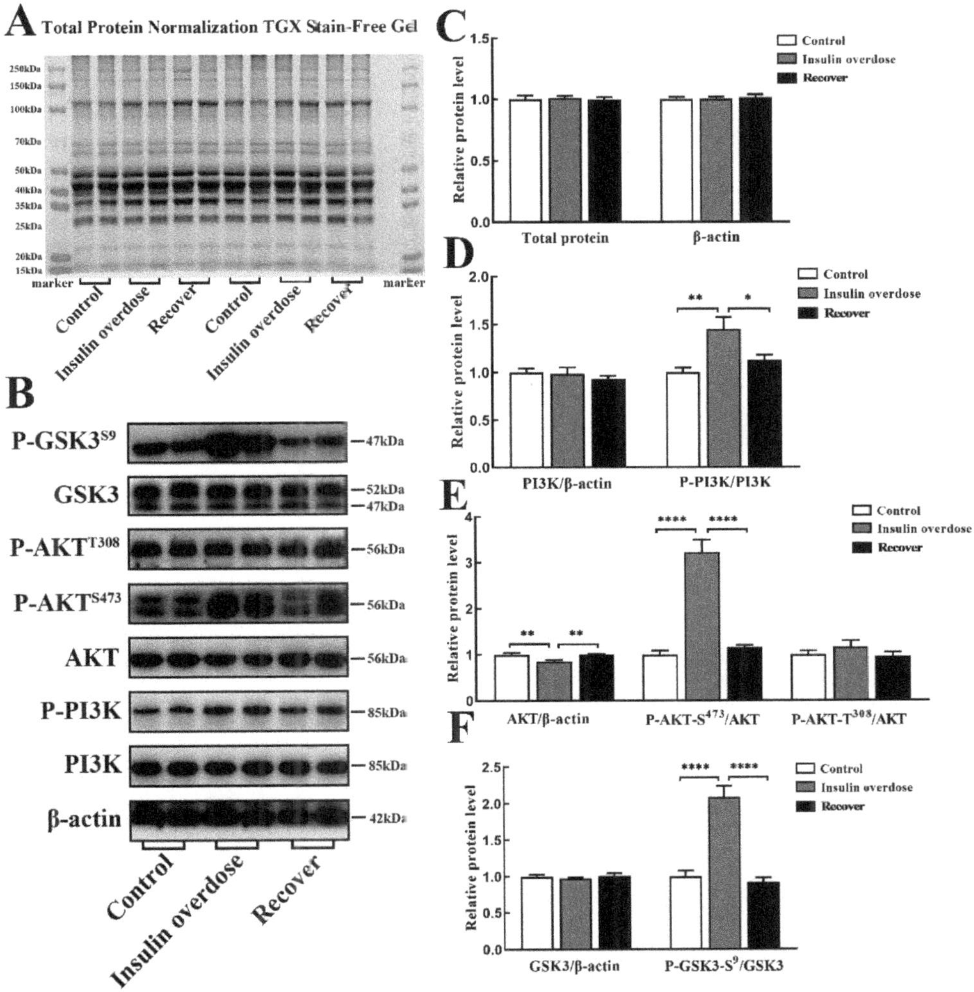

Figure 8. Protein levels of insulin signaling pathway in skeletal muscle. (**A**) Total protein normalization and β-actin internal reference in each group; (**B**) Band images of key proteins in each group; (**C–F**) Relative levels of key proteins in each group. Data are expressed as mean ± SEM, * $p < 0.05$, ** $p < 0.01$, **** $p < 0.0001$, One-way ANOVA.

3.6. Insulin Overdose Promotes GLUT4 and Na^+-K^+-ATPase Translocation in Skeletal Muscle

WB results, as shown in Figure 9A–C, with GLUT4 and Na^+-K^+-ATPase expression levels were not significantly different among all groups ($p > 0.05$). However, compared with the other groups, confocal microscopy immunofluorescence images, as shown in Figure 10, indicated that the signals of GLUT4 and Na^+-K^+-ATPase on the sarcolemma were significantly increased in the insulin overdose group. The above data and the phosphorylation of PI3K-AKT suggest that insulin overdose stimulates GLUT4 and Na^+-K^+-ATPase translocation to the sarcolemma through the PI3K-AKT signaling pathway. Figure 11 shows the schematic diagram of the membrane translocation of GLUT4 and Na^+-K^+-ATPase stimulated by insulin overdose, which was drawn by ourselves.

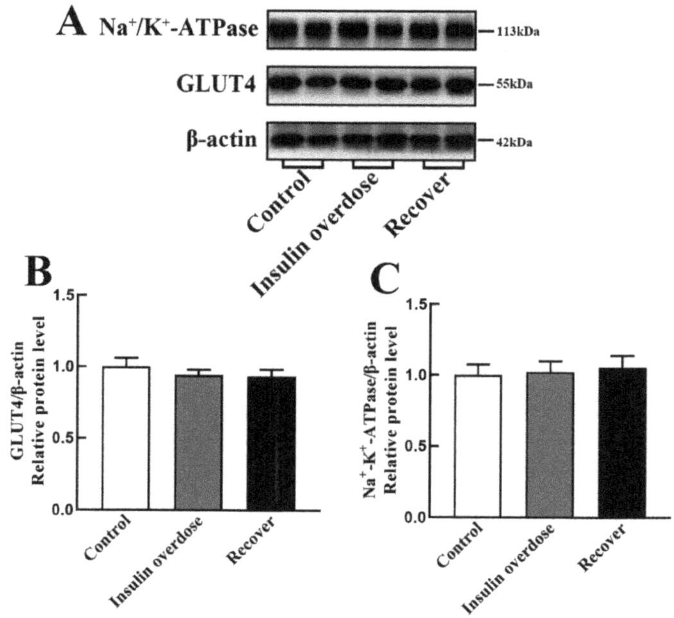

Figure 9. GLUT4 and Na^+/K^+-ATPase in skeletal muscle. (**A**) Band images of GLUT4 and Na^+/K^+-ATPase in each group; (**B**,**C**) Relative levels of GLUT4 and Na^+/K^+-ATPase in each group. Data are expressed as mean ± SEM, One-way ANOVA.

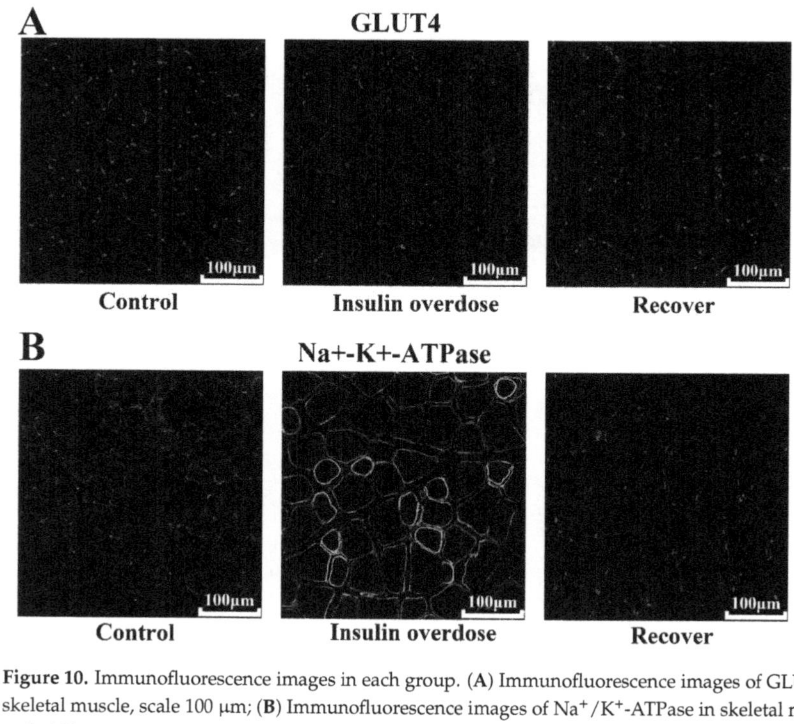

Figure 10. Immunofluorescence images in each group. (**A**) Immunofluorescence images of GLUT4 in skeletal muscle, scale 100 μm; (**B**) Immunofluorescence images of Na^+/K^+-ATPase in skeletal muscle, scale 100 μm.

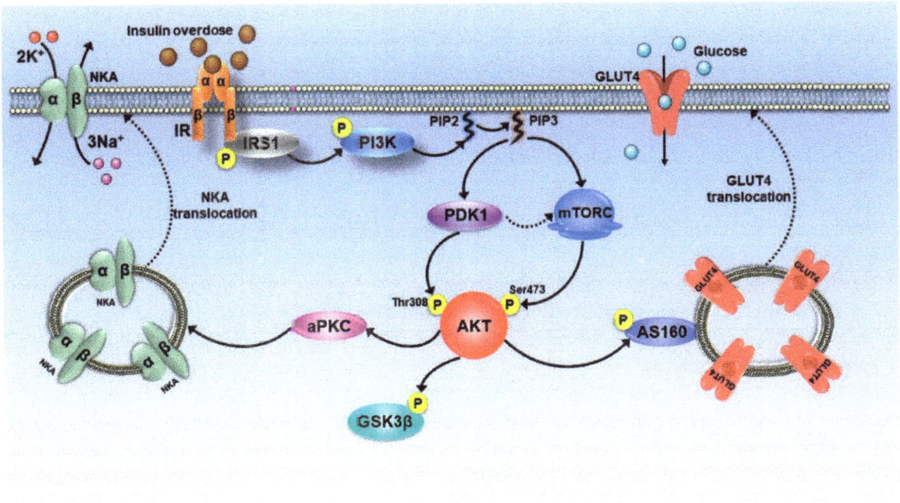

Figure 11. Schematic diagram of the regulation of GLUT4 translocation, Na^+/K^+-ATPase translocation, and glycogen synthase kinase phosphorylation after insulin overdose in skeletal muscle. IR: insulin receptor; IRS1: insulin receptor substrate 1; PI3K: Phosphoinositide-3-Kinase; PIP2: phosphatidylinositol-4,5-bisphosphate; PIP3: phosphatidylinositol-3,4,5-bisphosphate; PDK1: Phosphoinositide-dependent kinase; mTORC: Mammalian Target of Rapamycin; AKT: Protein kinase B; aPKC: atypical Protein kinase C; AS160: TBC1D4, TBC1 domain family, member 4; GSK3β: glycogen synthase kinase 3 beta; NKA: Na^+/K^+ ATPase 1; GLUT4: solute carrier family 2 (facilitated glucose transporter), member 4.

4. Discussion

Insulin has a variety of effects on peripheral tissues, such as promoting glucose transport from extracellular to intracellular, regulating cellular glucose metabolism, promoting substance synthesis, inhibiting glycogenolysis, inhibiting gluconeogenesis, etc. [24,25]. The physiological effects of insulin are mainly realized through the PI3K-AKT signaling pathway, in which AKT plays an important role in substance metabolism [24,26,27]. As shown in Figure 11, insulin binds to the insulin receptor (IR), phosphorylates the tyrosine site of insulin receptor substrate 1 (IRS1) in the skeletal muscle, and then activates Phosphoinositide-3-Kinase (PI3K). Activated PI3K catalyzes Phosphatidylinositol-4,5-bisphosphate (PIP2) to Phosphatidylinositol-3,4,5-bisphosphate (PIP3), which acts as a second messenger to activate Protein kinase B (AKT) through phosphoinositide-dependent kinase (PDK1) and the Mammalian Target of Rapamycin (mTORC), respectively [26–28]. Phosphorylation at Thr308 is required for AKT activation, while phosphorylation at Ser473 is required for complete AKT activation [27,29]. In this study, as shown in Figure 8, we found that the phosphorylation levels of PI3K and Akt were significantly increased in skeletal muscle cells after insulin overdose, which verified that insulin overdose also exerts its effects mainly through the PI3K-Akt signaling pathway in skeletal muscle cells.

Glucose transporter 4, as an insulin-sensitive glucose transporter, is mainly distributed in the skeletal muscle and adipose tissue [30,31]. Without insulin stimulation, more than 95% glut4 is stored in cells as vesicle GSV [30,32,33]. When insulin stimulates the cells, the downstream proteins are activated through the PI3K-Akt signaling pathway [33,34]. This leads to GLUT4 vesicles losing their anchoring function and translocating to the cell membrane in the form of vesicles, thereby promoting glucose absorption and playing a vital role in lowering blood glucose levels [30,33,35]. The half-life of insulin in the body is only 4–6 min [2,25]. After insulin binds to the receptor, the signaling pathway is activated, and the insulin–receptor complex is rapidly degraded after internalization [2,32].

Therefore, physiological doses of insulin do not cause the sustained translocation of GLUT4 to the membrane of skeletal muscle cells [32,33]. In this study, as shown in Figure 9B, we found no significant difference in the expression of GLUT4 between the insulin overdose group and the control group. However, as shown in Figures 8B and 10A, the intensified immunofluorescence signal of GLUT4 on the skeletal sarcolemma and the activation of the PI3K-Akt signaling pathway following insulin overdose suggested that excessive insulin facilitated the translocation of GLUT4 to the muscle membrane, leading to increased glucose absorption in the skeletal muscle. Furthermore, excess insulin can maintain the continuous translocation of GLUT4 to skeletal sarcolemma, and considering the specific effect of insulin on GLUT4, the detection of GLUT4 signal intensity in skeletal sarcolemma could be useful for the forensic diagnosis of insulin overdose.

Skeletal muscle stores more than 70% of the total body K^+, with a total amount of about 2600 mmol, which is 46 times the total extracellular K^+ and 236 times the total plasma K^+, and contains abundant Na^+-K^+-ATPase [36,37]. Therefore, slight K^+ changes in skeletal muscle can cause significant changes in plasma K^+ [36,38]. K^+ homeostasis on a moment-to-moment basis is mainly achieved by the transmembrane transport of extracellular K^+ to skeletal muscle [38–40]. Studies have shown that insulin may activate the PI3K-Akt signaling pathway and promote the translocation of intracellular vesicles containing Na^+-K^+-ATPase to the skeletal sarcolemma through atypical protein kinase C (aPKC) [40,41]. Interestingly, it has also been shown that muscle contractions during intense exercise or during epilepsy promote the diffusion of K+ from the muscles to the capillaries, thereby raising blood potassium levels [36,41]. In this study, as shown in Figure 9C, we found no significant difference in the expression level of Na^+-K^+-ATPase between the insulin overdose group and the control group. However, as shown in Figure 10B, there was an enhanced immunofluorescence signal of Na^+-K^+-ATPase on the skeletal sarcolemma, suggesting that excessive insulin activates the PI3K-Akt signaling pathway, leading to the translocation of Na^+-K^+-ATPase to the skeletal sarcolemma and subsequently increasing the transport of blood potassium into the muscles. It is important to emphasize that the decrease in blood potassium levels after insulin overdose is primarily attributed to the skeletal muscle-mediated translocation of potassium rather than absolute potassium loss. Clinical cases have provided evidence that aggressively supplementing potassium in response to initial hypokalemia during the early stages of an insulin overdose can lead to hyperkalemia once the underlying cause of the insulin overdose is resolved [42,43]. Therefore, it is necessary to prolong the monitoring of the plasma potassium level and consider conservative potassium supplementation in clinical practice for the decrease in plasma potassium induced by insulin overdose. In addition, due to the relatively specific effect of insulin on Na^+-K^+-ATPase, it is worthwhile to further investigate the detection of the signal intensity of Na^+-K^+-ATPase in skeletal sarcolemma for the forensic diagnosis of insulin overdose.

Studies have shown that the body activates counterregulatory systems to prevent hypoglycemia in response to decreased blood glucose levels [44–46]. After an exogenous insulin overdose, the secretion of endogenous insulin decreases, and the release of glucose-raising hormones increases, among which glucagon plays a major role [44,45,47]. Furthermore, hypoglycemia can increase the ability of glucagon to produce glucose in the liver [48,49], and the dual effect of hypoglycemia and glucagon surpasses the inhibitory impact of insulin, resulting in enhanced glycogen decomposition but has no significant effect on gluconeogenesis [45,48,50]. In this study, as shown in Figure 4A,D, plasma insulin levels and glucagon levels were significantly increased after insulin overdose, while liver glycogen and glucose contents were significantly decreased, confirming the hepatic glycogen depletion caused by insulin overdose. Previous studies have shown that, during intense exercise, glucose is the only fuel for muscles, while muscles produce large amounts of lactate that diffuse along the concentration gradients [51–54]. In this study, symptoms such as persistent muscle twitching during insulin overdose may lead to substantial glucose consumption and the production of significant amounts of lactic acid in the skeletal muscle. Although insulin overdose promotes GLUT4 cell membrane translocation and glycogen synthase kinase activation in the skeletal muscle, it eventually leads to glycogen consumption in the skeletal muscle under the dual effects of energy consumption and the negative feedback regulation mechanism after insulin overdose. Therefore, the detection of glycogen levels in the liver and skeletal muscle is beneficial for the forensic diagnosis of insulin overdose, but it needs to be differentiated from other causes of death.

When endogenous insulin is released from the pancreas, equimolar amounts of the C-peptide are released simultaneously, and the C-peptide is metabolized and cleared more slowly than insulin, so the C-peptide can be used to assess the level of endogenous insulin secretion [55–57]. In the normal body, the ratio of insulin to C-peptide (I:C) is less than 1 [55]. When hyperinsulinemia occurs, such as pancreatic β-cell tumors and the rare insulin autoimmune syndrome, the insulin level and C-peptide level increase simultaneously, and the ratio of insulin to C-peptide (I:C) is still less than one [55,58]. However, when exogenous insulin is injected into the body, endogenous insulin secretion is inhibited, resulting in a decrease in the C-peptide level, and the ratio of the insulin level to C-peptide (I:C) is greater than one [55,57]. In this study, as shown in Figure 4C, the level of C-peptide decreased significantly after insulin overdose, and the ratio of insulin to the C-peptide (I:C) was much greater than one, which could be diagnosed as an exogenous insulin overdose. Therefore, both forensically and clinically, measurements of insulin and the C-peptide, as well as the ratio of insulin to the C-peptide (I:C), can be used to determine whether an insulin overdose is endogenous or exogenous.

For the immunological detection of insulin, it is necessary to consider the influence of insulin analog cross-reactions [59,60]. In this study, the Mercodia Iso-Insulin Elisa kit validated by an insulin analog cross-reaction was used for detection to exclude the interference of a cross-reaction on the detection value. Studies have shown that insulin is easily distributed widely throughout the body through blood vessels [61,62]. Clinically, hypoglycemia caused by an exogenous insulin overdose can be diagnosed via the simultaneous detection of an absolute increase in insulin, a decrease in the C-peptide level, and a decrease in the blood glucose level of <2.8 mmol/L (50 mg/dL) [63]. However, in forensic practice, insulin in postmortem blood is easily degraded by hemolysis, corruption, and other influences, which makes it extremely difficult to detect insulin in postmortem blood [64]. In addition, postmortem blood glucose shows a wide range of fluctuations, resulting in blood glucose parameters that are also of no value in forensic pathology [65]. Interestingly, Duckworth found that the muscle is the third major organ for insulin metabolism [66], and Bryant confirmed that insulin is more stable in acidic media [67]. In this study, as shown in Figures 2E and 4B, both insulin and lactate levels were increased in the skeletal muscle after insulin overdose. Given the ample sample size of the muscle and the acidic environment provided by postmortem glycolysis, there is great potential for forensic insulin detection from muscle.

Glycogenic hepatopathy is a rare complication of poor glycemic control in patients with type 1 diabetes mellitus [68,69], which is pathologically characterized by elevated liver transaminase, hepatomegaly, and glycogen deposition [70,71]. In this study, rats developed glycogenic hepatopathy similar to those in type 1 diabetes after resuscitation and insulin overdose. In the recovery group, as shown in Figure 3C,D, Figures 5 and 6, AST and ALT were significantly increased, the liver weight and liver coefficient were significantly increased, HE staining showed hepatomegaly and ballooning degeneration, and PAS staining and glycogen measurement confirmed that liver glycogen was significantly increased. Studies have shown that transient glycogenic hepatopathy generally does not cause persistent liver damage, but it is easily misdiagnosed by clinicians as non-alcoholic fatty liver disease (NAFLD) in patients with type 2 diabetes [70,72], which requires differential diagnosis by clinicians.

5. Conclusions

In conclusion, our study shows that insulin overdose also plays a role in skeletal muscle cells mainly through the PI3K-Akt signaling pathway, and the detection of GLUT4 and Na^+-K^+-ATPase signals in the skeletal muscle cell membrane is helpful for the forensic diagnosis of insulin overdose. Glycogen detection in the liver and skeletal muscle is helpful for the forensic diagnosis of insulin overdose, but it needs to be differentiated from other causes of death. Skeletal muscle has great potential as a substitute for blood to detect an insulin overdose, and the ratio of insulin to C-peptide (I:C) can be used to determine whether it is an exogenous insulin overdose.

Author Contributions: C.B. and J.L. conceived and designed the study. C.B., X.H., Z.Z., Y.Z., H.X., Q.W. and Y.L. performed and assisted with the experiments. All authors analyzed and interpreted the results. C.B. and X.H. drafted the manuscript, and all authors critically revised it for the final version. J.L. is the guarantor of this work and, as such, had full access to all the data in the study and takes responsibility for the integrity of the data and the accuracy of the data analysis. All authors have read and agreed to the published version of the manuscript.

Funding: This research received no external funding.

Institutional Review Board Statement: This study was approved by the Ethics Committee of Chongqing Medical University (IACUC-CQMU-2023-07023).

Informed Consent Statement: Not applicable.

Data Availability Statement: Data are available upon request to the corresponding author.

Acknowledgments: The authors would like to thank Chongqing Medical University for providing the experimental animals.

Conflicts of Interest: The authors declare no conflict of interest.

References

1. Kramer, C.K.; Retnakaran, R.; Zinman, B. Insulin and insulin analogs as antidiabetic therapy: A perspective from clinical trials. *Cell Metab.* **2021**, *33*, 740–747. [CrossRef] [PubMed]
2. De Meyts, P. Insulin and its receptor: Structure, function and evolution. *BioEssays News Rev. Mol. Cell. Dev. Biol.* **2004**, *26*, 1351–1362. [CrossRef] [PubMed]
3. Sims, E.K.; Carr, A.L.J.; Oram, R.A.; DiMeglio, L.A.; Evans-Molina, C. 100 years of insulin: Celebrating the past, present and future of diabetes therapy. *Nat. Med.* **2021**, *27*, 1154–1164. [CrossRef]
4. Niswender, K.D. Basal insulin: Physiology, pharmacology, and clinical implications. *Postgrad. Med.* **2011**, *123*, 17–26. [CrossRef] [PubMed]
5. Kristensen, P.L.; Hansen, L.S.; Jespersen, M.J.; Pedersen-Bjergaard, U.; Beck-Nielsen, H.; Christiansen, J.S.; Nørgaard, K.; Perrild, H.; Parving, H.H.; Thorsteinsson, B.; et al. Insulin analogues and severe hypoglycaemia in type 1 diabetes. *Diabetes Res. Clin. Pract.* **2012**, *96*, 17–23. [CrossRef] [PubMed]
6. Johansen, N.J.; Christensen, M.B. A Systematic Review on Insulin Overdose Cases: Clinical Course, Complications and Treatment Options. *Basic Clin. Pharmacol. Toxicol.* **2018**, *122*, 650–659. [CrossRef]
7. Rzepczyk, S.; Dolińska-Kaczmarek, K.; Uruska, A.; Żaba, C. The Other Face of Insulin-Overdose and Its Effects. *Toxics* **2022**, *10*, 123. [CrossRef]
8. Graveling, A.J.; Frier, B.M. Hypoglycaemia: An overview. *Prim. Care Diabetes* **2009**, *3*, 131–139. [CrossRef]
9. McNeilly, A.D.; McCrimmon, R.J. Impaired hypoglycaemia awareness in type 1 diabetes: Lessons from the lab. *Diabetologia* **2018**, *61*, 743–750. [CrossRef]
10. McCrimmon, R.J.; Frier, B.M. Hypoglycaemia, the most feared complication of insulin therapy. *Diabete Metab.* **1994**, *20*, 503–512.
11. Binder, G.; Bosk, A.; Gass, M.; Ranke, M.B.; Heidemann, P.H. Insulin tolerance test causes hypokalaemia and can provoke cardiac arrhythmias. *Horm. Res.* **2004**, *62*, 84–87. [CrossRef] [PubMed]
12. Reno, C.M.; Skinner, A.; Bayles, J.; Chen, Y.S.; Daphna-Iken, D.; Fisher, S.J. Severe hypoglycemia-induced sudden death is mediated by both cardiac arrhythmias and seizures. *Am. J. Physiol. Endocrinol. Metab.* **2018**, *315*, E240–E249. [CrossRef] [PubMed]
13. Robinson, R.T.; Harris, N.D.; Ireland, R.H.; Lee, S.; Newman, C.; Heller, S.R. Mechanisms of abnormal cardiac repolarization during insulin-induced hypoglycemia. *Diabetes* **2003**, *52*, 1469–1474. [CrossRef] [PubMed]
14. Manetti, A.C.; Visi, G.; Spina, F.; De Matteis, A.; Del Duca, F.; Turillazzi, E.; Maiese, A. Insulin and Oral Hypoglycemic Drug Overdose in Post-Mortem Investigations: A Literature Review. *Biomedicines* **2022**, *10*, 2823. [CrossRef] [PubMed]
15. Marks, V.; Wark, G. Forensic aspects of insulin. *Diabetes Res. Clin. Pract.* **2013**, *101*, 248–254. [CrossRef]
16. Baumgartner, K.; Devgun, J. Toxicology of Medications for Diabetes Mellitus. *Crit. Care Clin.* **2021**, *37*, 577–589. [CrossRef]

17. Tong, F.; Wu, R.; Huang, W.; Yang, Y.; Zhang, L.; Zhang, B.; Chen, X.; Tang, X.; Zhou, Y. Forensic aspects of homicides by insulin overdose. *Forensic Sci. Int.* **2017**, *278*, 9–15. [CrossRef]
18. Birkinshaw, V.J.; Gurd, M.R.; Randall, S.S.; Curry, A.S.; Price, D.E.; Wright, P.H. Investigations in a Case of Murder by Insulin Poisoning. *Br. Med. J.* **1958**, *2*, 463. [CrossRef]
19. Haibach, H.; Dix, J.D.; Shah, J.H. Homicide by insulin administration. *J. Forensic Sci.* **1987**, *32*, 208–216. [CrossRef]
20. Beastall, G.H.; Gibson, I.H.; Martin, J. Successful suicide by insulin injection in a non-diabetic. *Med. Sci. Law* **1995**, *35*, 79–85. [CrossRef]
21. Marks, V. Murder by insulin: Suspected, purported and proven-a review. *Drug Test. Anal.* **2009**, *1*, 162–176. [CrossRef] [PubMed]
22. Kleebauer, A. 'Caring' nurse goes on trial for murder. *Nurs. Stand.* **2015**, *29*, 7. [CrossRef]
23. Bottinelli, C.; Cartiser, N.; Bévalot, F.; Fanton, L.; Guitton, J. Is insulin intoxication still the perfect crime? Analysis and interpretation of postmortem insulin: Review and perspectives in forensic toxicology. *Crit. Rev. Toxicol.* **2020**, *50*, 324–347. [CrossRef] [PubMed]
24. Tokarz, V.L.; MacDonald, P.E.; Klip, A. The cell biology of systemic insulin function. *J. Cell Biol.* **2018**, *217*, 2273–2289. [CrossRef] [PubMed]
25. Mayer, J.P.; Zhang, F.; DiMarchi, R.D. Insulin structure and function. *Biopolymers* **2007**, *88*, 687–713. [CrossRef] [PubMed]
26. Engelman, J.A.; Luo, J.; Cantley, L.C. The evolution of phosphatidylinositol 3-kinases as regulators of growth and metabolism. *Nat. Rev. Genet.* **2006**, *7*, 606–619. [CrossRef] [PubMed]
27. Manning, B.D.; Toker, A. AKT/PKB Signaling: Navigating the Network. *Cell* **2017**, *169*, 381–405. [CrossRef]
28. Bozulic, L.; Hemmings, B.A. PIKKing on PKB: Regulation of PKB activity by phosphorylation. *Curr. Opin. Cell Biol.* **2009**, *21*, 256–261. [CrossRef]
29. Risso, G.; Blaustein, M.; Pozzi, B.; Mammi, P.; Srebrow, A. Akt/PKB: One kinase, many modifications. *Biochem. J.* **2015**, *468*, 203–214. [CrossRef]
30. Richter, E.A.; Hargreaves, M. Exercise, GLUT4, and skeletal muscle glucose uptake. *Physiol. Rev.* **2013**, *93*, 993–1017. [CrossRef]
31. Klip, A.; McGraw, T.E.; James, D.E. Thirty sweet years of GLUT4. *J. Biol. Chem.* **2019**, *294*, 11369–11381. [CrossRef] [PubMed]
32. Leto, D.; Saltiel, A.R. Regulation of glucose transport by insulin: Traffic control of GLUT4. *Nat. Rev. Mol. Cell Biol.* **2012**, *13*, 383–396. [CrossRef] [PubMed]
33. Sylow, L.; Tokarz, V.L.; Richter, E.A.; Klip, A. The many actions of insulin in skeletal muscle, the paramount tissue determining glycemia. *Cell Metab.* **2021**, *33*, 758–780. [CrossRef] [PubMed]
34. Jaldin-Fincati, J.R.; Pavarotti, M.; Frendo-Cumbo, S.; Bilan, P.J.; Klip, A. Update on GLUT4 Vesicle Traffic: A Cornerstone of Insulin Action. *Trends Endocrinol. Metab. TEM* **2017**, *28*, 597–611. [CrossRef]
35. Hoffman, N.J.; Elmendorf, J.S. Signaling, cytoskeletal and membrane mechanisms regulating GLUT4 exocytosis. *Trends Endocrinol. Metab. TEM* **2011**, *22*, 110–116. [CrossRef]
36. Clausen, T. Hormonal and pharmacological modification of plasma potassium homeostasis. *Fundam. Clin. Pharmacol.* **2010**, *24*, 595–605. [CrossRef]
37. Clausen, T. Na^+-K^+ pump regulation and skeletal muscle contractility. *Physiol. Rev.* **2003**, *83*, 1269–1324. [CrossRef]
38. Galuska, D.; Kotova, O.; Barrès, R.; Chibalina, D.; Benziane, B.; Chibalin, A.V. Altered expression and insulin-induced trafficking of Na+-K+-ATPase in rat skeletal muscle: Effects of high-fat diet and exercise. *Am. J. Physiol. Endocrinol. Metab.* **2009**, *297*, E38–E49. [CrossRef]
39. Nguyen, T.Q.; Maalouf, N.M.; Sakhaee, K.; Moe, O.W. Comparison of insulin action on glucose versus potassium uptake in humans. *Clin. J. Am. Soc. Nephrol. CJASN* **2011**, *6*, 1533–1539. [CrossRef]
40. Ho, K. A critically swift response: Insulin-stimulated potassium and glucose transport in skeletal muscle. *Clin. J. Am. Soc. Nephrol. CJASN* **2011**, *6*, 1513–1516. [CrossRef]
41. Mohammadi, K.; Kometiani, P.; Xie, Z.; Askari, A. Role of protein kinase C in the signal pathways that link Na^+/K^+-ATPase to ERK1/2. *J. Biol. Chem.* **2001**, *276*, 42050–42056. [CrossRef] [PubMed]
42. Miyakuni, Y.; Nakajima, M.; Kaszynski, R.H.; Tarui, T.; Goto, H.; Yamaguchi, Y. A Case Involving Massive Insulin Overdose: Direct and Indirect Conditions Requiring Extended Management of Serum Potassium. *Am. J. Case Rep.* **2020**, *21*, e920078. [CrossRef] [PubMed]
43. Thewjitcharoen, Y.; Lekpittaya, N.; Himathongkam, T. Attempted suicide by massive insulin injection: A case report and review of the literature. *J. Med. Assoc. Thail. = Chotmaihet Thangphaet* **2008**, *91*, 1920–1924.
44. Dobbins, R.L.; Connolly, C.C.; Neal, D.W.; Palladino, L.J.; Parlow, A.F.; Cherrington, A.D. Role of glucagon in countering hypoglycemia induced by insulin infusion in dogs. *Am. J. Physiol.* **1991**, *261*, E773–E781. [CrossRef] [PubMed]
45. Ramnanan, C.J.; Edgerton, D.S.; Kraft, G.; Cherrington, A.D. Physiologic action of glucagon on liver glucose metabolism. *Diabetes Obes. Metab.* **2011**, *13* (Suppl. 1), 118–125. [CrossRef] [PubMed]
46. Cryer, P.E. Glucose counterregulation: Prevention and correction of hypoglycemia in humans. *Am. J. Physiol.* **1993**, *264*, E149–E155. [CrossRef] [PubMed]
47. Boyle, P.J.; Shah, S.D.; Cryer, P.E. Insulin, glucagon, and catecholamines in prevention of hypoglycemia during fasting. *Am. J. Physiol.* **1989**, *256*, E651–E661. [CrossRef]
48. Rivera, N.; Ramnanan, C.J.; An, Z.; Farmer, T.; Smith, M.; Farmer, B.; Irimia, J.M.; Snead, W.; Lautz, M.; Roach, P.J.; et al. Insulin-induced hypoglycemia increases hepatic sensitivity to glucagon in dogs. *J. Clin. Investig.* **2010**, *120*, 4425–4435. [CrossRef]

49. Bolli, G.; De Feo, P.; Perriello, G.; De Cosmo, S.; Ventura, M.; Campbell, P.; Brunetti, P.; Gerich, J.E. Role of hepatic autoregulation in defense against hypoglycemia in humans. *J. Clin. Investig.* **1985**, *75*, 1623–1631. [CrossRef]
50. Wasserman, D.H.; Spalding, J.A.; Lacy, D.B.; Colburn, C.A.; Goldstein, R.E.; Cherrington, A.D. Glucagon is a primary controller of hepatic glycogenolysis and gluconeogenesis during muscular work. *Am. J. Physiol.* **1989**, *257*, E108–E117. [CrossRef]
51. Wolfe, R.R.; Nadel, E.R.; Shaw, J.H.; Stephenson, L.A.; Wolfe, M.H. Role of changes in insulin and glucagon in glucose homeostasis in exercise. *J. Clin. Investig.* **1986**, *77*, 900–907. [CrossRef] [PubMed]
52. Brooks, G.A. The Precious Few Grams of Glucose During Exercise. *Int. J. Mol. Sci.* **2020**, *21*, 5733. [CrossRef] [PubMed]
53. Arogyasami, J.; Conlee, R.K.; Booth, C.L.; Diaz, R.; Gregory, T.; Sephton, S.; Wilson, G.I.; Winder, W.W. Effects of exercise on insulin-induced hypoglycemia. *J. Appl. Physiol.* **1990**, *69*, 686–693. [CrossRef] [PubMed]
54. Bangsbo, J.; Johansen, L.; Graham, T.; Saltin, B. Lactate and H^+ effluxes from human skeletal muscles during intense, dynamic exercise. *J. Physiol.* **1993**, *462*, 115–133. [CrossRef] [PubMed]
55. DeWitt, C.R.; Heard, K.; Waksman, J.C. Insulin & C-peptide levels in sulfonylurea-induced hypoglycemia: A systematic review. *J. Med. Toxicol. Off. J. Am. Coll. Med. Toxicol.* **2007**, *3*, 107–118. [CrossRef]
56. Abellan, R.; Ventura, R.; Palmi, I.; di Carlo, S.; di Giovannandrea, R.; Bellver, M.; Olive, R.; Pascual, J.A.; Pacifici, R.; Segura, J.; et al. Evaluation of immunoassays for the measurement of insulin and C-peptide as indirect biomarkers of insulin misuse in sport: Values in selected population of athletes. *J. Pharm. Biomed. Anal.* **2009**, *49*, 793–799. [CrossRef]
57. Uezono, T.; Shiono, H.; Shimizu, K.; Ogawa, K.; Saito, O.; Yoshida, M.; Mizukami, H.; Matsubara, K. Simultaneous analyses of hypoglycemic agents and C-peptide are essential in a homicide case with the combined dosing insulin and insulin-releasing drug. *Leg. Med.* **2002**, *4*, 34–36. [CrossRef]
58. Labay, L.M.; Bitting, C.P.; Legg, K.M.; Logan, B.K. The Determination of Insulin Overdose in Postmortem Investigations. *Acad Forensic Pathol.* **2016**, *6*, 174–183. [CrossRef]
59. Owen, W.E.; Roberts, W.L. Cross-reactivity of three recombinant insulin analogs with five commercial insulin immunoassays. *Clin. Chem.* **2004**, *50*, 257–259. [CrossRef]
60. Dayaldasani, A.; Rodríguez Espinosa, M.; Ocón Sánchez, P.; Pérez Valero, V. Cross-reactivity of insulin analogues with three insulin assays. *Ann. Clin. Biochem.* **2015**, *52*, 312–318. [CrossRef]
61. Elgee, N.J.; Williams, R.H.; Lee, N.D. Distribution and degradation studies with insulin I131. *J. Clin. Investig.* **1954**, *33*, 1252–1260. [CrossRef] [PubMed]
62. Williams, I.M.; Valenzuela, F.A.; Kahl, S.D.; Ramkrishna, D.; Mezo, A.R.; Young, J.D.; Wells, K.S.; Wasserman, D.H. Insulin exits skeletal muscle capillaries by fluid-phase transport. *J. Clin. Investig.* **2018**, *128*, 699–714. [CrossRef] [PubMed]
63. Roberge, R.J.; Martin, T.G.; Delbridge, T.R. Intentional massive insulin overdose: Recognition and management. *Ann. Emerg. Med.* **1993**, *22*, 228–234. [CrossRef] [PubMed]
64. Wunder, C.; Kauert, G.F.; Toennes, S.W. Factors leading to the degradation/loss of insulin in postmortem blood samples. *Forensic Sci. Int.* **2014**, *241*, 173–177. [CrossRef] [PubMed]
65. Hess, C.; Musshoff, F.; Madea, B. Disorders of glucose metabolism-post mortem analyses in forensic cases: Part I. *Int. J. Leg. Med.* **2011**, *125*, 163–170. [CrossRef] [PubMed]
66. Duckworth, W.C.; Bennett, R.G.; Hamel, F.G. Insulin degradation: Progress and potential. *Endocr. Rev.* **1998**, *19*, 608–624. [CrossRef]
67. Bryant, C.; Spencer, D.B.; Miller, A.; Bakaysa, D.L.; McCune, K.S.; Maple, S.R.; Pekar, A.H.; Brems, D.N. Acid stabilization of insulin. *Biochemistry* **1993**, *32*, 8075–8082. [CrossRef]
68. Khoury, J.; Zohar, Y.; Shehadeh, N.; Saadi, T. Glycogenic hepatopathy. *Hepatobiliary Pancreat. Dis. Int. HBPD INT* **2018**, *17*, 113–118. [CrossRef]
69. Sherigar, J.M.; Castro, J.; Yin, Y.M.; Guss, D.; Mohanty, S.R. Glycogenic hepatopathy: A narrative review. *World J. Hepatol.* **2018**, *10*, 172–185. [CrossRef]
70. Mukewar, S.; Sharma, A.; Lackore, K.A.; Enders, F.T.; Torbenson, M.S.; Kamath, P.S.; Roberts, L.R.; Kudva, Y.C. Clinical, Biochemical, and Histopathology Features of Patients With Glycogenic Hepatopathy. *Clin. Gastroenterol. Hepatol. Off. Clin. Pract. J. Am. Gastroenterol. Assoc.* **2017**, *15*, 927–933. [CrossRef]
71. van den Brand, M.; Elving, L.D.; Drenth, J.P.; van Krieken, J.H. Glycogenic hepatopathy: A rare cause of elevated serum transaminases in diabetes mellitus. *Neth. J. Med.* **2009**, *67*, 394–396. [PubMed]
72. Imtiaz, K.E.; Healy, C.; Sharif, S.; Drake, I.; Awan, F.; Riley, J.; Karlson, F. Glycogenic hepatopathy in type 1 diabetes: An underrecognized condition. *Diabetes Care* **2013**, *36*, e6–e7. [CrossRef] [PubMed]

Disclaimer/Publisher's Note: The statements, opinions and data contained in all publications are solely those of the individual author(s) and contributor(s) and not of MDPI and/or the editor(s). MDPI and/or the editor(s) disclaim responsibility for any injury to people or property resulting from any ideas, methods, instructions or products referred to in the content.

toxics

MDPI

Review

The Perils of Methanol Exposure: Insights into Toxicity and Clinical Management

Mohammed Alrashed [1,2,3,*], Norah S. Aldeghaither [1], Shatha Y. Almutairi [1], Meshari Almutairi [1], Abdulrhman Alghamdi [4], Tariq Alqahtani [3,5], Ghada H. Almojathel [6], Nada A. Alnassar [6], Sultan M. Alghadeer [6], Abdulmajeed Alshehri [1,2,3], Mohammed Alnuhait [7] and Omar A. Almohammed [6,8]

1 Department of Pharmacy Practice, College of Pharmacy, King Saud bin Abdulaziz University for Health Sciences, Riyadh 14611, Saudi Arabia; aldeghaither263@ksau-hs.edu.sa (N.S.A.); almoteri040@ksau-hs.edu.sa (S.Y.A.); almutairi0217@ksau-hs.edu.sa (M.A.); shehriabdul@ksau-hs.edu.sa (A.A.)
2 Pharmaceutical Care Department, King Abdulaziz Medical City, National Guard Health Affairs, Riyadh 11426, Saudi Arabia
3 King Abdullah International Medical Research Center, Riyadh 11481, Saudi Arabia; qahtanita@ksau-hs.edu.sa
4 Emergency Medical Services Department, College of Applied Medical Sciences, King Saud bin Abdulaziz University for Health Sciences, Riyadh 14611, Saudi Arabia; ghamdia@ksau-hs.edu.sa
5 Department of Pharmaceutical Sciences, College of Pharmacy, King Saud bin Abdulaziz University for Health Sciences, Riyadh 14611, Saudi Arabia
6 Department of Clinical Pharmacy, College of Pharmacy, King Saud University, Riyadh 12371, Saudi Arabia; 439200038@student.ksu.edu.sa (G.H.A.); 439200129@student.ksu.edu.sa (N.A.A.); salghadeer@ksu.edu.sa (S.M.A.); oalmohammed@ksu.edu.sa (O.A.A.)
7 Pharmaceutical Practices Department, College of Pharmacy, Umm Al-Qura University, Makkah 21955, Saudi Arabia; manuhait@uqu.edu.sa
8 Pharmacoeconomics Research Unit, College of Pharmacy, King Saud University, Riyadh 12371, Saudi Arabia
* Correspondence: alrashidm@ksau-hs.edu.sa; Tel.: +966-114299999 (ext. 95029)

Abstract: Methanol is a widely used industrial and household alcohol that poses significant health risks upon exposure. Despite its extensive use, methanol poisoning remains a critical public health concern globally, often resulting from accidental or intentional ingestion and outbreaks linked to contaminated beverages. Methanol toxicity stems from its metabolic conversion to formaldehyde and formic acid, leading to severe metabolic acidosis and multiorgan damage, including profound CNS effects and visual impairments. Epidemiological data underscore the widespread impact of methanol poisoning, with alarming case fatality rates reported in various countries. Comprehensive prevention and effective management strategies are urgently needed to address the significant morbidity and mortality associated with methanol poisoning. The clinical manifestations of methanol toxicity vary between adult and pediatric populations and between acute and chronic exposure. Adults typically present with gastrointestinal and neurological symptoms, whereas pediatric patients often exhibit more severe outcomes due to differences in metabolism and body weight. The diagnosis of methanol poisoning involves a combination of clinical evaluation, laboratory testing, and advanced diagnostic techniques. The identification of metabolic acidosis, elevated anion and osmolal gaps, and confirmation through methanol and formate levels are critical for accurate diagnosis. Timely intervention is crucial, and the management of methanol poisoning includes securing the airway, breathing, and circulation; addressing metabolic acidosis with sodium bicarbonate; administering antidotes such as fomepizole or ethanol; and administering hemodialysis, which plays a pivotal role in eliminating methanol and its toxic metabolites, especially in severe cases. The complexity of methanol poisoning necessitates a comprehensive approach encompassing early recognition, prompt intervention, and coordinated care among healthcare providers. Increased awareness, effective prevention strategies, and timely treatment protocols are essential to mitigate severe health consequences and improve patient survival and recovery.

Keywords: methanol; toxicity; pathophysiology; clinical presentation; diagnostics; management

1. Introduction

Methanol is a toxic alcohol found in various products. Methanol poisoning occurs through accidental or intentional ingestion, leading to outbreaks. This global health concern contributes to significant morbidity and mortality. Common products containing methanol include windshield washer fluid, gas line antifreeze, carburetor cleaner, copy machine fluids, perfumes, food warming fuels, and other types of fuel. A variety of detrimental consequences are associated with methanol poisoning, necessitating measures such laboratory monitoring, antidotal therapy, and emergency dialysis. The severity of methanol poisoning highlights the urgent need for comprehensive preventive measures and effective management strategies to address its consequences, including permanent neurological damage, blindness, and even death [1].

The global consumption of methanol exceeds 225 million liters per day, and in recent years, methanol poisoning outbreaks in many developed countries have increased alarmingly [2]. Methanol poisoning presents differently in adult and pediatric populations and varies between acute and chronic exposure. Although uncommon among pediatric patients, methanol toxicity has been reported with varying severity. In mild cases, there is a minimal decrease in central nervous system (CNS) activity, accompanied by weakness, dizziness, and nausea. Severe cases lead to metabolic acidosis, which manifests as blurred vision, bilateral mydriasis, gastrointestinal (GI) symptoms, disorientation, visual abnormalities, photophobia, and sporadic blindness [3]. Adults may present symptoms such as nausea, vomiting, abdominal pain, and neurological disturbances, whereas pediatric patients pose unique challenges due to differences in metabolism and body weight, potentially resulting in more severe manifestations and poorer outcomes [4]. Acute poisoning typically involves a single large ingestion, resulting in rapid onset of symptoms such as metabolic acidosis, visual disturbance, and CNS depression. Conversely, chronic poisoning results from repeated low-level exposures over time, leading to insidious symptoms such as chronic headaches, dizziness, and progressive visual impairment [5].

This review aims to examine methanol toxicity, focusing on the proper evaluation of methanol poisoning cases, the contributing factors and circumstances leading to exposure, the effectiveness of current treatment protocols, challenges in diagnosis and management, and preventive strategies to reduce methanol-related incidents in various regions. Understanding these aspects is crucial for improving outcomes and implementing effective public health measures.

2. Pathophysiology

Methanol poisoning manifests as a complex pathophysiological sequence. Methanol is rapidly absorbed through the GI tract, causing nausea, vomiting, and abdominal pain, and subsequently enters the CNS, causing confusion and drowsiness. Methanol undergoes metabolism through several enzymatic processes in the liver. This series of oxidation reactions results in the accumulation of more toxic metabolites (Figure 1) [1].

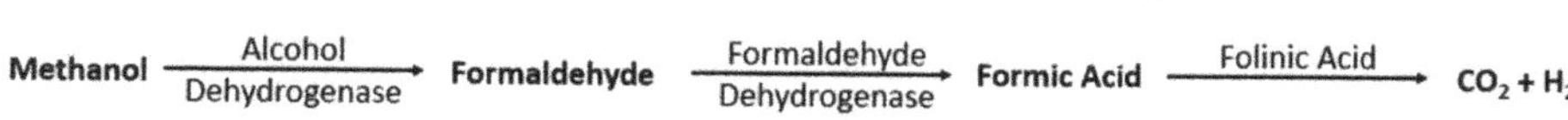

Figure 1. The metabolism of methanol in the liver.

The key driver of the pathophysiological effects of methanol poisoning is the accumulation of formic acid, which leads to metabolic acidosis. This condition interferes with normal cellular metabolism and can result in harmful consequences for various organ systems. The CNS is particularly vulnerable to the consequences of methanol poisoning. Formic acid and formaldehyde can lead to neurological symptoms, including headache, confusion, seizures, and, in severe cases, coma. These CNS effects contribute to direct damage to brain tissues and neurotransmitter imbalances. Another hallmark of methanol poisoning pathophysiology is visual impairment, including blindness. If not promptly addressed, this damage can become irreversible [1,6].

Methanol poisoning is not limited to the CNS; it can impact multiple other organ systems. The cardiovascular system may experience hemodynamic instability, and acute kidney injury may occur because of the systemic influence of acidosis and the accumulation of toxic metabolites. Timely intervention is crucial when managing methanol poisoning cases. Antidotes such as ethanol or fomepizole are administered to inhibit the activity of alcohol dehydrogenase (ADH), effectively halting the further breakdown of methanol. This intervention reduces the formation of toxic metabolites and mitigates acidosis, CNS effects, and multiorgan dysfunction [4,6]. Ethanol administration plays a crucial role in inhibiting methanol metabolism due to its competitive binding with ADH. Ethanol has a higher affinity (lower Km) for ADH compared to methanol, effectively outcompeting methanol for enzymatic binding. This prevents the oxidation of methanol into its toxic metabolites, such as formaldehyde and formic acid, thereby reducing their harmful effects. Fomepizole, on the other hand, is a direct inhibitor of ADH and works by completely halting the enzymatic activity of ADH. Both interventions are essential for mitigating metabolic acidosis, CNS effects, and multiorgan dysfunction associated with methanol poisoning [4,6].

3. Toxicokinetic

Methanol toxicity primarily occurs through ingestion, although exposure can also happen via inhalation or skin absorption. For an adult, a potentially fatal dose is approximately 1 g per kilogram of body weight [1,7]. Once ingested, methanol is rapidly absorbed from the GI tract, reaching peak concentrations within 30 to 90 min. Due to its small molecular size and lipophilic nature, methanol readily crosses the blood–brain barrier, leading to severe CNS effects in poisoning cases [8].

The liver plays a critical role in methanol pharmacokinetics as the primary site for its metabolism. Hepatic alcohol dehydrogenase (ADH) oxidizes methanol into formaldehyde, a highly toxic intermediate metabolite [9]. Formaldehyde is then rapidly oxidized into formic acid [10]. At physiological pH, formic acid dissociates into formate and a hydrogen ion. A folate-dependent system further metabolizes formate, ultimately producing water and carbon dioxide (Figure 1). This metabolic pathway begins with the interaction of formate and tetrahydrofolate, leading to the formation of 10-formyl tetrahydrofolate [11].

Formate oxidation depends on hepatic tetrahydrofolate levels, which are regulated by two key factors: the availability of dietary folic acid and the efficiency of tetrahydrofolate regeneration during formate oxidation [12]. The enzyme 10-formyl tetrahydrofolate dehydrogenase plays a pivotal role in recycling tetrahydrofolate and catalyzing the final step of formate oxidation [11]. Studies have shown that folic acid supplementation can reduce the toxic effects of methanol and enhance formate oxidation in various species, including humans and monkeys [13]. These findings highlight the critical role of formic acid in methanol toxicity and suggest that folate supplementation may be beneficial in treating methanol poisoning [14]. Methanol oxidation leads to the formation of formaldehyde, which is subsequently converted into formic acid.

Formic acid, a primary toxic metabolite of methanol, inhibits cytochrome oxidase, a critical enzyme in the electron transport chain responsible for oxidative phosphorylation. This inhibition disrupts mitochondrial energy production, leading to reduced ATP synthesis and cellular energy failure. High-energy-demand organs, such as the brain and retina, are particularly vulnerable to this effect. Furthermore, cytochrome oxidase inhibition contributes to the accumulation of lactate and exacerbates metabolic acidosis, further impairing cellular function. These highly reactive metabolites can also quickly bind to tissue proteins [8]. During methanol metabolism, the osmolar gap decreases while the anion gap increases. The development of anion gap metabolic acidosis due to formic acid accumulation is a complex process. It involves the buildup of organic acids, such as formic acid and formate, which are difficult to eliminate. Moreover, formate disrupts oxidative phosphorylation by inhibiting cytochrome oxidase, thereby impairing mitochondrial respiration. This disruption can lead to elevated lactate levels, which facilitates the passage of formic acid across the blood–brain barrier [1,15,16].

The half-life of methanol is approximately eight minutes, with peak blood levels reached rapidly after ingestion, before declining [17]. Methanol elimination generally follows zero-order kinetics due to the saturation of ADH. Limited data indicate elimination rates ranging from 2.7 mmol/L/h (8.5 mg/dL/h) to 6.3 mmol/L/h (20 mg/dL/h). However, when methanol metabolism is inhibited by antidotes such as ethanol or fomepizole, elimination transitions to first-order kinetics, with a half-life extending from 22 to 87 h. Half-life appears to increase with higher serum methanol concentrations, although the underlying reasons remain unclear [18].

4. Clinical Presentation

Like ethanol, methanol acts as a central nervous system depressant. Early symptoms include a general feeling of malaise, accompanied by weakness, headache, and nausea. In some cases, severe symptoms may develop. Most of the methanol in the body is converted into formaldehyde, which is then rapidly metabolized into the highly toxic formic acid and its anion, formate. Extremely high doses can cause severe acidosis, leading to multiorgan failure, brain damage, blindness, and even death [1].

Methanol poisoning can be identified through a range of clinical signs and symptoms, often occurring in distinct phases. In the early stages, which occur within the first few hours following exposure, individuals may experience nonspecific symptoms, such as headache and dizziness, and GI disturbance, such as nausea and vomiting. These early manifestations can be misleading or confusing and may not be immediately recognized as methanol poisoning. However, as toxic metabolites accumulate, more severe and specific symptoms arise. Systemic toxicity includes metabolic acidosis, increased respiratory rate (hyperpnea), loss of appetite (anorexia), headache, and nausea. Hyperventilation may lead to the initial complaint of shortness of breath in many patients. Some individuals may experience chest pain and, as a result, could be initially diagnosed with acute myocardial infarction. The neurological symptoms of these patients often include altered mental status, confusion, and, in severe cases, seizures or coma. Delayed treatment can lead to lasting consequences such as impaired vision and brain damage [1,4,19]. A comprehensive understanding of these clinical signs and symptoms is critical for timely diagnosis and intervention, emphasizing the need for early treatment to mitigate the potentially life-threatening consequences of methanol poisoning (Figure 2).

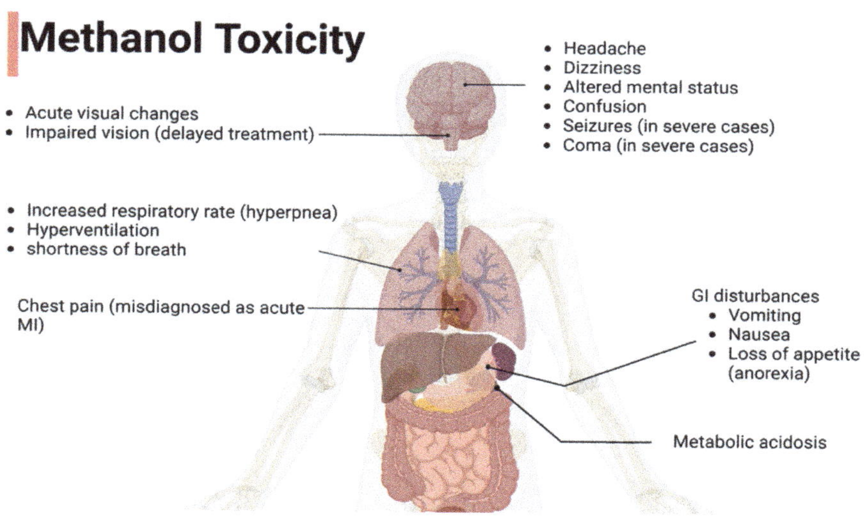

Figure 2. Clinical manifestations of methanol poisoning across various organ systems.

5. Evaluation and Diagnostic Testing

Diagnosing methanol poisoning becomes challenging in the absence of exposure history, particularly when ethanol coingestion occurs, leading to an extended latency period. A comprehensive evaluation approach is needed to assess the severity of methanol toxicity. Clinical evaluation plays a crucial role in the initial assessment, with healthcare professionals considering symptoms such as headache, nausea, vomiting, and visual disturbances. Vital signs are typically normal, and Kussmaul respirations are uncommon even in cases of severe acidosis [20]. Patients who experience severe abdominal pain may exhibit rigidity of the abdominal wall, although rebound tenderness is not usually present [20].

Performing visual acuity and fundoscopy examinations is essential in cases of methanol poisoning. Signs of ocular toxicity include dilated pupils that are partially reactive or nonreactive, as well as optic disc hyperemia with blurred margins resembling pseudopapillitis [20,21]. Microscopic analysis of optic nerves from methanol-poisoned individuals may reveal generalized swelling of intra-axonal mitochondria and clear spaces within the myelin sheath in the retrolaminar portion. These ocular changes are attributed to the direct toxic effects of formate, which inhibits cytochrome oxidase, leading to decreased ATP production and impaired ATP-dependent functions. Inhibition of the sodium–potassium membrane pump disrupts electrical conduction, resulting in early but potentially reversible visual disturbances [22].

A definitive diagnosis of methanol poisoning is made by detecting methanol and formic acid in the blood or urine. A patient who has ingested methanol may present with symptoms ranging from being asymptomatic with an elevated osmolar gap to experiencing severe illness with end-organ toxicity, high anion gap metabolic acidosis, and potentially elevated lactic acid levels. Urinalysis results are generally normal, with no crystals found in the sediment [4]. Advanced diagnostic techniques, such as gas chromatography, can be employed to quantify methanol and its metabolites in biological fluids. Arterial blood gas analysis may reveal metabolic acidosis, a hallmark of methanol poisoning in severe cases. The osmolar gap, which measures the difference between the measured and calculated serum osmolarity, can also be a valuable diagnostic tool [4]. To evaluate neurological complications, which are a hallmark of methanol poisoning, radiological imaging, particularly brain imaging, may be necessary. Multidisciplinary team collaboration in evaluations is essential to confirm the diagnosis and guide appropriate therapeutic interventions.

All toxicology patients suspected of self-harm should receive a complete toxicological screening, an electrocardiogram, and a basic metabolic panel. Additional tests to consider include complete blood count; transaminase, lipase, and amylase levels; pregnancy status; and serum or urine ketone, lactate, ethanol, and salicylate concentrations. White blood cell counts, hemoglobin, and hematocrit are typically normal, but the mean corpuscular volume may be higher, which could be a sign of more serious poisoning and widespread cellular swelling. Elevated serum amylase levels can also indicate acute pancreatitis. Salicylate toxicity must be eliminated, particularly in patients who have metabolic acidosis. Because ethanol prevents methanol from being metabolized, the concentration of ethanol is also required. Although gas chromatography is a confirmatory method for measuring toxic alcohol concentrations, it is not readily available in all healthcare facilities. These concentrations, reported in mg/dL, typically peak soon after absorption and decrease via zero-order kinetics. The time of ingestion is important because the toxic alcohol concentration may not reflect toxicity levels if metabolism has progressed, as the metabolites are primarily responsible for the toxic effects. Assessing the formate concentration for methanol can be related to clinical signs of end-organ damage or acidosis. While a diagnosis is typically required sooner, obtaining dangerous alcohol concentrations frequently necessitates sending a serum sample to an external institution, which could take hours or days for findings. A patient with normal acid–base status shortly after methanol ingestion should be observed for at least 12 h, with serial basic metabolic panels performed every 2 to 4 h to monitor for the onset of metabolic acidosis and an elevated anion gap. This observation period should begin only after confirming that the patient's ethanol concentration is undetectable. The 12 h observation period is considered the standard of care, based more on clinical experience than specific data, as acidosis typically develops within this timeframe following ingestion [3]. Diagnosing methanol poisoning can be challenging, particularly when the patient's history is unclear, necessitating a high degree of clinical suspicion. Prompt detection and timely therapeutic interventions, including the use of ADH inhibitors, are critical for assessing and potentially reversing the damage caused by formic acid.

6. Diagnostic Testing

Methanol levels are typically assessed via gas chromatography or radioimmunoassay methods [4]. Laboratory assessments for methanol poisoning should include arterial blood gas analysis alongside blood samples. Urinalysis with microscopy is essential for detecting crystalluria, which may indicate ethylene glycol poisoning, although the absence of crystals has no diagnostic significance. When encountering patients with unexplained metabolic acidosis, especially after diabetic ketoacidosis and renal failure are ruled out, calculating the anion and osmolal gaps (OGs) can provide diagnostic clues [4,21]. Methanol increases serum osmolality at toxicity-related doses. This effect can be evaluated by calculating the OG with the following common formula:

$$\text{Osmolal Gap} = [\text{Measured Osmolality}] - [\text{Calculated Osmolality}]$$

$$\text{Calculated osmolality} = [1.86 \times \text{sodium concentration (mmol)}] + [\text{glucose concentration (mg/dL)}/18] + [\text{BUN concentration (mg/dL)}/2.8] + [1.25 \times \text{ethanol (mmol/L)}]$$

The normal range for OG in acute patients is 5 ± 14 mOsm/kg H_2O [23]. An OG above 10 indicates the presence of exogenous osmoles. However, a cutoff value of 25 mOsm/kg H_2O is considered effective [23,24]. In the initial stages or with ethanol coingestion, only OG may be elevated, as methanol has not yet been metabolized into formate. In the later stages, when methanol is converted to formate, the anion gap increases, whereas the OG may normalize. Detecting formate might then be necessary for confirmation. Additionally, brain scans such as CT or MRI might reveal late-stage findings such as necrosis in the putamenal areas due to methanol poisoning [4].

7. Treatment

Methanol poisoning is a medical emergency that can lead to severe complications such as permanent neurological damage, blindness, and death. Therefore, prompt recognition and intervention are needed. Treatment decisions are based only upon clinical suspicion and readily available laboratory data (Figure 3).

7.1. Airways, Breathing, and Circulation

The first step in managing methanol toxicity is to secure the patient's airway, breathing, and circulation. Advanced cardiac life support measures are considered in cases of severe metabolic acidosis, complications that threaten cardiac and respiratory functions, or standard treatments for methanol toxicity that have proven ineffective in stabilizing patients' condition [6,25]. In hyperventilated patients with existing or suspected significant metabolic acidosis, endotracheal intubation is needed. In addition, it is crucial to monitor arterial/venous blood gases closely to evaluate pH and ensure adequate ventilation and oxygenation [7].

7.2. Gastrointestinal Decontamination

Gastrointestinal decontamination is not commonly used when treating methanol poisoning, as methanol is rapidly absorbed. However, gastric aspiration via flexible nasogastric tubing can be an option if a patient ingests a large amount of methanol within 60 min of admission. Other methods, such as activated charcoal, gastric lavage, and syrup with ipecac, do not have a role in alcohol toxicity [8].

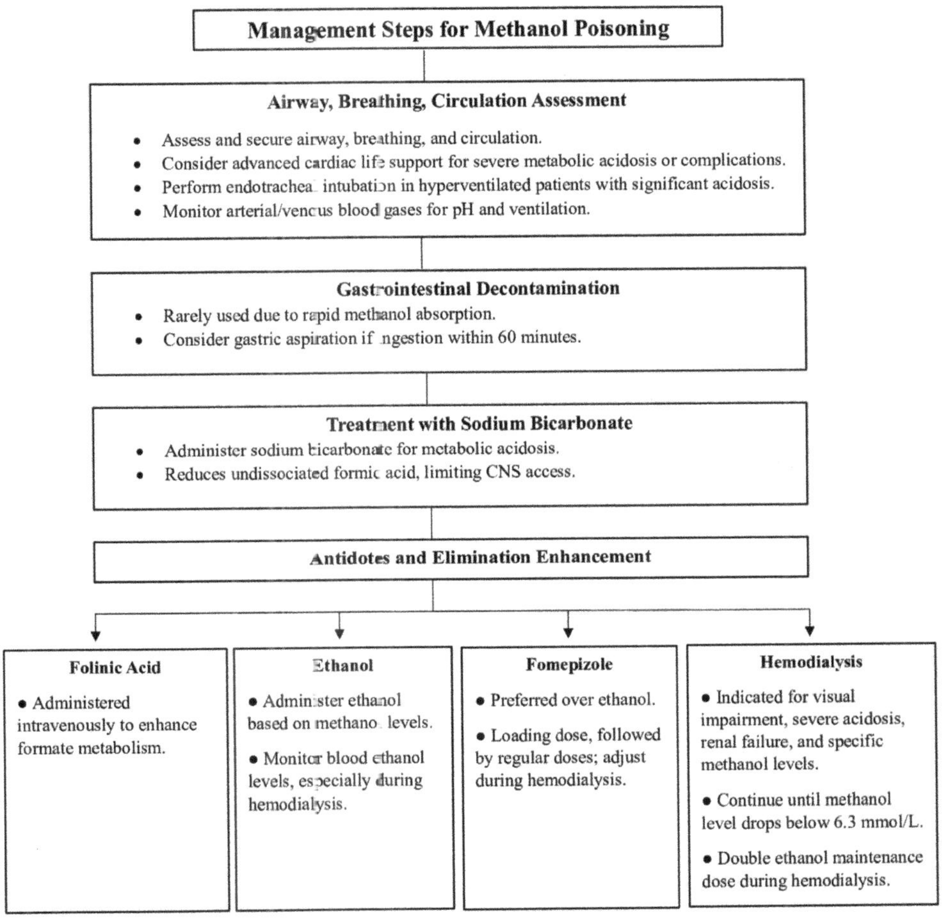

Figure 3. The clinical management of methanol poisoning.

7.3. Treatment with Sodium Bicarbonate

The immediate and aggressive treatment of methanol poisoning involves the administration of sodium bicarbonate with the aim of completely correcting acidosis. Notably, bicarbonate treatment lowers the quantity of undissociated formic acid to diminish the access of formate to the CNS and thereby reduce toxicity [25]. It also treats metabolic acidosis. Initial infusion may require as many as 400 to 600 milliequivalents (mEq) within the first few hours. The final goal of treatment is to maintain the arterial/venous pH above 7.35 when infusion is discontinued.

7.4. Antidotes and Elimination Enhancement

The inhibition of ADH prevents the metabolism of methanol into its more toxic metabolites. The ADH inhibitors used for managing methanol toxicity are fomepizole and ethanol. They are indicated if the serum methanol level is >20 mg/dL, there is a recent history of ingesting toxic amounts of methanol and a serum osmol gap > 10, or there is strong clinical suspicion of methanol toxicity with at least two of the following criteria: arterial pH < 7.3, serum bicarbonate < 20 meq/L (mmol/L), an osmol gap > 10, and the presence of urinary oxalate crystals. If obtaining a methanol level is challenging and interpreting anions and OG is difficult, initiating ethanol or fomepizole therapy is recommended for any patient with metabolic acidosis and symptoms or a history of potential toxic alcohol ingestion [1,6,26].

7.4.1. Folinic Acid

Increasing additional formate metabolism may be facilitated by intravenous folinic acid administration at doses ranging from 1 mg/kg to 50 mg every 4 h. If folinic acid is not available, folic acid at the same dosage can serve as an alternative [4].

7.4.2. Ethanol

A therapeutic blood ethanol level of about 22 mmol/L (100 mg/dL) is recommended. However, because there is dynamic competition with the liver's ADH enzyme, the amount of ethanol needed to block methanol metabolism is dependent on the level of methanol present at the time. The molar ethanol concentration should be at least one-fourth of the molar methanol concentration if the blood methanol level is known [1,4,25,26]. By giving a bolus dose of 600–800 mg/kg of 10% ethanol in D5W, followed by a maintenance dose of 66–154 mg/kg/h as an intravenous infusion of the 10% ethanol in D5W, or by taking 20% ethanol diluted in orange juice orally, for instance, a blood ethanol level of 100 mg/dL can be achieved. Monitoring blood ethanol levels is crucial, especially during hemodialysis. If ethanol was coingested with methanol and the blood ethanol level initially was >22 mmol/L (100 mg/dL), the bolus dose of ethanol can be skipped. Typically, the maintenance dose of ethanol should be doubled during hemodialysis to prevent the resumption of methanol metabolism when ethanol levels decrease, leading to worsening toxicity despite hemodialysis [1,25–27]. Ethanol therapy should continue until the diagnosis of toxic alcohol ingestion is ruled out or specific criteria related to blood pH and the serum alcohol concentration are met. In addition, owing to associated risks, patients should be treated in a critical care setting, ideally with a central venous catheter and an infusion pump. In the absence of fomepizole and pharmaceutical-grade IV ethanol, oral ethanol administration can be considered with appropriate dilutions, but it may lead to side effects such as gastritis and vomiting. Combining ethanol with fomepizole therapy offers no added benefit in methanol and ethylene glycol poisoning cases [28].

7.4.3. Fomepizole

Fomepizole is a commercially available treatment for methanol poisoning and is preferred over ethanol. A loading dose of fomepizole (15 mg/kg IV) followed by four maintenance doses 12 h apart (10 mg/kg IV) and 15 mg/kg every 12 h thereafter is the recommended dosing regimen for fomepizole. If hemodialysis is initiated, the fomepizole dosing frequency should be increased every 4 h [29–31]. Fomepizole therapy should continue until the diagnosis of toxic alcohol ingestion is ruled out or a controlled blood pH and decreased serum alcohol concentration to <20 mg/dL is achieved.

Fomepizole, due to its higher affinity for ADH compared to ethanol, offers several clinical advantages. These include a broader therapeutic index, longer duration of action, simplified dosing, and more consistent pharmacokinetics. Additionally, fomepizole is associated with fewer side effects compared to ethanol [8]. However, its primary drawback is its high cost. Despite this, significant cost savings can be achieved by reducing the need for hemodialysis, ethanol infusions, prolonged hospital stays, and intensive care unit admissions [15].

7.4.4. Hemodialysis

Hemodialysis is a highly effective method for eliminating methanol and formate while correcting metabolic acidosis. The primary indication for hemodialysis is any degree of visual impairment in a patient with metabolic acidosis or detectable methanol levels. Other indications include severe metabolic acidosis (especially if unresponsive to previous therapies), deteriorating vital signs and electrolyte imbalances despite optimal treatment, renal failure, a blood methanol level exceeding 15.6 mmol/L (50 mg/dL), and ingestion of more than 1 g/kg methanol. In severe poisonings characterized by marked metabolic acidosis (base deficit > 20 mmol/L) and visual disturbances, hemodialysis is strongly recommended to rapidly remove methanol and formate [4,27].

Hemodialysis is typically continued until the blood methanol level falls below 6.3 mmol/L (20 mg/dL) and metabolic acidosis resolves. In cases where methanol level testing is unavailable, hemodialysis should proceed for at least 8 h or until the osmolar gap normalizes in two consecutive samples taken 1 h apart (after accounting for any osmolal contribution from ethanol) [1,26,27]. This method has proven effective in optimizing dialysis time, particularly during large outbreaks or when dialysis resources are limited. Serum formate concentrations may also serve as an alternative guide for determining the need for hemodialysis. Additionally, doubling the maintenance dose of ethanol during hemodialysis is generally recommended, as failing to do so may allow methanol metabolism to resume when ethanol levels drop, potentially worsening toxicity despite ongoing hemodialysis [27].

8. Conclusions

Methanol (CH_3OH) is a widely used industrial and household alcohol that poses significant health risks upon exposure. Despite its extensive use, methanol poisoning remains a critical public health concern globally, often resulting from accidental or intentional ingestion and outbreaks linked to contaminated beverages. Methanol toxicity stems from its metabolic conversion to formaldehyde and formic acid, leading to severe metabolic acidosis and multiorgan damage, including profound CNS effects and visual impairments.

Epidemiological data underscore the widespread impact of methanol poisoning, with alarming case fatality rates reported in various countries. Comprehensive prevention and effective management strategies are urgently needed to address the significant morbidity and mortality associated with methanol poisoning.

The clinical manifestations of methanol toxicity vary between adult and pediatric populations and between acute and chronic exposure. Adults typically present with gastrointestinal and neurological symptoms, whereas pediatric patients often exhibit more severe outcomes due to differences in metabolism and body weight. Acute poisoning generally involves a large, single ingestion, leading to rapid symptom onset, whereas chronic poisoning results from small, repeated exposures, causing insidious, progressive symptoms.

The diagnosis of methanol poisoning involves a combination of clinical evaluation, laboratory testing, and advanced diagnostic techniques. The identification of metabolic acidosis, elevated anion and OG levels, and confirmation through methanol and formate levels are critical for accurate diagnosis. Timely intervention is crucial, and the management of methanol poisoning includes securing the airway, breathing, and circulation; addressing metabolic acidosis with sodium bicarbonate; and administering antidotes, such as fomepizole or ethanol. Hemodialysis plays a pivotal role in eliminating methanol and its toxic metabolites, especially in severe cases with significant metabolic acidosis or visual disturbances.

In conclusion, the complexity of methanol poisoning necessitates a comprehensive approach encompassing early recognition, prompt intervention, and coordinated care among healthcare providers. Increased awareness, effective prevention strategies, and timely treatment protocols are essential to mitigate severe health consequences and improve patient survival and recovery.

Author Contributions: M.A. (Mohammed Alrashed) conceptualized the study and was the primary author responsible for drafting the manuscript. G.H.A. and N.A.A. contributed to the literature review as well as drafting specific sections of the manuscript related to the introduction and pathophysiology. N.S.A. and S.Y.A. contributed to the literature review as well as drafting specific sections of the manuscript related to the clinical presentation and toxicokinetics. M.A. (Meshari Almutairi) contributed to the literature review as well as drafting specific sections of the manuscript related to the evaluation and diagnostic testing and treatment. T.A. was responsible for developing the methodological approach used in the study as well as the review and editing of the manuscript. A.A. (Abdulrhman Alghamdi), S.M.A., M.A. (Mohammed Alnuhait) and A.A. (Abdulmajeed Alshehri) provided expertise in emergency medicine and helped with the interpretation of the clinical data and management strategies, as well as the review and editing of the manuscript. O.A.A. supervised the project, critically reviewed the manuscript, and provided guidance throughout the writing process. All authors have read and agreed to the published version of the manuscript.

Funding: This research received no external funding.

Institutional Review Board Statement: Ethics approval and consent to participate were not required for this study as it is a review article that does not involve direct research with human or animal subjects.

Informed Consent Statement: Consent for publication is not applicable to this article as it is a review of previously published literature and does not include any individual data or images requiring consent.

Conflicts of Interest: The authors declare no conflicts of interest.

References

1. Ashurst, J.V.; Nappe, T.M. *Methanol Toxicity;* StatPearls Publishing: Treasure Island, FL, USA, 2023; StatPearls Web Site. Available online: https://www.ncbi.nlm.nih.gov/books/NBK482121/ (accessed on 2 July 2024).
2. World Health Organization (WHO). *Methanol Poisoning Outbreaks;* World Health Organization (WHO): Geneva, Switzerland, 2014. Available online: https://www.methanol.org/wp-content/uploads/2016/06/WHO-Methanol-Poisoning-Fact-Sheet.pdf (accessed on 2 July 2024).
3. Loza, R.; Rodriguez, D. A case of methanol poisoning in a child. *Case Rep. Nephrol.* **2014**, *2014*, 652129. [CrossRef] [PubMed] [PubMed Central]
4. Nekoukar, Z.; Zakariaei, Z.; Taghizadeh, F.; Musavi, F.; Banimostafavi, E.S.; Sharifpour, A.; Ebrahim Ghuchi, N.; Fakhar, M.; Tabaripour, R.; Safanavaei, S. Methanol poisoning as a new world challenge: A review. *Ann. Med. Surg.* **2021**, *66*, 102445. [CrossRef]
5. Bateman, N.; Jefferson, R.; Thomas, S.; Thompson, J.; Vale, A. (Eds.) Common complications of poisoning. In *Oxford Desk Reference: Toxicology;* Oxford University Press: Oxford, UK, 2014.
6. Hantson, P.E. Acute methanol intoxication: Physiopathology, prognosis and treatment. *Bull. Mem. Acad. R. Med. Belg.* **2005**, *160*, 294–300.
7. Moon, C.S. Estimations of the lethal and exposure doses for representative methanol symptoms in humans. *Ann. Occup. Environ. Med.* **2017**, *29*, 44. [CrossRef] [PubMed]
8. Dorokhov, Y.L.; Shindyapina, A.V.; Sheshukova, E.V.; Komarova, T.V. Metabolic methanol: Molecular pathways and physiological roles. *Physiol. Rev.* **2015**, *95*, 603–644. [CrossRef] [PubMed]
9. Teschke, R. Alcoholic Liver Disease: Alcohol Metabolism, Cascade of Molecular Mechanisms, Cellular Targets, and Clinical Aspects. *Biomedicines* **2018**, *6*, 106. [CrossRef] [PubMed]
10. Quiroz Torres, J.; Royer, S.; Bellat, J.-P.; Giraudon, J.-M.; Lamonier, J.-F. Formaldehyde: Catalytic Oxidation as a Promising Soft Way of Elimination. *ChemSusChem* **2013**, *6*, 578–592. [CrossRef]
11. Eells, J.T.; Makar, A.B.; Noker, P.E.; Tephly, T.R. Methanol poisoning and formate oxidation in nitrous oxide-treated rats. *J. Pharmacol. Exp. Ther.* **1981**, *217*, 57–61. [PubMed]
12. Baumbach, G.L.; Cancilla, P.A.; Martin-Amat, G.; Tephly, T.R.; McMartin, K.E.; Makar, A.B.; Hayreh, M.S.; Hayreh, S.S. Methyl alcohol poisoning. IV. Alterations of the morphological findings of the retina and optic nerve. *Arch. Ophthalmol.* **1977**, *95*, 1859–1865. [CrossRef] [PubMed]
13. Pietzke, M.; Meiser, J.; Vazquez, A. Formate metabolism in health and disease. *Mol. Metab.* **2020**, *33*, 23–37. [CrossRef]
14. Jacobsen, D.; Webb, R.; Collins, T.D.; McMartin, K.E. Methanol and formate kinetics in late diagnosed methanol intoxication. *Med. Toxicol. Adverse. Drug Exp.* **1988**, *3*, 418–423. [CrossRef] [PubMed]
15. Skrzydlewska, E. Toxicological and metabolic consequences of methanol poisoning. *Toxicol. Mech. Methods* **2003**, *13*, 277–293. [CrossRef]
16. Cederbaum, A.I. Alcohol metabolism. *Clin. Liver Dis.* **2012**, *16*, 667–685. [CrossRef] [PubMed]
17. Graw, M.; Haffner, H.T.; Althaus, L.; Besserer, K.; Voges, S. Invasion and distribution of methanol. *Arch. Toxicol.* **2000**, *74*, 313–321. [CrossRef]
18. Haffner, H.T.; Wehner, H.D.; Scheytt, K.D.; Besserer, K. The elimination kinetics of methanol and the influence of ethanol. *Int. J. Legal Med.* **1992**, *105*, 111–114. [CrossRef] [PubMed]
19. Centers for Disease Control and Prevention (CDC). Methanol: Systemic Agent. Available online: https://www.cdc.gov/niosh/ershdb/emergencyresponsecard_29750029.html (accessed on 27 January 2024).
20. Bennett, I.L., Jr.; Cary, F.H.; Mitchell, G.L., Jr.; Cooper, M.N. Acute methyl alcohol poisoning: A review based on experiences in an outbreak of 323 cases. *Medicine* **1953**, *32*, 431–463. [CrossRef] [PubMed]
21. Klein, K.A.; Warren, A.K.; Baumal, C.R.; Hedges, T.R. Optical coherence tomography findings in methanol toxicity. *Int. J. Retin. Vitr.* **2017**, *3*, 36. [CrossRef] [PubMed]

22. Liberski, S.; Kaluzny, B.J.; Kocięcki, J. Methanol-induced optic neuropathy: A still-present problem. *Arch. Toxicol.* **2022**, *96*, 431–451. [CrossRef]
23. Aabakken, L.; Johansen, K.S.; Rydningen, E.B.; Bredesen, J.E.; Ovrebø, S.; Jacobsen, D. Osmolal and anion gaps in patients admitted to an emergency medical department. *Hum. Exp. Toxicol.* **1994**, *13*, 131–134. [CrossRef] [PubMed]
24. Lynd, L.D.; Richardson, K.J.; Purssell, R.A.; Abu-Laban, R.B.; Brubacher, J.R.; Lepik, K.J.; Sivilotti, M.L. An evaluation of the osmole gap as a screening test for toxic alcohol poisoning. *BMC Emerg. Med.* **2008**, *8*, 5. [CrossRef]
25. Kleiman, R.; Nickle, R.; Schwartz, M. Medical toxicology and public health--update on research and activities at the Centers for Disease Control and Prevention, and the Agency for Toxic Substances and Disease Registry inhalational methanol toxicity. *J. Med. Toxicol.* **2009**, *5*, 158–164. [CrossRef] [PubMed]
26. Barceloux, D.G.; Bond, G.R.; Krenzelok, E.P.; Cooper, H.; Vale, J.A. American Academy of Clinical Toxicology practice guidelines on the treatment of methanol poisoning. *J. Toxicol. Clin. Toxicol.* **2002**, *40*, 415–446. [CrossRef]
27. Driscoll, D.; Bleecker, G.; Francis, J.; Jaberi, A. Acute Hemodialysis for Treatment of Severe Ethanol Intoxication. *Kidney Med.* **2020**, *2*, 793–796. [CrossRef]
28. Gallagher, N.; Edwards, F.J. The Diagnosis and Management of Toxic Alcohol Poisoning in the Emergency Department: A Review Article. *Adv. J. Emerg. Med.* **2019**, *3*, e28. [CrossRef]
29. Mégarbane, B. Treatment of patients with ethylene glycol or methanol poisoning: Focus on fomepizole. *Open Access Emerg. Med.* **2010**, *2*, 67–75. [CrossRef]
30. Shannon, M.W.; Borron, S.W.; Burns, M.J. (Eds.) Emergency Management of Poisoning. In *Haddad and Winchester's Clinical Management of Poisoning and Drug Overdose*, 4th ed.; Elsevier: Amsterdam, The Netherlands, 2007; pp. 13–61.
31. Beatty, L.; Green, R.; Magee, K.; Zed, P. A Systematic Review of Ethanol and Fomepizole Use in Toxic Alcohol Ingestions. *Emerg. Med. Int.* **2013**, *2013*, 638057. [CrossRef] [PubMed]

Disclaimer/Publisher's Note: The statements, opinions and data contained in all publications are solely those of the individual author(s) and contributor(s) and not of MDPI and/or the editor(s). MDPI and/or the editor(s) disclaim responsibility for any injury to people or property resulting from any ideas, methods, instructions or products referred to in the content.

MDPI AG
Grosspeteranlage 5
4052 Basel
Switzerland
Tel.: +41 61 683 77 34

Toxics Editorial Office
E-mail: toxics@mdpi.com
www.mdpi.com/journal/toxics

Disclaimer/Publisher's Note: The title and front matter of this reprint are at the discretion of the Guest Editors. The publisher is not responsible for their content or any associated concerns. The statements, opinions and data contained in all individual articles are solely those of the individual Editors and contributors and not of MDPI. MDPI disclaims responsibility for any injury to people or property resulting from any ideas, methods, instructions or products referred to in the content.

www.ingramcontent.com/pod-product-compliance
Lightning Source LLC
Chambersburg PA
CBHW061453210926
51850CB00008B/1705
* 9 7 8 3 7 2 5 8 5 1 8 9 8 *